MANUAL OF PEDIATRIC ANESTHESIA

Third Edition

MANUAL OF PEDIATRIC ANESTHESIA

Third Edition

DAVID J. STEWARD,
M.B., F.R.C.P.(C)

Anaesthetist-in-Chief
Department of Anaesthesia
British Columbia's Children's Hospital
Vancouver, British Columbia, Canada

Professor
Department of Anaesthesia
University of British Columbia
Vancouver, British Columbia, Canada

Churchill Livingstone
New York, Edinburgh, London, Melbourne, Tokyo

Library of Congress Cataloging-in-Publication Data

Steward, David J., date
    Manual of pediatric anesthesia / David J. Steward. — 3rd ed.
       p.   cm.
    Includes bibliographical references.
    ISBN 0-443-08573-0
    1. Pediatric anesthesia — Handbooks, manuals, etc.   I. Title.
    [DNLM: 1. Anesthesia — in infancy & childhood — handbooks. WO 231
S849m]
    RD139.S84   1990
    617.9′6798 — dc20
    DNLM / DLC
    for Library of Congress   89-22315
                                                       CIP

Distributed in the United Kingdom by Churchill Livingstone, Robert Stevenson
House, 1–3 Baxter's Place, Leith Walk, Edinburgh EH1 3AF, and by
associated companies, branches, and representatives throughout the world.

Accurate indications, adverse reactions, and dosage schedules for drugs are
provided in this book, but it is possible that they may change. The reader is
urged to review the package information data of the manufacturers of the
medications mentioned.

The Publishers have made every effort to trace the copyright holders for
borrowed material. If they have inadvertently overlooked any, they will be
pleased to make the necessary arrangements at the first opportunity.

Copy Editor: *Bridgett Dickinson*
Production Designer: *Charlie Lebeda*
Production Supervisor: *Christina Hippeli*

Printed in the United States of America

First published in 1990   7 6 5 4 3 2

Preface to the Third Edition

The objectives of the third edition of *Manual of Pediatric Anesthesia* remain unchanged from previous editions—to provide a compact but informative guide to pediatric anesthesia with suggestions for further reading. Much new information relating to pediatric anesthesia has become available since this manual first appeared—reflecting a very welcome increase in clinical studies relating to our subspecialty. Many of the practices we adopted "because they worked" can now be continued with the knowledge of why they worked, while some have been modified to improve their effectiveness or abandoned because they are not as effective as was once thought.

This manual is written without much padding; my aim is to provide facts and suggested methods that I hope will serve the reader well. Though some readers may find the style too dogmatic, I have tried to include as many options as possible while providing a manual that can be easily carried.

The first and second editions of this book were written with the invaluable aid of my colleagues at the Hospital for Sick Children in Toronto. I am grateful to them all. Particularly I must thank Dr. Robert Creighton, the current Department Chairman, and Drs. David Pelton, John Relton, and Sharon Nabeta. During the preparation of this edition I have relied on my new colleagues to assist me. I am particularly grateful to Drs. Derek Blackstock, Gerard O'Conner, and Michael Smith.

I hope readers will find that the *Manual of Pediatric Anesthesia* helps them to meet the not insignificant challenge of caring for their pediatric patients.

David J. Steward, M.B., F.R.C.P.(C)

Preface to the Second Edition

The objectives of the second edition of *Manual of Pediatric Anesthesia* remain unchanged from those of the first edition: to discuss important features of the anatomy and physiology of pediatric patients, to present the principles of pediatric anesthesia management, and to describe the techniques which we have found successful in our Hospital.

In this edition the text has been expanded and new knowledge gained since publication of the first edition has been added. A rationale is provided for selecting specific anesthesia techniques. We have been criticized for dogmatism and failure to present alternative methods for anesthesia management. In this edition, we compromise sightly and outline some alternatives, but our main objective is unchanged—to detail the methods that we, in our everyday practice, find most successful.

In the few years since the first edition was published, numerous textbooks of pediatric anesthesia have appeared. Our objective is to supplement rather than to compete with these books. This book is designed for easy reference, to help the reader in his everyday practice and to point the way to further reading.

All the members of staff of the Department of Anesthesia have contributed something to this handbook. Special thanks are due those who contributed sections to the first edition: Drs. Blackwood, Brummitt, Creighton, Davies, Johnston, Nabeta, Pelton, Relton, Sheehan, Sloan, and Whalen, and the late Dr. Norman Park.

Dr. David Pelton has continued to assist in adding to the section on syndromes, and Dr. Robert Creighton has been a special help with his critical reviews of my additions to this volume.

I thank Miss Jane Court for her editorial assistance with the second edition.

David J. Steward, M.B., F.R.C.P.(C)

Abbreviations

$A\text{-}aDO_2$	alveolar arterial oxygen tension gradient
ACT	activated clotting time
AS	aortic stenosis
ASD	atrial septal defect
BP	blood pressure
BPD	bronchopulmonary dysplasia
CBF	cerebral blood flow
CF	cystic fibrosis
CHD	congenital heart disease
CK	creatine kinase
C_L	lung compliance
CNS	central nervous system
CPAP	constant positive airway pressure
CPB	cardiopulmonary bypass
CPK	creatine phosphokinase
CSF	cerebrospinal fluid
CVP	central venous pressure
CVS	cardiovascular system
DIC	disseminated intravascular coagulation
DN	dibucaine number
2,3-DPG	2,3-diphosphoglycerate
EBV	estimated blood volume
ECF	extracellular fluid
ECG	electrocardiogram
ED_{95}	effective dose in 95% of patients
EEG	electroencephalogram
EMG	electromyogram
ETT	endotracheal tube
EUA	examination under anesthesia
FN	fluoride number
FRC	functional residual capacity
GFR	glomerular filtration rate
GI	gastrointestinal
GU	genitourinary

Hb	hemoglobin
HbA	adult hemoglobin
3-HBDH	3-hydroxybutyrate dehydrogenase
HbF	fetal hemoglobin
Hct	hematocrit
HME	heat and moisture exchanger
ICF	intracellular fluid
ICP	intracranial pressure
ICU	intensive care unit
ID	internal diameter
IM	intramuscular
IMV	intermittent mandatory ventilation
IOP	intraocular pressure
IPPB	intermittent positive-pressure breathing
IPPV	intermittent positive-pressure ventilation
ITP	idiopathic thrombocytopenia purpura
IV	intravenous
IVC	inferior vena cava
IVH	intraventricular hemorrhage
L/S	lecithin/sphingomyelin
LA	left atrium
LDH	lactate dehydrogenase
LES	lower esophageal pressure
LV	left ventricle
MAC	minimal alveolar concentration
MH	malignant hyperthermia or hyperpyrexia
NICU	neonatal intensive care unit
NPO	nothing by mouth
OR	operating room
PA	pulmonary artery
PAR	postanesthetic room (recovery room)
PCA	patient controlled analgesia
PDA	patent ductus arteriosus
PEEP	positive end-expiratory pressure
PGE$_1$	prostaglandin E_1
PNF	protamine neutralization factor
PO	per os (by mouth)
PS	pulmonary stenosis
PT	prothrombin time
PTT	partial thromboplastin time
PVC	polyvinyl chloride
PVOD	pulmonary vascular obstructive disease

PVR	pulmonary vascular resistance
RA	right atrium
RBC	red blood cell
RDS	respiratory distress syndrome
REM	rapid eye movement
ROP	retinopathy of prematurity
RV	respiratory volume
RV	right ventricle
SBE	subacute bacterial endocarditis
SGA	small for gestational age
SGOT	serum aspartate aminotransferase; EC 2.6.1.7 (serum glutamic-oxaloacetic transaminase)
SNP	sodium nitroprusside
SSEP	somatosensory evoked potential
SVC	superior vena cava
SVR	systemic vascular resistance
SVT	supraventricular tachycardia
TCPO$_2$	transcutaneous oxygen tension
TEF	tracheoesophageal fistula
TGA	transposition of great arteries
TLC	total lung capacity
URI	upper respiratory infection
$\dot{V}/\dot{Q}$	ventilation/perfusion ratio
VA	alveolar ventilation
V$_C$	vital capacity
V$_D$	dead space volume
VSD	ventricular septal defect
V$_T$	tidal volume

Contents

Psychological Aspects of Anesthesia in Pediatric Patients

EFFECTS OF HOSPITALIZATION AND MEDICAL INTERVENTION

Hospitalization and medical procedures may have profound emotional consequences for children. Some patients demonstrate behavior disturbances that persist long after the event. The extent of the upset is determined by several factors, the most important of which is the child's age.

Infants less than 6 months old are not upset by separation from parents and readily accept a nurse as a substitute mother. From a psychological viewpoint, this is probably a good age for major surgery, although prolonged separation may impair parent-child bonding. Older infants and young children (6 months to 4 years) are much more upset by a hospital stay, principally because of the separation from family and home. Explanations are difficult at this age, and not surprisingly these children show the most severe behavior regression following hospitalization. School-age children are usually less upset at separation and are more concerned with the surgical procedure and its possible multilating effect. Adolescents fear the process of narcosis, the loss of control, and the possibility of not being able to cope with their illness. Teenagers who can be helped to cope with a serious illness may, however, gain significant self-esteem from this experience.

The type and extent of the surgical procedure is obviously a factor; major surgery, craniofacial surgery, or amputation must be expected to have significant effects, and appropriate psychiatric support should be provided. Surgery of the genitalia may also have significant psychological implications and is probably best performed before 18 months of age.

Other factors also influence the child's emotional response. For example, long hospitalization is much more disturbing than a brief admission, and day surgery has a negligible effect on most patients. Repeated hospitalization and surgery deserve special attention with regard to psychological needs. The ethnic origin and family background are important. Some children are much more upset than others of similar age; this probably reflects the extent to which they have been coddled at home. Those from higher socioeconomic groups are generally more upset, as are those children of separated parents. Parental anxiety is readily perceived and reacted on by the child.

ROLE OF THE ANESTHESIOLOGIST

Anesthesia, particularly the induction period, is recognized as a potential cause of psychological trauma. Studies indicate that anesthesiologists vary in their ability to minimize this upset. Preoperative psychological preparation is very important and has been clearly demonstrated to be beneficial. Usually, this must be done by the parents, and the extent of preparation necessary is determined by the child's age. The basic objective is to explain to the child in simple, understandable, and reassuring terms what will happen at the hospital. Older children and adolescents should be prepared well in advance, as soon as hospitalization is arranged. Younger children should not be prepared as far in advance—it is unnecessary and will be a continuing source of worry for them.

Some books that may help parents to prepare their child are listed at the end of this chapter. Hospital tours, puppet shows, and audiovisual presentations are easy to arrange and have all been demonstrated to be beneficial. In some cities, it has been possible to deliver prehospital preparation programs for children via community television stations on a regular weekly basis. By this means, a whole population of children can be prepared for the possibility of hospitalization, rather than just those who are already booked for surgery.

PREPARING PATIENTS FOR AN OPERATION

1. Try to meet the young child with his parents so that the child can see them accept you.
2. Direct most of your attention to the child at all times and try to maintain eye contact.
3. Talk to the child in simple terms that the child can understand.
4. Pay special attention to the silent child and recognize that this child may be very upset. Beware also of the nonchalant child—the nonchalance usually disappears at the "moment of truth."
5. Truthfully explain all the procedures to be undertaken but avoid unnecessary alarming details. Some children may ask about the operation; try to help them understand what is to be done, using drawings if necessary. In many cases, children grossly overestimate the extent of the procedure and must be reassured about the small size of the incision, etc.
6. Do not use the phrase "put you to sleep"—this may worry some children if they recall a family pet who never came back. It may also cause the child to worry about waking up from "sleep" while the operation is still in progress.
7. Do not present the child with unpleasant and difficult choices. For example, avoid questions such as: "Do you want the needle or the mask?" Tell the child what you intend to do and then try to meet any special requests (e.g., "I want to go to sleep with the mask").

8. Avoid uncovering the child more than is necessary to complete your examination; many children get upset at being disrobed.
9. Allow the child to bring a favorite toy or other security object to the operating room (OR). Label the toy with the child's name, and if it is a doll, suggest that perhaps the doll should also get a cast or a dressing applied during the operation. If the child is able, let the child walk to the OR rather than be carried or wheeled.
10. If possible, allow parents of young children to accompany their child to an induction area and to stay with the child during the induction. If this is not possible, it is sometimes very useful to start an intravenous (IV) infusion away from the OR with the parents present. This can then be used for an IV induction as soon as the child is taken to the OR. Always use local analgesia (0.5% lidocaine) to insert the IV cannula. Small children who are crying during venipuncture will often be calmed by telling them "We will put on a bandaid in a minute."
11. Reassure older children and adolescents and provide them with careful explanations. They may be quite scared and have many questions. It is important to reassure them of the safety of the procedure and to emphasize that they *will not* wake up during the operation but *will definitely wake up* when it is over. Older children may benefit from a carefully selected premedicant drug (*see below*).
12. Select the most appropriate induction technique for each child and proceed without undue delay (*see* page 47). Do not allow a child to lie waiting on the OR table longer than is absolutely necessary for the positioning of basic monitors.
13. Talk to the child throughout the induction period to explain or distract the child from the procedures that are required. Ensure that all extraneous noise and conversation is excluded during this time.
14. Use premedicant drugs only when indicated and always select the *appropriate* premedicant for each individual child. Premedicant drugs per se have not been proved to minimize psychological upset. However, if they facilitate a smooth induction of anesthesia, they may be beneficial. There is no place for routine premedication schedules.
15. Tell the child what to expect upon awakening: where he will be and what discomfort he will have. Carefully explain such items as eye patches, nasogastric tubes, etc.
16. Plan for optimal postoperative pain relief for every patient.

POSTOPERATIVE CARE

The parents should be allowed to be with their child as soon as is practical—as the child awakens if possible. Every effort should be made to provide good, but safe, analgesia. Regional nerve blocks, narcotic infusions, epidural narcotics, and all ancillary techniques used for adults should be considered and provided for infants and children when appropriate.

In the intensive care unit, the pediatric patient's problems are very similar to those described for adults: pain, lack of sleep, and, later, boredom. In addition, children have their own special problems, for example, separation from the family. Special attention should be directed to pain relief, regular visiting by the parents, and the provision of toys, games, and other distractions (e.g., television) as the child's condition improves.

Suggested Additional Reading

Bothe A, and R Galdston: The child's loss of consciousness: a psychiatric view of pediatric anesthesia. Pediatrics 50:252, 1972.

Manley CB: Elective genital surgery at one year of age: psychological and surgical considerations. Surg Clin North Am 62:941, 1982.

*Pinkerton P: Preventing psychotrauma in childhood anaesthesia. *In*: Paediatric Anaesthesia, Trends in Current Practice (GJ Rees and TC Gray, eds). London, Butterworth, 1981, p. 1–18.

Roberts MC, SK Wurtele, and RR Boone, et al: Reduction of medical fears by use of modeling: a preventive application in a general population of children. J Pediatr Psychiatry 6:293, 1981.

Seeman RG, and MA Rockoff: Preoperative anxiety: the pediatric patient. Int Anesthesiol Clin 24(4):1–15, 1986.

*Smith RM: Children, hospitals and parents. Anesthesiology 25:461, 1964.

Steward DJ: Psychological considerations in the pediatric patient. *In*: Emotional and Psychological Responses to Anesthesia and Surgery (F Guerra and JA Aldrete, eds). Orlando, FL, Grune & Stratton, 1979.

Vernon DTA, and WC Bailey: The use of motion pictures in the psychological preparation of children for induction of anesthesia. Anesthesiology 40:68, 1974.

*Vernon DTA, JL Schulman, and JM Foley: Changes in children's behavior after hospitalization: some dimensions of response and their correlates. Am J Dis Child 111:581, 1966.

Recommended Reading for Professionals

"Preparing Children and Families for Health Care Encounters." Association for the Care of Children's Health, 3615 Wisconsin Avenue N.W., Washington, DC 20016.

Suggested Reading for Parents and Children

Rey M, and H Rey: Curious George Goes to Hospital. Houghton-Mifflin, Boston, 1966. (For preschool age.)

My Trip to the Hospital. A coloring book prepared by the ASA Committee

---

* Key Article

on Communications and Dr. Frederick Berry. Available from the American Society of Anesthesiologists, 515 Busse Highway, Park Ridge, IL 60068.

Howe J, and M Warshaw: The Hospital Book. New York, Crown Publishers, 1981. (For school age.)

Richter E: The Teenage Hospital Experience: You Can Handle It. Coward, McCann, and Geoghegan, New York, 1982. (For adolescents.)

Videotape Presentation

"Preop Jitters." Rainbow Remedies Inc., P.O. Box 1253, Cape Girardeau, MO 63702-1253.

2

Outline of Pediatric Anatomy and Physiology in Relation to Anesthesia

CENTRAL NERVOUS SYSTEM
The cranium
Cerebral blood flow
Cerebrospinal fluid
Hydrocephalus
Suggested additional reading

THE EYES
Retinopathy of prematurity (retrolental fibroplasia)
Suggested additional reading

RESPIRATORY SYSTEM
Anatomy
Physiology
Control of ventilation in the newborn
Mechanics of ventilation
Lung volumes in the newborn
The work of breathing
Ventilation-perfusion ($\dot{V}/\dot{Q}$) relationships in the newborn lung
Lung surfactant
Changes with anesthesia
Suggested additional reading

CARDIOVASCULAR SYSTEM
The fetus
Changes at birth
Transitional circulation
Newborn cardiovascular system
Suggested additional reading

METABOLISM; FLUID AND ELECTROLYTE BALANCE
Glucose metabolism
Calcium metabolism
Bilirubin metabolism
Suggested additional reading

COMPOSITION AND REGULATION OF BODY FLUIDS
Body water
Neonatal renal function and water balance
Maintenance requirements
Suggested additional reading

PHYSIOLOGY OF TEMPERATURE HOMEOSTASIS
Suggested additional reading

CENTRAL NERVOUS SYSTEM

The central nervous system (CNS) in the newborn differs from that in the older child in several ways. Myelination of nerve fibers is incomplete, muscle tone and reflexes are different, and the cerebral cortex is less developed (its cellular elements increase during the first years of life).

Newborn infants, even preterm, can appreciate pain and will react with tachycardia, hypertension, increased intracranial pressure (ICP), and a measurable neuroendocrine response. This knowledge of their pain sensitivity dictates that we should provide analgesia or anesthesia for all babies during *any* painful procedure with the same care as we do for adult patients. The pain threshold for young children is lower than that for older children or adults.

THE CRANIUM

The intact skull is less rigid in infants than in adults. As a result, an increase in the volume of the contents (blood, cerebrospinal fluid [CSF], and brain tissue) can be accommodated to some extent by expansion of the fontanelles and separation of the suture lines. Thus, palpation of the fontanelle can be used to assess the ICP in infants.

CEREBRAL BLOOD FLOW

Autoregulation of the cerebral blood flow (CBF) is impaired in sick newborn infants. Thus, blood flow is pressure dependent, and increased blood pressure is transmitted to the capillaries. In the preterm infant, the cerebral vessels are very fragile, especially in the region of the germinal matrix overlying the caudate nucleus. Rupture of these vessels leads to intracerebral hemorrhage, which often ruptures into the ventricular system, causing intraventricular hemorrhage (IVH). Factors predisposing to IVH include hypoxia, hypercarbia, hypernatremia, fluctuations in arterial or venous pressures and/or CBF, and possibly the rapid administration of hypertonic fluids (e.g., sodium bicarbonate). Airway manipulations, including awake endotracheal intubation and suctioning, have been demonstrated to increase anterior fontanelle pressure in some infants, but the significance of this is uncertain at present.

CEREBROSPINAL FLUID

Cerebrospinal fluid, which occupies the cerebral ventricles and the subarachnoid spaces surrounding the brain and spinal cord, is formed by choroid plexuses in the temporal horns of the lateral ventricles, the posterior portion of the third ventricle, and the roof of the fourth ventricle. Meningeal and ependymal vessels and blood vessels of the brain and spinal cord also contribute a small amount of CSF.

The choroid plexuses are cauliflowerlike structures consisting of blood vessels covered by thin epithelium through which CSF continuously exudes. The rate of secretion is about 750 ml/day in the adult, that is, about five times the intracavity volume. Except for the active secretion of a few substances by the choroid plexus, CSF is similar to interstitial fluid.

Cerebrospinal fluid flow is initiated by pulsation in the choroid plexus. From the lateral ventricles it passes into the third ventricle via the foramen of Monro and along the aqueduct of Sylvius into the fourth ventricle, each ventricle contributing more fluid by secretion from its choroid plexus. Cerebrospinal fluid then flows through the two lateral foramina of Luschka and the midline foramen of Magendie into the cisterna magna and throughout the subarachnoid spaces.

Cerebrospinal fluid is reabsorbed into the blood by hydrostatic filtration through the arachnoid villi, which project from the subarachnoid space into the venous sinuses.

HYDROCEPHALUS

Hydrocephalus is an abnormal accumulation of CSF within the cranium that may be obstructive or nonobstructive.

Obstructive hydrocephalus is due to blockage in the fluid pathway of the CSF. It may be communicating (i.e., the CSF pathway into the subarachnoid space is open, as after chronic arachnoiditis) or noncommunicating (i.e., the result of obstruction of the fluid's pathway proximal to the subarachnoid space, e.g., in aqueduct stenosis or Arnold-Chiari syndrome).

Nonobstructive hydrocephalus is due either to a reduction in the volume of brain substance, with secondary dilation of the ventricles, or to overproduction of CSF, for example, as in choroid plexus papilloma.

Suggested Additional Reading

*Berry FA, and GA Gregory: Do premature infants require anesthesia for surgery? Anesthesiology 67:291–293, 1987.
Harper AM: General physiology of cerebral circulation. Int Anesthesiol Clin 7:473, 1969.

---

* Key article

Jay SM, M Ozolins, and CH Elliot: Assessment of children's distress during painful medical procedures. Health Psychiatry 2:133–137, 1983.

Langfitt TW, NF Kassell, and JD Weinstein: Cerebral blood flow with intracranial hypertension. Neurology 15:761, 1965.

McDowall DG: Physiology of the cerebrospinal fluid. Int Anesthesiol Clin 7:507, 1969.

Milhorat TH: The third circulation revisted. J Neurosurg 42:628–645, 1975.

Miller JD: The effect of space-occupying lesions on cerebral circulation. Int Anesthesiol Clin 7:617, 1969.

Perlman JM, S Goodman, KL Kreusser, and JJ Volpe: Reduction in intraventricular hemorrhage by elimination of fluctuating cerebral blood flow velocity in infants with respiratory distress syndrome. N Engl J Med 312:1353–1357, 1985.

Stow, PJ, ME Mcleod, and FA Burrows: Anterior fontanel pressure response to endotracheal intubation in neonates and young infants. Anesth Analg 66S:169, 1987.

Tarby TJ, and JJ Volpe: Intraventricular hemorrhage in the premature infant. Pediatr Clin North Am 29:1077, 1982.

Williamson, PS, and ML Williamson: Physiologic stress reduction by a local anesthetic during newborn circumcision. Pediatrics 71:36–40, 1983.

Yaster M: Analgesia and anesthesia in neonates. J Pediatr 111:394, 1987.

THE EYES

In the past, visual acuity was believed to develop in infants when they were a few weeks old, but it is now recognized that term infants can recognize and respond to objects.

RETINOPATHY OF PREMATURITY (RETROLENTAL FIBROPLASIA)

Retinopathy of prematurity (ROP) may occur in the immature retina of the preterm infant. Increased oxygen tension in the retinal arteries is thought to be the principal etiologic factor, but occasionally ROP occurs in infants who have never been given additional oxygen. Hyperoxia leads to vasoconstriction, capillary endothelial swelling, and degeneration in the peripheral region of the retina with a visible demarcation line (stage 1 ROP). These changes are later followed by the formation of a ridge at this line (stage 2 ROP), extraretinal fibrovascular proliferation (stage 3 ROP), and retinal detachment (stage 4 ROP). Other risk factors in ROP may possibly include hypercarbia or hypocarbia, blood transfusion, and recurrent apnea.

ROP is most common in the preterm infant of <35 weeks gestational age and ≤1,500 g body weight. The risk of developing ROP is increased in direct proportion to the duration of exposure to oxygen. It has been suggested that ROP follows oxygen administered solely during anesthesia and postoperative recovery, but the evidence is not conclusive. Undoubtedly, many infants at risk have been given additional inspired oxygen during anesthesia and have not developed ROP.

All preterm infants should be examined regularly by an ophthalmologist. The inspired oxygen concentration should be carefully controlled to avoid unnecessary hyperoxia. The safe level of PaO_2 is now considered to be 50–70 mmHg. The transcutaneous oxygen electrode has greatly facilitated oxygen therapy in the neonatal intensive care unit (NICU) but does not perform as well in the operating room (OR). Monitoring of transcutaneous pulse oximetry is more reliable in the OR. Maintaining the SaO_2 at 90–95% will usually result in a safe level of oxygenation. Vitamin E administered regularly while the infant is receiving O_2 therapy may confer some protection against ROP and reduce the severity of the disease. In the OR, the anesthesiologist should certainly avoid unnecessary hyperoxia; systemic oxygenation should be monitored in all patients at risk of ROP. Obviously, it may still be necessary, on occasion, to err on the side of safety (*see* Chapter 3). Major surgery does not appear to predispose to ROP (Flynn 1984).

Suggested Additional Reading

Baum JD: Retrolental fibroplasia. Dev Med Child Neurol 21:385, 1979.

Betts EK, JJ Downes, DB Schaffer, and R Johns: Retrolental fibroplasia and oxygen administration during general anesthesia. Anesthesiology 47:518, 1977.

Flynn JT: Oxygen and retrolental fibroplasia: update and challenge. Anesthesiology 60:397–399, 1984.

James L, and J Lanman (eds): History of oxygen therapy and retrolental fibroplasia. Pediatrics 57:681, 1976.

Johnson L, D. Schaffer, and T Boggs: The premature infant, vitamin deficiency, and retrolental fibroplasia. Am J Clin Nutr 27:1158, 1974.

Patz A: Observations on the retinopathy of prematurity. Am J Ophthalmol 100:164–168, 1985.

Phelps DL: Neonatal oxygen toxicity—is it preventable? Pediatr Clin North Am 29:1233, 1982.

Phibbs RH: Oxygen therapy: a continuing hazard to the premature infant. Anesthesiology 47:486, 1977.

RESPIRATORY SYSTEM

The respiratory system is of very special interest to the anesthesiologist. It is the route of administration of inhaled anesthetic agents, and its functions may be significantly altered during and after anesthesia. Changes occur continuously from infancy to about age 12 as the system grows to maturity. This section describes the respiratory system of the newborn and its subsequent development.

ANATOMY

There are major anatomic differences in the neonate that are important to the anesthesiologist.

1. The head is relatively large and the neck is short.
2. The tongue is relatively large and readily blocks the pharynx during anesthesia; hence, an oropharyngeal airway may be required. The large tongue may also hamper attempts to visualize the glottis at laryngoscopy.
3. The nasal passages are narrow and are readily blocked by secretions or edema. Nasal obstruction may cause serious problems because many infants will not immediately switch to mouth-breathing. Neonates were previously described as "obligate nose-breathers," but whether this is always true has recently been questioned. It is certain that many infants will not easily convert to mouth-breathing if the nasal passages are obstructed.
4. The larynx is situated more cephalad (C4) and anteriorly, and its long axis is directed inferiorly and anteriorly.
5. The airway is narrowest at the level of the cricoid cartilage just below the vocal cords. Here it is lined with pseudostratified, ciliated epithelium that is loosely bound to areolar tissue. Trauma to these tissues results in edema, which reduces the lumen and greatly increases resistance to airflow (stridor). Even a small amount of circumferential edema significantly encroaches on the small area of the infant airway, raising resistance markedly.
6. The epiglottis is relatively long and stiff. It is U-shaped and projects posteriorly at an angle of 45° above the glottis. It must be elevated by the tip of a laryngoscope before the glottis can be seen; hence, the use of a straight-blade laryngoscope is recommended.
7. The trachea is short (approximately 5 cm); therefore, precise placement and firm fixation of endotracheal tubes are essential. The tracheal cartilages are soft and can easily be compressed by the anesthetist's fingers

while holding a mask or can be collapsed by vigorous attempts of the patient to breathe against an obstructed airway.

8. Because the ribs are almost horizontal, ventilation is primarily diaphragmatic. The abdominal viscera are bulky and can readily hamper diaphragmatic excursion, especially if the gastrointestinal tract is distended.

PHYSIOLOGY

Breathing movements begin in utero and are characteristically rapid, irregular, and episodic during late pregnancy. Normally, they are present for 30–60% of the time and are subject to diurnal variation. Fetal breathing movements may help to develop the respiratory muscles, and monitoring of these movements may provide information on fetal health. The fetal lung is filled with fluid, which is moved by this respiratory activity. After 26–28 weeks of gestation, production of surface-active substances (surfactant) is established in the type II pneumocytes. Surfactant is secreted into the lung and can be detected in amniotic fluid samples; thus providing a diagnostic index of lung maturity and hence neonatal prognosis (*see* page 19).

Passage of the fetus through the birth canal compresses the thorax, forcing fluid from the lungs via the nose and mouth. On delivery, this compression is relieved and some air is sucked into the lungs. The first breath is initiated by peripheral (cold, touch, etc.) and biochemical (respiratory and metabolic acidosis) stimuli. The first few spontaneous breaths are characterized by high transpulmonary pressures (over 50 cm H_2O) and establish the functional residual capacity (FRC) of the neonate's lungs. Remaining lung fluid is removed within hours by the pulmonary lymphatics and blood vessels. The stability of the alveolar matrix in the newborn is dependent on the presence of adequate amounts of surfactant, which may be deficient in the premature infant. Lack of surfactant leads to collapse of alveoli, maldistribution of ventilation, impaired gas exchange, decreased compliance, and increased work of breathing—the respiratory distress syndrome (RDS). Not surprisingly, pneumothorax occurs more commonly during the neonatal period than at any other age.

CONTROL OF VENTILATION IN THE NEWBORN

Observations of neonatal control of ventilation are difficult to interpret. First, the intervention necessary to obtain measurements (e.g., placing a mask on the face) may itself induce a change in ventilation. Second, the use of measurements of ventilation to assess "respiratory drive" assumes that respiratory muscles are performing optimally to convert this "drive" into work, and such may not be the case.

The newborn's muscles of ventilation are subject to fatigue, a tendency that is determined by the types of muscle fiber present. In preterm infants, less than 10% of the fibers in the diaphragm are type I (i.e., slow-twitch, highly oxidative, fatigue resistant). In term infants, 30% of these fibers are type I, and the percentage increases to 55% (the adult level) over the first year of life. Thus, the preterm infant is very prone to ventilatory muscle fatigue, a predisposition that progressively disappears with advancing maturity. Ventilation is also affected by changes that occur during changing sleep states. The preterm infant spends 50–60% of his time in rapid eye movement (REM) sleep during which intercostal muscle activity is inhibited and paradoxical movement of the soft chest wall occurs. This lack of intercostal activity is compensated by an increase in diaphragmatic activity, much of which is wasted when the ribs move paradoxically, and it may lead to diaphragmatic fatigue.

Control of ventilation, which involves biochemical and reflex mechanisms, is well developed in the healthy full-term neonate. The ventilatory response to increased concentrations of inspired CO_2 is proportionally similar to that in adults; however, ventilation relative to body mass is greater for any given $PaCO_2$, reflecting a higher metabolic rate. The response of the preterm infant to increased inspired CO_2 is not well sustained, and the slope of the CO_2 response curve is decreased in infants displaying episodes of apnea.

The newborn is also sensitive to changes in arterial oxygen tension. Administration of 100% O_2 decreases ventilation, indicating the existence of chemoreceptor activity. The ventilatory response of the newborn to hypoxia is modified by many factors, including gestational and postnatal age, body temperature, and sleep state. Preterm and full-term infants less than 1 week old who are awake and normothermic usually demonstrate a biphasic response, a brief period of hyperpnea followed by ventilatory depression. Hypothermic infants respond to hypoxia with ventilatory depression without initial hyperpnea. This depression of ventilation is thought to be due to the central effects of hypoxia on the cortex and medulla. The peripheral chemoreceptors, though demonstrated to be active in newborns, are presumably unable to maintain a significant influence on this response. Infants may be even less responsive to hypoxia during REM sleep. However, during non-REM sleep increased ventilation is sustained. The arousal response to hypoxia during sleep is not seen in newborns but normally develops over the first few weeks of life. Hypoxia that occurs during sleep usually results in arousal. During hypoxia, the ventilatory response to CO_2 is depressed in the newborn (in contrast to that in infants and adults). Infants over 2–3 weeks old demonstrate hyperpnea in response to hypoxia, probably owing to maturing of the chemoreceptor function.

Reflexes arising from the lung and chest wall are probably more important in maintaining ventilation in the newborn, primarily determining the rate (f) and tidal volume (V_T). The Hering-Breuer inflation reflex, which is active in the newborn, is even more powerful in the premature infant. This reflex disappears during REM sleep and progressively fades during the early weeks of life. The paradoxical "Head" reflex, a large inspiration triggered by a small lung inflation, is active in the newborn. It may play a role in maintaining the lung volume of the newborn and persists even during deep halothane anesthesia.

Periodic breathing (rapid ventilation alternating with periods of apnea lasting 5–10 second) occurs in many preterm and some term infants. It is thought to result from incoordination with the feedback loops controlling ventilation. During episodes of periodic breathing, the $PaCO_2$ level is above normal, but the heart rate does not change significantly. Periodic breathing seems to have no serious physiologic consequences and usually ceases by 6 weeks of age.

Some preterm infants demonstrate far more serious and indeed life-threatening episodes of apnea. These commonly exceed 20 seconds and are accompanied by bradycardia. The pathogenesis of apnea in preterm infants is not clearly understood. It is suggested that apnea may reflect excessive physiologic demands on an immature respiratory control system. A variety of pathophysiologic mechanisms seem to be involved, however. Apneic episodes may result from failure to respond to hypoxia, but may also be due to airway obstruction or failure of the ventilatory muscles. Many apneic episodes occur during REM sleep, when it is possible that ventilatory muscle fatigue may be an important factor.

While neonatal apnea may be idiopathic, it may also be symptomatic of an underlying disease; sepsis, intracranial bleeding, anemia, and patent ductus arteriosus may precipitate episodes of apnea.

Preterm infants must be carefully monitored to detect apneic episodes. Treatment is by tactile stimulation or, if this fails, by bag-and-mask resuscitation. The incidence of apneic episodes is decreased by therapy with aminophylline (central stimulation) or by instituting continuous positive airway pressure (CPAP) (increased reflex activity of lung and chest wall reflexes and "splinting" of the airway).

MECHANICS OF VENTILATION

The specific compliance of the lung increases slowly after birth as fluid is removed from the lung and at 1 week is similar to that in the adult. The chest wall compliance of the infant (especially the preterm infant) is very high, so that total compliance approximates lung compliance (CL). This highly compliant chest wall provides only a relatively weak force to maintain the FRC and oppose the effect of the diaphragm. Intercostal muscle inhibition during REM sleep or resulting from inhaled anesthetic agents compounds this weakness and results in paradoxical movement of the chest wall and a fall in FRC. This paradoxical chest wall movement is, of course, markedly increased by any obstruction to ventilation. As the child grows through infancy and childhood, the rib cage stiffens so that it becomes better able to oppose the action of the diaphragm.

The transpulmonary pressure to achieve lung inflation is remarkably similar in healthy infants and adults. During artificial ventilation, peak inspiratory pressures of 15–20 cm H_2O are normal. Total airway resistance is high in newborn infants. The restricted lumen of the nasal passages, the diameter of the small airways, and the low lung volume all contribute to this.

LUNG VOLUMES IN THE NEWBORN

In the term infant, total lung capacity (TLC) is approximately 160 ml, and the FRC is about one-half this volume. The V_T is approximately 16 ml, and the dead space volume (V_D) is about 5 ml (0.3 of the V_T). Relative to body size, all these volumes are similar to adult values. Note, however, that any dead space in anesthesia or ventilator circuits is much more significant when related to the small volumes of the infant (i.e., a 5-ml apparatus dead space would increase the total effective V_D by 100%).

In contrast to the static lung volumes, alveolar ventilation ($\dot{V}_A$) is proportionally much larger in the newborn (100–150 ml/kg of body weight*/min) than in the adult (60 ml/kg/min). This high $\dot{V}_A$ in the infant results in a $\dot{V}_A$:FRC ratio of 5:1, compared with 1.5:1 in the adult. Consequently, the FRC is a much less effective "buffer" in the infant, so that changes in the concentration of inspired gases (including anesthetic gases) are more rapidly reflected in alveolar and arterial levels.

The closing volume (CV) is higher in infants and young children than in young adults and may exceed the FRC to encroach on the V_T during normal ventilation. Airway closure during normal ventilation may explain the lower normal values for PaO_2 during infancy and childhood (Table 2-1). A fall in FRC, which usually occurs during general anesthesia and persists into the postoperative period, may be expected to further increase the significance of the high CV and further increase the A-aDO_2. The

---

* **Note.** Hereafter, throughout this manual, "kilograms of body weight" is expressed simply as kilograms (kg).

TABLE 2-1.   ARTERIAL OXYGEN
TENSION IN HEALTHY INFANTS AND
CHILDREN

Age	Normal Arterial Oxygen (mmHg) in Room Air
0–1 week	70
1–10 months	85
4–8 years	90
12–16 years	96

younger the infant or child, the larger is this fall in FRC. Hence, there is a requirement to increase the oxygen concentration of inspired gases. The perioperative fall in FRC may be less during operations with the patient prone and the abdomen hanging free, and it may be partially reversed by CPAP.

The total surface area of the air-tissue interface of the alveolae is small in the infant (2.8 m^3). When this area is related to the metabolic rate for O_2 (VO_2), it is apparent that the infant is dependent on a smaller air-tissue interface: VO_2 ratio than the adult and as a result has a reduced reserve capability for gas exchange. This may assume great significance if congenital defects (e.g., diaphragmatic hernia) interfere with lung growth or the lungs become damaged (e.g., from meconium aspiration). Then the remaining healthy lung tissue may be inadequate to sustain life.

THE WORK OF BREATHING

The muscles of ventilation generate the force necessary to overcome the resistance to air flow as well as the elastic recoil of the lungs and chest wall. These two factors dictate an optimal rate of ventilation and V_T for each child that delivers a given alveolar ventilation while expending minimal muscular energy. As the time constant of the infant's lung is relatively short, efficient alveolar ventilation can be achieved at high respiratory rates. In the newborn, a respiratory rate of 37/min has been calculated to be most efficient; this is close to the rate observed in the healthy newborn. The term infant is similar to the adult, requiring 1% of his metabolic energy to maintain ventilation; the oxygen cost of breathing is 0.5 ml/0.5 L of ventilation. The preterm infant has a higher oxygen cost of breathing (0.9 ml/0.5 L) that is greatly increased if the lungs are diseased, for example, as in RDS or bronchopulmonary dysplasia (BPD).

VENTILATION-PERFUSION ($\dot{V}/\dot{Q}$)
RELATIONSHIPS IN THE NEWBORN LUNG

Ventilation and perfusion are imperfectly matched in the neonatal lung. This may be partly due to gas trapping in the lungs. $\dot{V}/\dot{Q}$ mismatch is evident in the A-aN$_2$ difference, which is 25 mmHg immediately after birth and declines to about 10 mmHg within the first week. The normal arterial oxygen tension (PaO$_2$) in an infant breathing room air is about 50 mmHg just after birth and increases to 70 mmHg by 24 hours of age. The high A-aO$_2$ difference in infants is also due to persisting anatomic shunts (*see* page 23) and the relatively high CV.

LUNG SURFACTANT

Surfactants, or surface-active substances, in the alveolar lining layer stabilize the alveoli, preventing their collapse on expiration. Lowering the surface tension at the air-liquid interface in the alveoli also reduces the force required for their reexpansion. The principal surfactant in the lung is lecithin, which is produced by type II pneumocytes. The quantity of lecithin produced in the fetal lung rises progressively, beginning at 22 weeks gestational age and increasing sharply at 35 to 36 weeks as the lung matures. The lecithin production of the lung can be assessed by determining the lecithin/sphingomyelin (L/S) ratio in amniotic fluid.

The L/S ratio is less than 1 until 32 weeks gestation, 2 by 35 weeks, and 4–6 at term. Premature infants with inadequate pulmonary lecithin production suffer from RDS. The biochemical pathways for surfactant production may also be depressed by hypoxia, hyperoxia, acidosis, or hypothermia. Hence, early correction of these abnormalities in the sick neonate is vitally important. Inhaled anesthetic agents seem to have little effect on surfactant production. Maturation of biochemical processes in the lungs of the fetus in utero may be accelerated by the administration of corticosteroids to the mother.

CHANGES WITH ANESTHESIA

The following is a summary of some of the major changes that occur in the respiratory system during and after anesthesia.

1. Spontaneous ventilation is decreased. This is thought to be due to the combined effects of anesthetic drugs on the chemical control of ventilation and on the muscles of ventilation. Intercostal muscle activity in inhibited by potent volatile anesthetic agents (e.g., halothane); consequently, diaphragmatic breathing predominates and the chest wall

may move paradoxically, especially if the airway is obstructed. Surgical stimulation tends to increase ventilation toward normal levels.

2. The FRC is reduced. This reduction is greatest in the youngest patients and is due to elevation of the diaphragm and loss of chest wall stability. As the FRC falls, airway closure may occur during tidal ventilation with consequent impaired oxygen transfer in the lung.

3. The dead space:tidal volume ($V_D : V_T$) ratio remains constant in patients breathing spontaneously but may increase in those whose ventilation is controlled.

4. Compliance is little changed, and airway resistance is generally reduced by the bronchodilator action of potent volatile anesthetic agents. Insertion of an endotracheal tube will increase total flow resistance (*see* page 67), especially in patients under 5 years old.

5. During controlled ventilation, major alterations in gas distribution within the lungs occur as a result of changes in the action of the diaphragm. This effect tends to markedly unbalance the matching of ventilation and perfusion of the lungs.

6. The efficiency of gas exchange may be impaired by the effect of anesthetic drugs on the physiologic processes that normally control the regional distribution of gases and blood throughout the lung.

7. Laryngospasm occurs more frequently in association with pediatric anesthesia, especially during induction and after extubation (*see* Chapter 3). Laryngeal closure results from apposition of the vocal cords and supraglottic structures. The reason for the increased incidence of laryngospasm in children is unknown.

Suggested Additional Reading
Respiratory System: Anatomy

*Crelin ES: Development of the lower respiratory system. Clin Symp 28:1, 1976.

*Crelin ES: Development of the upper respiratory system. Clin Symp 29:1, 1977.

*Eckenhoff JE: Some anatomic considerations of the infant larynx influencing endotracheal anesthesia. Anesthesiology 12:401, 1951.

Pelton DA, and JS Whalen: Airway obstruction in infants and children. Int Anesthesiol Clin 10:123, 1972.

Respiratory System: Physiology

*Bryan AC, and MH Bryan: Control of respiration in the newborn. Clin Perinatol 5:269, 1978.

Dawes GS, HE Fox, BM Leduc, GC Liggins, and RT Richards: Respi-

---

* Key article

ratory movements and rapid eye movement sleep in the foetal lamb. J Physiol (Lond) 220:119, 1972.

Gerhardt T, and E Bancalari: Apnea of prematurity. I. Lung function and regulation of breathing. Pediatrics 74:58, 1984.

Gerhardt T, E Bancalari: Apnea of prematurity. II. Respiratory reflexes. Pediatrics 74:63, 1984.

Gluck L, MV and Kulovich, AL Eidelman, L Cordero, and AF Khazin: Biochemical development of surface activity in mammalian lung. IV. Pulmonary lecithin synthesis in the human fetus and newborn and etiology of the respiratory distress syndrome. Pediatr Res 6:81, 1972.

Gregory GA, JA Kitterman, and WH Tooley: Lung volume in newborn infants after cardiovascular surgery. In: Abstracts of Scientific Papers Presented at the Annual Meeting of the American Society of Anesthesiologists, Atlanta, GA, 1971, p. 45.

Henderson-Smart DJ, AG Pettygrew, and DJ Campbell: Clinical apnea and brainstem neural function in preterm infants. N Engl J Med 308:353, 1983.

Hogg JC, J Williams, JB Richardson, PT Macklem, and WM Thurlbeck: Age as a factor in the distribution of lower-airway conductance and in the pathologic anatomy of obstructive lung disease. N Engl J Med 282:1283, 1970.

Kitagawa M, A Hislop, EA Boyden, and L Reid: Lung hypoplasia in congenital diaphragmatic hernia: a quantitative study of airway, artery, and alveolar development. Br J Surg 58:342, 1971.

Lindahl SG, AP Yates, and DJ Hatch: Respiratory depression in children at different end-tidal halothane concentrations. Anaesthesia 42:1267–1275, 1987.

Mansell A, C Bryan, and H Levison: Airway closure in children. J Appl Physiol 33:711, 1972.

Martin RJ, MJ Miller, and AC Waldemar: Pathogenesis of apnea in preterm infants. J Pediatr 109:733–741, 1986.

Miller RN, and PA Thomas: Pulmonary surfactant: determinations from lung extracts of patients receiving diethyl ether or halothane. Anesthesiology 28:1089, 1967.

Nisbet HIA, H Levison, and DA Pelton: Static thoracic compliance in normal children under general anaesthesia. Acta Anaesthesiol Scand 15:179, 1971.

Owen-Thomas JB, F Meade, RS Jones, and GJ Rees: The measurement of oxygen uptake in infants with congenital heart disease during general anaesthesia and intermittent positive pressure ventilation. Br J Anaesth 43:746, 1971.

Reynolds RN, and BE Etsten: Mechanics of respiration in apneic anesthetized infants. Anesthesiology 27:13, 1966.

*Rigatto H: Apnea. Pediatr Clin North Am 29:1105, 1982.

Roy WL, and J Lerman: Laryngospasm in paediatric anaesthesia. Can Anaesth Soc J 35:93–98, 1987.

Woo SW, D Berlin, and J Hedley-Whyte: Surfactant function and anesthetic agents. J Appl Physiol 26:571, 1969.

CARDIOVASCULAR SYSTEM

THE FETUS

Much of our information about the fetal cardiovascular system (CVS) has been gained from studies conducted in lambs. However, a few studies in previable human fetuses indicate that these fetal CVSs are reasonably comparable.

The fetal CVS perfuses the low-resistance placental circulation, directing 36–42% of the combined ventricular output to this organ; only 5–10% goes to the lungs. Flow to the fetal lungs is limited by their high vascular resistance, and as a result, blood bypasses the lungs via the foramen ovale and the ductus arteriosus. Most of the blood returning from the placenta bypasses the liver via the ductus venosus. The pattern of flow from the inferior vena cava (IVC) into the right atrium (RA) ensures that about one-third of the oxygenated (PO_2 28–30 mmHg) placental blood is directed through the foramen ovale into the left atrium (LA). This blood, which combines with the limited venous return from the lungs, is pumped by the left ventricle (LV) into the ascending aorta and thence to the coronary, cerebral, and forelimb circulations. Blood returning via the superior vena cava (SVC) (PO_2 12–14 mmHg) passes through the RA into the right ventricle (RV), from which most of the output flows through the ductus arteriosus into the descending aorta. Thus, blood supplied to the heart and upper body has a higher O_2 content (saturation 65%, PO_2 26–28 mmHg) than that supplied to the abdominal organs, lower limbs, and placenta (saturation 55–60%, PO_2 20–22 mmHg). In utero the RV pumps about 66% of the combined ventricular output and the LV pumps the remaining 34%.

CHANGES AT BIRTH

At birth, pulmonary ventilation is established quickly, and blood flow to the lungs is greatly increased as placental flow ceases. When the lungs expand with air, pulmonary vascular resistance (PVR) falls markedly as a result of mechanical effects on the vessels and relaxation of pulmonary vasomotor tone when the PO_2 rises and the PCO_2 falls in alveolar gas. PVR falls by 80% from prenatal levels within a few minutes of normal initiation of ventilation. As PVR falls, blood flow to the lungs and then via the pulmonary veins into the LA increases, elevating LA pressure above that in the RA and closing the atrial septum over the foramen ovale.

Simultaneously, as flow to the placenta ceases (owing either to clamping or to umbilical artery constriction), a large low-resistance vascular bed is excluded from the systemic circulation. This results in a large increase in systemic vascular resistance (SVR) and a fall in IVC blood flow and RA pressure. The increase in SVR and simultaneous fall in PVR elevate the aortic pressure above that in the pulmonary artery (PA). Therefore, blood flow through the ductus arteriosus reverses (left to right), and the ductus fills with oxygenated blood. This increased local PO_2 (to >50–60 mmHg) causes the muscular wall of the ductus arteriosus to constrict. The entire sequence of biochemical events leading to closure of the ductus is not known, but a prostaglandin-mediated response has been suggested. Shunts may persist through the ductus for some hours after birth, producing audible murmurs. Normally, however, flow through the ductus is insignificant by 15 hours. Permanent histologic closure of the ductus is usually complete by 5–7 days but may not occur until 3 weeks have passed.

TRANSITIONAL CIRCULATION

During the early neonatal period, reversion to the fetal circulatory pattern is possible under some circumstances. If hypoxia occurs, PVR increases and the ductus arteriosus may reopen; a significant proportion of blood then again bypasses the (now high resistance) pulmonary circulation, causing a further fall in arterial oxygenation. Impaired tissue oxygenation then results in acidosis, which causes a further increase in PVR, establishing a vicious circle of hypoxemia → acidosis → impaired pulmonary blood flow → hypoxemia.

Reversion to a fetal pattern of circulation may complicate any condition that causes hypoxemia or acidemia (e.g., RDS or congenital diaphragmatic hernia).

NEWBORN CARDIOVASCULAR SYSTEM

Heart and Cardiac Output

In healthy neonates, the RV exceeds the LV in wall thickness; this preponderance is evident in the electrocardiogram (ECG), which shows an axis of up to +180° during the first week of life. After birth, the LV enlarges disproportionately. By about 3–6 months, the adult ratio of ventricular size is established (axis ≈ +90°). During the immediate newborn period, the heart rate is between 100 and 170 beats/min and the rhythm

TABLE 2-2. NORMAL HEART RATE

Age	Heart Rate (per Minute)	
	Average	Range
Newborn	120	100–170
1–11 months	120	80–160
2 years	110	80–130
4 years	100	80–120
6 years	100	75–115
8 years	90	70–110
10 years	90	70–110
14 years		
Boys	80	60–100
Girls	85	65–105
16 years		
Boys	75	55–95
Girls	80	60–100

is regular. As the child grows, the heart rate gradually decreases (Table 2-2).

Sinus arrhythmia is common in children. All other irregular rhythms must be considered abnormal.

Systolic blood pressure is approximately 60 mmHg in the term newborn, and the diastolic pressure is 35 mmHg. These pressures vary considerably and may be 10–15 mmHg higher if clamping of the cord is delayed or the cord is "stripped." In either case they fall to normal levels within 4 hours. Preterm infants have lower arterial pressures: as low as 45/25 in the 750-g baby (Table 2-3).

The myocardium of the newborn contains less contractile tissue and more connective tissue than is present in the adult heart. Consequently, the neonate's ventricles are less compliant when relaxed and generate less tension during contraction. Because the low compliance of the relaxed ventricle tends to limit the size of the stroke volume, the cardiac output of the newborn is to a large extent rate dependent; bradycardia is invariably accompanied by reduced cardiac output. Reduced compliance and contractility of the ventricles also predisposes the infant heart to failure with increased volume load. In the infant, failure of one ventricle rapidly compromises the function of the other and biventricular failure results. The autonomic innervation of the heart is incomplete in the newborn, with a relative lack of sympathetic elements. This may further compromise the ability of the less contractile neonatal myocardium to respond to stress.

TABLE 2-3. NORMAL BLOOD PRESSURE

Age	Blood Pressure (mmHg)[a]		
	Systolic	Diastolic	Mean
Newborn			
Preterm (750 g)	44	24	33
Preterm (1,000 g)	49	26	34.5
Full term	60	35	45
3–10 days	70–75		
6 months	95		
4 years	98	57	
6 years	110	60	
8 years	112	60	
12 years	115	65	
16 years	120	65	

[a] Reported normal blood pressure (BP) for infants and children must be considered in light of the method of determining the BP. These values should serve as a guide only (see Monitoring during Anesthesia, page 76).

The differences is the newborn's myocardium are all particularly marked in the preterm infant.

In the neonate, shunts hamper the precise measurement of cardiac output, which averages two to three times that of the adult on a milliliter per kilogram of body weight basis and is appropriate to the metabolic rate. The total SVR is low, reflecting the high proportion (19%) of vessel-rich tissue and permitting a high cardiac output despite a low systemic blood pressure.

Pulmonary Circulation

The changes in the pulmonary circulation that occurred at birth continue with a slower progressive decline in PVR over the first 3 months of life. This is associated with a parallel regression in the thickness of the medial muscle layer of the pulmonary arterioles. During the neonatal period PVR is still high and the muscular pulmonary vessels are highly reactive. Hypoxia, acidosis, and stress, for example, as caused by endotracheal suctioning, may all result in rapid elevation of PVR. If elevation of PVR is sustained by such stimuli, right-sided intracardiac pressures may exceed those on the left and R→L shunting may ensue via the ductus arteriosus or foramen ovale. Right ventricular failure rapidly progressing to biventricular failure may occur.

In some circumstances, the normal regression of the muscular layer of the pulmonary vessels and associated fall in PVR may not occur. Continued hypoxemia, for example, resulting from high altitude, or continued high pulmonary blood flow resulting from L→R shunts (ventricular septal defect, etc.) may result in persistence of a high PVR into childhood and beyond. Initially, this high PVR is reversible, for example, with pulmonary vasodilators, but later structural changes in the pulmonary vascular bed lead to irreversible pulmonary vascular obstructive disease (PVOD).

Blood Volume

Blood volume varies considerably during the immediate postnatal period and depends on the amount of blood drained from the placenta before the cord is clamped. Delay in clamping or stripping the cord may increase the blood volume by over 20%, resulting in transient respiratory distress. Conversely, fetal hypoxia during labor causes vasoconstriction and a shift of blood to the placental circulation. Therefore, asphyxiated neonates may be hypovolemic.

The response to hypovolemia and restoration of the blood volume is of great importance to the anesthesiologist, as surgery in the newborn is often accompanied by significant blood loss. Withdrawal of blood during exchange transfusion has been demonstrated to cause a progressive parallel decline in systolic blood pressure and cardiac output. Reinfusion of an equal volume of blood restores these parameters to their original values. Thus, changes in arterial blood pressure are proportional to the degree of hypovolemia. A newborn's capacity to adapt the intravascular volume to the available blood volume is very limited, perhaps as a result of less efficient control of capacitance vessels. Because the baroreflexes of the infant, especially the preterm infant, are inactive, this further compromises the response to hypovolemia.

In summary, the infant's systolic arterial blood pressure (BP) is closely related to the circulating blood volume. Therefore, the BP is an excellent guide to the adequacy of blood replacement during anesthesia, a fact that is amply confirmed by extensive clinical experience. The hypovolemic infant will be unable to maintain an adequate cardiac output; hence, accurate early volume replacement is essential.

Table 2-4 shows approximate normal values for blood volume in pediatric patients. Values may be higher, however, particularly in the preterm infant.

Response to Hypoxia

Because of its high metabolic rate for O_2, hypoxemia can develop rapidly in the neonate, in whom the first observed response is usually bradycardia (in contrast to tachycardia in the adult). The anesthesiologist

TABLE 2-4.   NORMAL BLOOD VOLUME
OF CHILDREN

Age	Blood Volume (ml/kg)
Newborn	80–85
6 weeks to 2 years	75
2 years to puberty	72

should treat any episode of unexplained bradycardia by immediately ventilating the patient with 100% O_2. During hypoxemia, pulmonary vasoconstriction occurs and the pulmonary artery pressure increases more than in adults. The ductus arteriosus may reopen simultaneously. Then a large right-to-left shunt develops, further decreasing arterial O_2 saturation. Changes in cardiac output and SVR in infants also differ from those in older children and adults. During hypoxemia the principal response in adults is systemic vasodilation, which, together with an increased cardiac output, helps to maintain O_2 transport to the tissues. The fetus and some neonates respond to hypoxemia with systemic vasoconstriction. During fetal life this directs more blood to the placenta. After birth, however, this response may reduce cardiac output, thereby further limiting O_2 transport and forcing the heart to work harder. In the infant, the early and pronounced bradycardia in response to hypoxia may be due to myocardial hypoxia and acidosis.

In summary, neonates exposed to hypoxemia suffer pulmonary and systemic vasoconstriction, bradycardia, and a decrease in cardiac output. Rapid intervention is necessary to prevent this state from proceeding to cardiac arrest.

Blood and Oxygen Transport

Neonatal blood volume is approximately 80 ml/kg at term and about 20% higher in the preterm infant. The hematocrit (Hct) is 60%, and the hemoglobin (Hb) content is 18–19 g/dl. The values for blood volume, Hct, and Hb content vary from infant to infant, depending on the time of clamping of the umbilical cord. There is little change in these values for the first week of life, after which the Hb level starts to fall; this change occurs more rapidly in the preterm infant.

Most (70–90%) of the Hb present at term birth is of the fetal type. The affinity of fetal Hb (HbF) for oxygen is greater than that of adult Hb (HbA), primarily owing to a lack of effect of 2,3-diphosphoglycerate (2,3-DPG) on the HbF-O_2 interaction. Thus, HbF combines with more oxygen but releases it less readily in the tissues than does HbA. The P_{50} (PO_2 with 50% hemoglobin saturation) for HbF is approximately 20 mmHg in contrast to 26–27 mmHg for HbA. Therefore, adequate oxygen transport to the tissues of the newborn infant demands a higher Hb concentration; less than 12 g/dl constitutes anemia, and higher levels are very desirable in hypoxic states. Correction of anemia by blood transfusion is indicated if the infant requires O_2 therapy or is experiencing apneic episodes.

Transfusion with HbA-containing erythrocytes may improve O_2 transport to the tissues in the sick preterm infant. However, this therapy has been reported to increase the risk of retrolental fibroplasia.

During the first weeks of life, the Hct and Hb levels decline steadily as a result of early suppression of erythropoiesis, with improved tissue oxygenation and a progressive increase in blood volume. This physiologic anemia of infancy reaches a low point at 2–3 months of age, with Hb levels of 9–11 g/dl. At this time the HbF content of the blood has been largely replaced by HbA, and as a result O_2 delivery at the tissues is improved. Provided nutrition is adequate, the Hb level now increases gradually over several weeks to a level of 12–13 g/dl, which is maintained during early childhood.

The preterm infant demonstrates an earlier and greater fall in Hb level, with levels reaching 7–8 g/dl in those under 1,500 g birth weight. This is due to a short erythrocyte life span, rapid growth, and a low level of erythropoietin production. The early "physiologic" anemia of the preterm infant is often followed by a continuing "late" anemia, which is secondary to nutritional deficiencies. Iron therapy is not effective in correcting this situation and may even cause other problems (e.g., hemolysis, infection). Anemia of the preterm infant may lead to tachycardia, tachypnea, poor feeding and growth, diminished activity, and apnea. In severe states, congestive heart failure may occur.

Suggested Additional Reading

Burrows FA, JR Klinck, M Rabinovitch, and DJ Bohn: Pulmonary hypertension in children: perioperative management. Can Anaesth Soc J 33:606–628, 1986.

Delivoria-Papadopoulos M, NP Roncevic, and FA Oski: Post-natal changes in oxygen transport of term, premature, and sick infants: the role of 2,3-diphosphoglycerate and adult hemoglobin. Pediatr Res 5:235, 1971.

Editorial: Anaemia in premature infants. Lancet 2:1371, 1987.

Friedman WF: The intrinsic properties of the developing heart. Prog Cardiovasc Dis 15:87, 1972.

Gregory GA: The baroresponses of preterm infants during halothane anaesthesia. Can Anaesth Soc J 29:105, 1982.

Holland BM, JG Jones, and CAJ Wardrup: Lessons from the anemia of prematurity. Hematol Oncol Clin North Am 1:355, 1987.

James LS, and RD Rowe: The pattern of response of pulmonary and systemic arterial pressures in newborn and older infants to short periods of hypoxia. J Pediatr 51:5, 1957.

Kaplan S: Evaluation of the heart and circulation in health and disease. *In*: Nelson Textbook of Pediatrics, 10th ed. (VC Vaughan, RJ McKay, and WE Nelson, eds). Philadelphia, WB Saunders, 1975, p. 1000.

Keith JD, RD Rowe, and P Vlad: Heart Disease in Infancy and Childhood, 3rd ed. New York, Macmillan, 1978, Ch. 4.

Moss AJ, and FH Adams (eds): Heart Disease in Infants, Children, and Adolescents. Baltimore, Williams & Wilkins, 1968.

O'Brien RT, and HA Pearson: Physiologic anemia of the newborn infant. J Pediatr 79:132, 1971.

Rowe MI, and MB Marchildon: Physiologic considerations in the newborn surgical patient. Surg Clin North Am 56:245, 1976.

*Rudolph AM: Congenital Diseases of the Heart. Chicago, Year Book Medical Publishers, 1974, Chs. 1 and 2.

Sabio H: Anemia in the high risk infant. Clin Perinatol 11:59, 1984.

Stockman JA: Anemia of prematurity. Clin Perinatol 4:239, 1977.

Swiet M, P Fayers, and EA Shinebourne: Systolic BP in a population of infants in the first year of life: the Brompton study. Pediatrics 65:1028, 1980.

Wallgren G, M Barr, and U Rudhe: Hemodynamic studies of induced acute hypo- and hypervolemia in the newborn infant. Acta Paediatr Scand 53:1, 1964.

Wallgren G, JS Hansen, and J Lind: Quantitative studies of the human neonatal circulation. III. Observations on the newborn infant's central circulatory responses to moderate hypovolemia. Acta Paediatr Scand [Suppl] 179:43, 1967.

Walsh SZ, WW Mayer, and J Lind: The Human Fetal and Neonatal Circulation. Function and Structure. Springfield, IL, Charles C Thomas, 1974.

METABOLISM: FLUID AND ELECTROLYTE BALANCE

GLUCOSE METABOLISM

At term, the neonate has stores of glycogen that are located mainly in the liver and myocardium. These are used during the first few hours of life until gluconeogenesis becomes established. Small-for-gestational-age

---

* Key article.

(SGA) and preterm infants may have inadequate glycogen stores and fail to establish adequate gluconeogenesis.

Hypoglycemia is common in the stressed neonate, especially in SGA and preterm infants, in infants of diabetic mothers, and in the Beckwith-Wiedemann syndrome (*see* page 232). Blood glucose levels should be measured in sick neonates, and levels below 40 mg/100 ml or 2.2 mmol/L should be corrected by continuous infusion of 10% dextrose (5 mg/kg/min). Symptoms of hypoglycemia should be treated immediately by injection of 1–2 ml/kg of 50% dextrose (diluted to 10% before injection). Neurologic damage may occur in up to 50% of infants with symptomatic hypoglycemia. Infants of diabetic mothers must be treated with particular care, as a therapeutic dose of intravenous (IV) glucose may precipitate hyperinsulinemia and a serious rebound hypoglycemia. A slow infusion of glucose (4–8 mg/kg/min) is recommended for these infants.

Hyperglycemia is a common iatrogenic problem of small infants receiving IV therapy. This is probably due to inadequate insulin release and continued hepatic glucose production. The effects of hyperglycemia can be serious. Osmotically induced cerebral fluid shifts may lead to cerebral hemorrhage, and glycosuria may result in water and electrolyte depletion. Recent evidence suggests that hyperglycemia may also increase the extent of neurologic damage suffered during a cerebral hypoxic-ischemic event. Thus, it is essential that glucose therapy be carefully controlled to avoid hyperglycemia.

Older infants and young children may become hypoglycemic during an excessively long preoperative fasting period.

CALCIUM METABOLISM

Calcium is actively transported across the placenta to meet the needs of the fetus. This transport accelerates near term and may cause a fall in maternal calcium levels. After birth, the infant must depend on its own calcium reserves. However, parathyroid function is not fully established, and vitamin D stores may be inadequate. As a result, hypocalcemia must be anticipated, especially in the preterm infant or after birth trauma, neonatal asphyxia, any severe neonatal illness, or blood transfusion. Correction of metabolic acidosis in the neonate with sodium bicarbonate may precipitate hypocalcemia.

Symptoms of hypocalcemia include twitching, increased muscle tone, and convulsions. (Obviously hypocalcemia is not always easily distinguished from hypoglycemia.) Chvostek's sign may be present, but confirmation depends on laboratory tests (total serum calcium <7 mg/dl or 1.75 mmol/L; ionized calcium <4 mg/dl or 1.0 mmol/L) or the response to therapy. The infant prone to hypocalcemia is treated by continuous calcium gluconate infusion containing 60 mg of calcium/kg/24 hr. Symptomatic hypocalcemia requires infusion of 10% calcium gluconate, 1 ml/min (maximum 3 ml/kg), with continuous ECG monitoring. Calcium-containing solutions may cause severe damage, leading to slough, if they leak from the IV line into the tissues.

BILIRUBIN METABOLISM

In the term infant, unconjugated hyperbilirubinemia during the first week of life (physiologic jaundice) is secondary to an increased bilirubin load, limited hepatic cell uptake of bilirubin, and deficient hepatic conjugation to the water-soluble glucuronide. Serum bilirubin levels seldom exceed 6 mg/dl (or 103 μmol/L). In preterm infants, higher levels (10–15 mg/dl or 170–255 μmol/L) are commonly reached. These levels persist for a longer period owing to a higher bilirubin load and delayed maturation of the hepatic conjugation pathway. Unfortunately, the preterm infant may sustain neurologic damage at lower serum bilirubin levels (6–9 mg/dl) than the term infant (20 mg/dl). This predisposition is a result of the less effective blood-brain barrier of the preterm infant and may be exacerbated by hypoxia, acidosis, hypothermia, or a low level of serum albumin (and hence decreased binding sites). Therefore, the preterm infant must be carefully monitored for increased serum bilirubin levels, and specific therapy should be administered as required. Treatment includes phototherapy and possibly exchange transfusion. Some drugs (e.g., diazepam, sulphonamides, furosemide) may displace protein-bound bilirubin and therefore increase the danger of toxicity. There are no reports of anesthetic drugs (except diazepam) producing adverse changes in bilirubin levels, but hypoxia, acidosis, hypothermia, and hypoalbuminemia may all increase the danger.

Suggested Additional Reading

Brodersen R: Prevention of kernicterus, based on recent progress in bilirubin chemistry. Acta Pediatr Scand 66:625, 1977.

Cashore WJ, and LJ Stern: Neonatal hyperbilirubinemia. Pediatr Clin North Am 29:1191, 1982.

Hall SC, HJ Przybylo and AG Roth: 5% and 10% dextrose intravenous solutions during neonatal surgery. Anesthesiology 69A:738, 1988.

Kwang-Sun L, LM Gartner, AI Eidelman, and S Ezhuthachan: Unconjugated hyperbilirubinemia in very low birth weight infants. Clin Perinatol 4:305, 1977.

Sieber FE, DS Smith, RJ Traystman, and H Wollman: Glucose: a reevaluation of its intraoperative use. Anesthesiology 67:72–81, 1987.

Tsang RC, JJ Steichen, and DR Brown: Perinatal calcium homeostasis: neonatal hypocalcemia and bone demineralization. Clin Perinatol 4:385, 1977.

Wald MK: Problems in metabolic adaptation: glucose, calcium, and magnesium. *In*: Care of the High Risk Neonate, 2nd ed. (MH Klaus and AA Fanaroff, eds). Philadelphia, WB Saunders, 1979, p. 224.

Watson BG: blood glucose levels in children during surgery. Br J Anaesth 44:712, 1972.

COMPOSITION AND REGULATION OF BODY FLUIDS

The management of fluid and electrolyte therapy demands a knowledge of the maturation of renal function in the infant and the differences in the volumes of the fluid compartments.

BODY WATER

The amount of total body water is relatively greater in neonates and infants than in adults. Its distribution also differs, the proportion of extracellular fluid (ECF) being greater in neonates and young children. In the preterm infant the ECF exceeds the intracellular fluid (ICF), whereas in the older child and adult the ECF is only half the volume of the ICF (Table 2-5). Normal levels of serum electrolytes in the newborn are listed in Table 2-6.

NEONATAL RENAL FUNCTION AND WATER BALANCE

In the newborn, and especially the preterm infant, renal function is determined by a relatively low glomerular filtration rate (GFR) and by limited tubular function. The relatively low GFR increases with fluid loading but only to limited capacity. Consequently, the infant cannot readily handle a large water load and may be unable to excrete excess electrolyte or other substances dependent on glomerular filtration. The GFR is further decreased by hypoxia, hypothermia, or congestive cardiac failure.

The limited tubular function impairs the infant's ability to modify the glomerular filtrate for conservation or excretion. Thus, sodium losses are large in the preterm infant and must be balanced by intake. They are further increased if the GFR is elevated by a high fluid intake. Glucose reabsorption is also limited by tubular function; hence, glycosuria may

TABLE 2-5. EXTRACELLULAR AND INTRACELLULAR FLUID

	% Body Weight			
	Neonate		Infant	
Fluid	Preterm	Term	(7–8 months)	Adult
ECF	50	35–40	30	20
ICF	30	35	35	45

occur. In the patient with marked hyperglycemia, the resultant osmotic diuresis may lead to severe dehydration. The ability of the tubule to excrete acid is reduced in the preterm infant; thus impairing renal compensation in acidosis. H^+ excretion capacity increases with gestational age. Newborn infants have a lower renal threshold for bicarbonate than adults, and this leads to lower serum bicarbonate levels The limitations of renal function summarized above necessitate careful fluid and electrolyte replacement therapy to approximate losses. Renal function matures rapidly over the first few weeks of life in the term infant. Preterm infants show less rapid changes in renal function.

Fluid loss (and hence replacement requirement) is related to insensible fluid loss, urine output, and metabolic rate. Insensible fluid losses are relatively high during infancy, a major factor being the high level of V_A. Fluid losses are increased by the use of radiant heat and phototherapy.

Because of the infant's proportionally higher water turnover and limited ability to concentrate urine and conserve water, dehydration develops rapidly when intake is restricted or losses occur.

MAINTENANCE REQUIREMENTS

Although maintenance requirements are directly related to O_2 consumption and caloric expenditure (and are more accurately expressed as milliliters per square meter of surface area), it is most convenient to relate

TABLE 2-6. NORMAL BLOOD CHEMISTRY

	Neonate		Over 2 Yrs
Parameter	Preterm	Term	to Adult
Serum chloride (mEq/L)	100–117	90–114	98–106
Serum potassium (mEq/L)	4.6–6.7	4.3–7.6	3.5–5.6
Serum sodium (mEq/L)	133–146	136–148	142
Blood glucose (mg/dl)	40–60	40–80	70–110
Total protein (g/dl)	3.9–4.7	4.6–7.7	5.5–7.8
$PaCO_2$ (mmHg)	30–35	33–35	35–40

TABLE 2-7. DAILY MAINTENANCE REQUIREMENTS FOR FLUID, ELECTROLYTES, AND CARBOHYDRATES IN RELATION TO WEIGHT

Weight	H_2O (ml/kg)	Na^+ (mEq/kg)	K^+ (mEq/kg)	Carbohydrate (g/kg)
Newborn[a] (g)				
1,000	up to 200	3.0	2.0–2.5	up to 10
1,000–1,499	up to 180	2.5	2.0–2.5	
1,500–2,500	up to 160	2.0	1.5–2.0	up to 8
2,500	up to 150	1.5–2.0	2.0	up to 5
4–10 kg	100–120	2.0–2.5	2.0–2.5	5–6
10–20 kg	80–100	1.6–2.0	1.6–2.0	4–5
20–40 kg	60–80	1.2–1.6	1.2–1.6	3–4
Adult (total)	2,500–3,000 ml	50 mEq	50 mEq	100–150 g

[a] Adjust according to postnatal age, exposure to phototherapy, reduced insensible losses with assisted ventilation, etc.

Reproduced with permission from The Hospital for Sick Children: Residents' Handbook of Pediatrics, 6th ed., 1979.

them to body weight. Table 2-7 shows the period of high metabolic activity in infants weighing 4–20 kg.

Fluid, Na, and K requirements can be met by the IV infusion of appropriate volumes of a solution of two-thirds 5% glucose and one-third 0.3% N saline, containing 20 mEq of K per liter.

Suggested Additional Reading

Albert MS, and RW Winters: Acid-base equilibrium of blood in normal infants. Pediatrics 37:728, 1966.

Arant BS: Fluid therapy in the neonate—concepts in transition. J Pediatr 101:387, 1982.

*Bennett EJ: Fluids for Anesthesia and Surgery in the Newborn and Infant. Springfield, IL, Charles C Thomas, 1975.

Cassels DE, and M Morse: Arterial blood gases and acid-base balance in normal children. J Clin Invest 32:824, 1953.

Guignard JP: Renal function in the newborn infant. Pediatr Clin North Am 29:777, 1982.

Leake RD: Perinatal nephrobiology: a development perspective. Clin Perinatol 4:321, 1977.

Winters RW (ed): Principles of Pediatric Fluid Therapy. Chicago, Abbott Laboratories, 1970.

Winters RW (ed): The Body Fluids in Pediatrics. Boston, Little, Brown, 1973.

* Key article

PHYSIOLOGY OF TEMPERATURE HOMEOSTASIS

Because of their large surface area relative to body weight and their lack of heat-insulating subcutaneous fat, infants tend to lose heat rapidly when placed in a cool environment. This heat is lost by radiation, conduction, and convection. Further heat is lost by evaporation of water in the respiratory tract and through the skin. Evaporative heat loss via the skin is a significant factor in the preterm infant and is related to increased skin permeability. Heat loss from the body surface by radiation is related to the temperature of surrounding objects (e.g., the wall of the incubator) and not to the surrounding air temperature. Hence, a single-walled incubator does not prevent radiant heat loss if the wall temperature is below that of the infant.

When heat loss occurs, heat production within the body must be increased to maintain a normal core temperature. In adults and older children, this heat production is principally a function of involuntary muscular activity (shivering) accompanied by increased oxygen uptake, both of which can be prevented by administering a neuromuscular blocking drug. Infants rely primarily on nonshivering thermogenesis to generate heat. This mechanism, which also results in increased oxygen uptake, is largely centered in the brown adipose tissue, which composes 2–6% of the term infant's body weight (less in the preterm infant) and is located around the scapulae, in the mediastinum, and surrounding the kidneys and adrenal glands. The cells of the "brown fat" have many mitochondria and fat vacuoles, and the tissue has a rich blood and autonomic nerve supply. Increased metabolic activity in brown fat is initiated by norepinephrine released at the sympathetic nerve endings. Hydrolysis of triglyceride to fatty acids and glycerol occurs with associated increased oxygen consumption and heat production. Brown fat deposits decline during the first weeks of extrauterine life.

It is now recognized that the mechanisms for controlling body temperature are well developed in the term newborn. A fall in rectal temperature results when compensatory increases in heat production cannot match heat losses. On exposure to a cool environment, increased metabolic activity is initiated in the brown fat to maintain the core (i.e., rectal) temperature. This is accompanied by increased oxygen and glucose utilization and by the formation of acid metabolites. A normal rectal temperature does not indicate that thermogenesis is inactive but may indeed be the result of intense activity of brown fat.

The physiologic responses to cooling lead to increased oxygen and glucose utilization and result in acidosis, all of which may compromise

TABLE 2-8. NEUTRAL THERMAL ENVIRONMENT TEMPERATURES

Age	Temperature (°C) by Weight			
	1,200 g	1,200–1,500 g	1,500–2,500 g	2,500 g
0–6 hr	34–35.4	33.9–34.4	32.8–33.8	32.0–33.8
6–12 hr	34–35.4	33.5–34.4	32.2–33.8	31.4–33.8
12–24 hr	34–35.4	33.3–34.3	31.8–33.8	31.0–33.7
24–36 hr	34–35	33.1–34.2	31.6–33.6	30.7–33.5
36–48 hr	34–35	33.0–34.1	31.4–33.5	30.5–33.3
48–72 hr	34–35	33.0–34.0	31.2–33.4	30.1–33.2
72–96 hr	34–35	33.0–34.0	31.1–33.2	29.8–32.8
4–12 days		33–34[a]	31–33.2	29.5–31.4
2–3 weeks		32.2–34[a]	30.5–33.0	
3–4 weeks		31.6–33.6[a]	30.0–32.7	

[a] 1,500 g.

the sick infant. The infant with chronic hypoxemia (e.g., cyanotic congenital heart disease) is unable to compensate if exposed to a low ambient temperature and will cool rapidly. To prevent the need for compensatory responses by the infant, sick neonates should be maintained in a neutral thermal environment, that is, in an ambient temperature that minimizes oxygen consumption (Table 2-8). During anesthesia the normal thermoregulatory response of the infant to cold stress is eliminated, and there is no increase in VO_2 or heat production. Thus, the patient may cool very rapidly. Measures to minimize heat loss and avoid cold stress are outlined on page 84.

Suggested Additional Reading

*Adamsons K, Jr, GM Gandy, and LS James: The influence of thermal factors upon oxygen consumption of the newborn human infant. J Pediatr 66:495, 1965.

Bennett EF, KP Patel, and EM Grundy: Neonatal temperature and surgery. Anesthesiology 46:303, 1977.

Hey EN, and G. Katz: The optimum thermal environment for naked babies. Arch Dis Child 45:328, 1970.

Heiser MS, and JJ Downes: Temperature regulation in the pediatric patient. Semin Anesth 3:37–42, 1984.

Lindahl SGE, EJ Grigsby, DM Meyer, and FMK Beynen: Oxygen uptake, body, skin, and room temperatures in anesthetised infants and children. Anesthesiology 69A:765, 1988.

---

* Key article

Levison H, and PR Swyer: Oxygen consumption and the thermal environment in newly born infants. Biol Neonate 7:305, 1964.

Ryan JF, RS Wilson, NG Goudsouzian, and MT Jasinka: Oxygen consumption as a measure of thermoregulation in children. *In*: Abstracts of Scientific Papers Presented at the Annual Meeting of the American Society of Anesthesiologists, San Francisco, 1973, p. 273.

*Silverman WA, and JC Sinclair: Temperature regulation in the newborn infant. N Engl J Med 274:92, 146, 1966.

3

Pediatric Anesthetic Techniques and Procedures, Including Pharmacology

PHARMACOLOGY OF ANESTHETIC DRUGS

ROUTES OF ADMINISTRATION

Intravenous. The intravenous (IV) route is the most certain route under all conditions and should be the principal route for all anesthetic drugs given parenterally. Be very careful to check all drugs and doses before administration. For less commonly used drugs (e.g., antibiotics), ensure that the manufacturer's directions as to speed of injection, dilution, etc., are carefully followed. Rapid injection of some drugs (e.g., erythromycin) may cause severe physiologic effects (e.g., hypotension).

Intramuscular. Drugs administered intramuscularly (IM) are quite rapidly absorbed, especially in small children. However, this route is much less certain, especially in patients with shock or hypovolemia, and there is a danger that repeated doses may have a cumulative effect when the muscle tissue perfusion improves. Intramuscular injections are painful and are universally disliked in a children's hospital.

Intralingual. Injections into the tongue have been suggested for use in an emergency (e.g., succinylcholine). It has not been my experience that this is ever necessary, and therefore I do not recommend it.

Intratracheal. Drugs sprayed into the trachea are very rapidly absorbed, and this may be a useful emergency route if an IV route is not available (i.e., to administer atropine or to give epinephrine during cardiopulmonary resuscitation).

N.B. Drugs should not be injected into central hyperalimentation lines, as infection or thrombosis of the line might result.

Rectal. Suppositories or rectal infusions of drugs (e.g., pentobarbital, methohexital) are usually well accepted by young children (under 4 years). Absorption is less certain than by other routes.

Oral. Premedication and postoperative analgesics may be given to selected patients by this route, which is pleasant but somewhat uncertain. Obviously, the oral route cannot be used if vomiting or other gastrointestinal malfunction is present or threatens.

DISTRIBUTION OF ADMINISTERED DRUGS

In infants and young children, the relative sizes of the body fluid compartments differ from those in the adult. The extracellular fluid (ECF) compartment is large, and hence drugs that are distributed throughout this space (e.g., succinylcholine) are required in larger doses.

Protein binding is less in neonates due to lower total serum protein levels; hence more of the administered drug will be free in the plasma to exert a clinical effect. Lower doses of such drugs as barbiturates are therefore indicated.

The composition of the body also has an influence on drug distribution; neonates have little fat or muscle tissue. Drugs normally distributed to these tissues will have a longer half-life.

METABOLISM AND ELIMINATION OF DRUGS

Drugs that are metabolized in the liver will generally have a longer half-life in the neonate compared with the adult (e.g, thiopental, diazepam). Older infants and young children may, however, demonstrate rapid elimination of some drugs, reflecting enhanced hepatic metabolism.

Excretion of drugs by the kidney (e.g., curare) depends on the glomerular filtration rate (GFR) or tubular secretion capacity, both of which are reduced in the first few weeks of life.

DRUGS USED IN PEDIATRIC ANESTHESIA

AGENTS FOR GENERAL ANESTHESIA

INHALATION AGENTS

Inhaled anesthetic drugs increase in concentration in the alveolus more rapidly in children than in adults; alveolar levels approach inspired levels most rapidly in infants. This is due to the high level of alveolar ventilation relative to the functional residual capacity (FRC), the higher proportion of vessel-rich tissues that rapidly equilibrate with blood levels, and the lower blood gas solubility coefficients for volatile anesthetics in infants. Therefore, induction of anesthesia is more rapid in infants and small children. The rapid rise in alveolar and blood levels of potent inhalation agents may partly account for the alarming blood pressure (BP) falls that sometimes occur when higher concentrations of these agents are given, especially during controlled ventilation.

Excretion of inhaled anesthetic agents, and therefore recovery, is also more rapid in infants and small children, provided ventilation is not depressed. The alveolar level of nitrous oxide falls to 10% within 2 minutes of discontinuing 70% N_2O, a level not reached until 10 minutes in adults.

The minimal alveolar concentration (MAC) for all anesthetic agents is higher in younger children than in older children or adults but is lower in newborn infants and especially preterm infants. The reasons for this are unknown.

Halothane

Halothane is an almost ideal anesthetic agent for children and is very widely used in pediatric anesthesia. It provides a smooth inhalation induction with minimal irritant effects on the respiratory system. The level of anesthesia is easily controlled and can be rapidly changed. The MAC for halothane is 0.87% in neonates, 1.2% in infants, and 0.75% in adults. If intubation of children under deep halothane anesthesia is planned, the MAC for endotracheal intubation without coughing (MAC-EI) is 40–50% higher than the values given above.

During halothane anesthesia a dose-dependent depression of spontaneous ventilation occurs; the tidal volume (V_T) decreases considerably, with an increase in respiratory rate. This is followed by an increase in the end-tidal CO_2. The level of ventilation returns toward normal during surgical stimulation and is quite variable throughout anesthesia. Halothane inhibits intercostal muscle activity; diaphragmatic ventilation predominates, and paradoxical movement of the chest wall may occur. Even very low blood levels of halothane cause severe depression of the ventilatory response to hypoxia in young volunteers, and it is likely that this effect occurs in all pediatric patients. Severe laryngeal spasm may occur during light planes of halothane anesthesia, especially on extubation of the trachea. This can be avoided by extubating children while they are still deeply anesthetized or completely awake. Alternatively, lidocaine, 1–2 mg/kg IV, given prior to extubation prevents laryngospasm. Halothane is a potent bronchodilator and is very useful in children with asthma.

Halothane depresses the myocardium. It also produces bradycardia, and hence causes a fall in cardiac output; an effect that can be largely reversed by the prior administration of atropine. Severe hypotension may result if high concentrations of halothane are administered to infants and children, especially when ventilation is controlled. This is likely to be due to myocardial depression and subsequent decreased cardiac output as the concentration of halothane rapidly increases in the child's myocardium. The infant's BP is very sensitive to changes in cardiac output, as vasoconstriction is less effective than in the adult. Inspired halothane concentrations should be limited to 0.5–1% during controlled ventilation, and the BP should be carefully monitored. In patients with cardiac failure, the myocardial depressant effects of halothane are prominent, and severe hypotension results. Halothane sensitizes the myocardium to catecholamines and arrhythmias may occur, but higher levels of exogenous epinephrine may be tolerated than in adults—epinephrine doses of 10 μg/kg in the tissues appear to be safe. Serious arrhythmias may occur in children receiving high-dose theophylline therapy if they are given halothane.

Shivering and muscle rigidity are common after halothane anesthesia. This may give rise to concern after orthopedic surgery and for patients in whom the additional oxygen demands of shivering might be detrimental; in such cases, an alternative anesthetic technique may be more appropriate.

Although halothane is a rare cause of hepatic failure in adults, only a few well-documented cases of hepatic dysfunction in children have been reported despite halothane's wide and often repeated use in this age group. Recent evidence suggests that halothane hepatitis does occur in children, supported by the fact that halothane-related antibodies have been detected in many of those affected. Significant episodes are extremely rare, however. Why prepubertal children are apparently much less at risk for halothane hepatitis is not known. Because halothane has proved to be such a satisfactory agent and because alternative regimens might introduce other more common hazards, many would advise against withholding halothane unless specific contraindications are present. Such contraindications would include a previous history of unexplained posthalothane jaundice.

Halothane, like most other potent inhalational anesthetic agents, increases cerebral blood flow (CBF) and thus may increase intracranial pressure (ICP). At low concentrations this effect is minimal, however, and if hyperventilation is employed the ICP does not increase significantly even in those with intracranial space-occupying lesions. In fact, halothane is widely used for pediatric neurosurgery and has proved most useful.

Complications after halothane are minimal. Most children who have had brief anesthesia with this agent for minor surgery are fully active very soon.

Enflurane

Enflurane was introduced into clinical practice in 1968. Compared with halothane, it produces a slower respiratory rate during anesthesia but has similar effects on the cardiovascular system (CVS). Enflurane is partly metabolized; it increases the levels of organic fluoride slightly (less than methoxyflurane) in the blood and urine. Electroencephalographic (EEG) recordings during deep enflurane anesthesia show excitatory changes, especially if respiratory alkalosis is present; epileptiform convulsions during enflurane anesthesia have been reported.

Induction of anesthesia with enflurane is not as smooth as with halothane, and breath-holding, coughing, and laryngospasm may occur. Although enflurane has a lower blood gas solubility coefficient, induction and recovery times are similar to those with halothane. The incidence of nausea and vomiting after enflurane seems to equal that with other agents. Enflurane has no clear advantages in pediatric anesthesia.

Isoflurane

Isoflurane has a lower blood gas solubility coefficient (1.43 versus 2.3 for halothane) than any other volatile anesthetic. It is a very stable compound and thus is not metabolized in the body to any significant degree. Because of the low solubility, induction and recovery times are predicted to be rapid. As the drug is virtually not metabolized but is almost all excreted unchanged by the lung, recovery should be very complete.

The MAC for isoflurane is 1.6% in neonates, 1.8% in infants 6–12 months old, and 1.6% in children 1–5 years of age. In the preterm infant, MAC is 1.3% for those under 32 weeks' gestation and 1.4% for those 32–37 weeks' gestation.

Unfortunately, isoflurane is more pungent in smell than halothane. This makes is less satisfactory for inhalation induction, during which coughing and breath-holding may occur and arterial oxygen saturation levels decline. However, isoflurane can be readily introduced following a barbiturate induction, provided the concentration is very slowly increased. Because of its pungency, induction of anesthesia is more prolonged with isoflurane (± 7 minutes) than with halothane (± 4 minutes). Recovery following isoflurane anesthesia is rapid, an effect that is most marked in infants. Postoperative analgesic drugs are required sooner after isoflurane if pain is present. Laryngospasm on extubation and during emergence is rare. Isoflurane has effects on the respiratory system similar to those of halothane. However, the cardiovascular effects are different. Isoflurane and halothane produce similar changes in the BP of children, but ventricular function and heart rate are better maintained with isoflurane; the hypotension being due to vasodilation. Isoflurane has less myocardial depressant effect in the presence of cardiac failure than halothane and thus is useful in many patients with congenital heart disease. Isoflurane does not sensitize the myocardium to the effects of catecholamines or theophylline.

Isoflurane has a marked potentiating effect on the nondepolarizing neuromuscular blocking drugs. This effect is reversible when isoflurane is withdrawn and allows lower doses of relaxant drugs to be used.

Summary

1. The MAC of anesthetic drugs is higher in infants and children than in neonates or adults (e.g., the MAC of halothane is >1% in children but only about 0.8% in adults).
2. The smaller the child, the more rapid is the uptake of anesthetics into the alveoli.
3. High concentrations of potent inhalation agents may cause serious hypotension in infants and young children, particularly when ventilation is controlled. **Beware: overdose of volatile agents is a leading cause of serious complications.**
4. Halothane-induced hepatic failure is very rare in children under 14 years but does occur.

INTRAVENOUS AGENTS

Intravenous administration is widely used for both induction and maintenance of anesthesia in children. Intravenous induction may cause fewer psychological sequelae than inhalation induction.

The anesthesiologist should be skilled in painless venipuncture, and the assistance of an experienced nurse should be available. A sharp, fine-gauge needle (no. 26 or 27) should be used with the smallest syringe that can accommodate the volume of induction agent. Needles and syringes should be kept out of the child's sight at all times, and the word "needle" should be specifically avoided. Veins on the dorsum of the hand are readily punctured with little discomfort in nearly all children. The prior application to the skin of a eutectic mixture of lidocaine and prilocaine (EMLA*) has been demonstrated to relieve the pain of venipuncture (*see* page 86). Music, pictures, television, bubble blowing will also help to distract the child during venipuncture. A disposable 26- or 27-gauge "butterfly" needle is easy to conceal during insertion and to leave in situ for short procedures. If the patient arrives in the operating room with a peripheral IV infusion running, this can of course be used as a route for induction drugs. Injections should not be made into central or IV hyperalimentation lines.

Induction
Thiopental

Thiopental is still the most commonly used IV induction agent in infants and children of all ages. The usual dose for healthy children is 4–5 mg/kg of 2.5% solution. Neonates are especially sensitive to barbiturates, so it is wise to reduce the dose accordingly (2–4 mg/kg). However, infants

---

* Astra Pharmaceuticals Inc., Missisauga, Ontario, Canada.

(1 month to 1 year) may require slightly higher doses of 6–7 mg/kg to ensure sleep. Contraindications to thiopental are similar to those for adults. Intravenous induction should not be used when there is a possible airway problem.

Methohexital

Methohexital is sometimes used for induction as an alternative to thiopental. Although some authors have reported faster recovery after methohexital than after thiopental, careful testing of coordination has shown little difference between the recovery times. In children, methohexital often causes muscle twitching or hiccups, effects that can be minimized by avoiding large doses. (The dosage is approximately 1.5 mg/kg.) Its IV injection in 1% solution commonly causes pain along the injected vein; this can be minimized by adding a small amount of 2% plain lidocaine (e.g., 1 mg of lidocaine/ml of solution).

Rectal Methohexital

Methohexital is effective by the rectal route: 15 mg/kg of a 1% solution will usually induce sleep in 6–8 minutes. Rarely, ventilatory obstruction or depression may occur; hence, the child must be observed closely until sleep is achieved. The anesthesiologist should be in attendance with equipment to establish an airway discreetly at hand. Once the child falls asleep, the induction may be continued with halothane; gently assisted ventilation may be needed at this stage. This is a pleasant method of induction, especially suitable for apprehensive patients under 3 years of age, who may remain in their mother's arms until they fall asleep. The drug should be administered from a syringe with a well-lubricated no. 10 catheter that should be inserted 3–4 cm. A small volume of air in the syringe will enable the total dose to be flushed into the rectum. A diaper should be placed under the child as sometimes soiling will occur.

Diprivan (Propofol)

Diprivan (2,6-diisopropylphenol) is a short-acting hypnotic reported to be followed by a very rapid full recovery. It has been suggested that Diprivan may have an antiemetic effect; postoperative nausea is reported to be rare. Cardiovascular effects of a sleep dose (2.5 mg/kg) are similar to those of thiopental. Unfortunately, excitatory effects are common, as is pain at the site of injection. This pain is less common if Diprivan is given into a free-flowing IV infusion or into a large vein, both of which are uncommon in the small child at induction. The addition of lidocaine to the solution of Diprivan may decrease local pain.

Diazepam

There have been reports of use of diazepam, a benzodiazepine tranquilizer, for induction and, with no adjuncts, for cardioversion and cardiac catheterization in children. As an induction agent, diazepam's principal advantage is the absence of cardiovascular side effects. However, very large IV doses are required to produce unconsciousness, and the dose required varies considerably from patient to patient. Recovery takes significantly longer than after thiopental or methohexital; therefore, we rarely use diazepam for anesthesia.

Midazolam

Midazolam is a water-soluble benzodiazapine that has been used for premedication and for sedation during endoscopic procedures. A dose of 0.2–0.3 mg/kg has been used for this purpose. There is usually little ventilatory depression and good cardiovascular stability. Midazolam has also been used as a continuous infusion to produce postoperative sedation following heart surgery; following a loading dose of 0.2 mg/kg, an infusion of 0.4 μg/kg/min is commenced. It has been suggested as a possibly useful agent for induction of anesthesia, but at present there are few reported data to support this.

Summary

Of the IV induction agents available, thiopental remains the most popular and widely used in pediatric practice. All of the newer agents have problems relating to administration that render their supplanting thiopental unlikely. However, ketamine may have advantages in a few selected cases (*see below*).

Maintenance
Narcotic Analgesic Drugs

Fentanyl, morphine, and meperidine have been extensively used as part of balanced anesthesia in children. The newer agents alfentanil and sufentanil have also been used in pediatric patients. Administration by infusion following a loading dose is optimal (for dosage, *see* page 101). In addition to providing analgesia, fentanyl and sufentanil, if given in adequate dosage, may block neuroendocrine and pulmonary vascular responses to stress.

Fentanyl

Fentanyl is potent but short-acting. Its metabolism in infants depends on age—neonates, and especially preterm infants, metabolize fentanyl more slowly than older infants. A raised intra-abdominal pressure (e.g., omphalocele, diaphragmatic hernia) slows the clearance of fentanyl by reducing hepatic blood flow. As a sole analgesic agent during anesthesia, doses of 12–15 μg/kg will prevent CVS responses to surgery in infants; no supplement will be required for 60–90 minutes. If it is planned to extubate the patient after surgery, 2–4 μg/kg/hr may be used to supplement N_2O during balanced anesthesia. Larger doses should not be given to small infants unless the patient will be ventilated or can be closely monitored postoperatively. Rebound of fentanyl blood levels may occur and cause depression of ventilation; therefore, if large doses have been given, the patient must be carefully watched. Older infants (>3 months) may be less sensitive to fantanyl-induced ventilatory depression and have been demonstrated to metabolize the drug more rapidly. Bradycardia may occur after fentanyl administration unless it is preceded by a vagal blocking drug (e.g., atropine or pancuronium). Muscle rigidity may occur with the potent analgesics but is rare in infants and children.

Alfentanil

Alfentanil has a more rapid onset and shorter duration of action than fentanyl. It is less lipid soluble than fentanyl and is highly protein bound. Most of the drug is metabolized in the liver, and only <1% is excreted via the kidney unchanged. Clearance of the drug is slower and more variable in young infants, especially those who are preterm. Otherwise, in older infants and children, the pharmacokinetics are similar to those in adults. The drug has minimal cardiovascular effects. Alfentanil, 35 μg/kg as a bolus, followed by intermittent doses of 10 μg/kg every 10–15 minutes, has been suggested as a suitable for children. A continuous infusion may be preferred. It is reported that recovery is very rapid and complete following alfentanil, but as this is a very potent drug, the patient should be closely observed for any signs of residual or recurring respiratory depression.

Sufentanil

Sufentanil is ten times as potent as fentanyl with a shorter elimination half-life. Clearance rates are slower in infants under 1 month old. It has been used in high doses for cardiac surgery, producing good cardiovascular stability with minimal depression of ventricular function. Sufentanil in large doses may favorably influence the metabolic and neuroendocrine response to major cardiovascular surgery in infants.

Morphine

Morphine has a longer duration of action and is suitable for supplementation of N_2O during many abdominal and thoracic procedures. Neonates are very sensitive to the ventilatory depressant effects of morphine but less so to meperidine (pethidine). Various factors have been postulated to account for this, including differences in permeability of the blood-brain barrier. Because of this sensitivity to morphine, it is prudent to avoid the drug and substitute fentanyl or meperidine for patients under 1 year of age or 10 kg body weight (unless postoperative ventilation is planned).

Neuroleptics

Droperidol is a powerful tranquilizer that potentiates sedatives and hypnotics. It has a potent antiemetic effect and has been found most useful to decrease vomiting following pediatric ophthalmic surgery.

Droperidol and fentanyl are sometimes given together to produce tranquility and analgesia during procedures performed under local analgesia (neuroleptanalgesia) or to supplement N_2O (neuroleptanesthesia).

Neuroleptanalgesia is most useful when the patient's cooperation is required during major surgery (*see* page 158). The patient should be monitored very closely afterwards as droperidol potentiates all other depressant drugs and its effects may continue for some hours.

Ketamine Hydrochloride

Ketamine, a phencyclidine derivative for general anesthesia, came into clinical use in 1964. It has been used extensively in pediatric anesthesia for a wide variety of situations, but with further knowledge the indications for its use have been limited to a few well-defined areas.

Ketamine's effects on the central nervous system (CNS) are unlike those of any other anesthetic agent in common use. It produces profound analgesia, unconsciousness, a cataleptic state, and amnesia; it increases CBF, ICP, and the cerebral metabolic rate. The airway is usually well maintained, but airway obstruction or laryngospasm may occur. Some degree of respiratory depression with brief periods of apnea may follow induction; also, because the protective laryngeal reflexes are depressed, gastric contents may be regurgitated and aspirated. Ketamine increases both heart rate and mean arterial pressure (although its direct effect on the isolated heart is a depressant one). In healthy subjects, cardiac output is increased and peripheral vascular resistance is little changed; these indirect cardiovascular responses are mediated by adrenergic pathways.

The drug has minimal gastrointestinal effects, although nausea and vomiting may occur. There have been no reports of hepatic or renal damage after its administration. Its most serious disadvantage is the very high incidence of emergence phenomena, ranging from hallucinations and bad dreams to frank psychosis. Although these phenomena can be significantly reduced by adequate premedication with a tranquilizing drug (e.g., diazepam) and by allowing the patient to recover in a quiet area, and although they may seem less common in children, the high incidence of these phenomena and other effects have limited ketamine's use. The effects on ICP and CBF have led most centers to abandon use of this drug during neuroradiologic or similar procedures, but some still use it for cardiac catheterization. Ketamine has no effect on visceral pain and therefore is unsatisfactory for abdominal surgery.

We believe that the principal indication at present for using ketamine in pediatric practice is severe burns that require numerous skin-grafting procedures; in such cases, the advantage of an early return to normal nutrition outweighs any of the disadvantages. It is also useful for minor superficial procedures in infants.

Ketamine may also be valuable for anesthesia during surgical procedures in the rare patient with epidermolysis bullosa or Stephens-Johnson syndrome, for induction of anesthesia in severely shocked patients, for general anesthesia when facilities are limited (as in some underdeveloped countries), or in the case of large-scale disasters.

Antagonist to Narcotics

There may be a need for an antagonist after the administration of narcotics as adjuncts to general anesthesia.

Naloxone hydrochloride (*Narcan*), an *N*-allyl derivative of oxymorphone HCl, antagonizes narcotics, but unlike previous agents it has no narcotic effects. In addition (unlike *N*-allylnormorphine or -levallorphan, it is also an antagonist to the narcotic effects of pentazocine. Naloxone does not increase barbiturate-induced respiratory depression and thus is useful when one does not know which drugs might be contributing to the depression. The dose is 0.01 mg/kg for infants and older children. It is preferable to avoid the necessity to administer naloxone; reversal of narcosis is accompanied by reversal of analgesia, and the patient may become very restless and upset. Always titrate the naloxone dosage slowly to achieve the desired effect.

NEUROMUSCULAR BLOCKING DRUGS

Neuromuscular blocking drugs are often used in pediatric anesthesia practice. They require special attention, as their effects in infants may differ from those in adults. The infant neuromuscular junction has less reserve than that of the adult; fade occurs at high rates of stimulation. This led to the suggestion that infants show a myasthenic response and would be sensitive to nondepolarizing relaxants. In fact, it has been found necessary to provide doses (milligrams per kilogram) for infants similar to those for adults to produce a similar degree of block. The reason for this is now recognized to be the combined effects of a larger volume of distribution in the infant and a greater degree of block at a given plasma concentration. It is important to note that while the average dose required of a nondepolarizing relaxant is similar in infants, the variability in dose requirement is much greater. Therefore, it is important to monitor the degree of neuromuscular block as a guide to dosage.

Succinylcholine

Infants require a relatively higher dose of succinylcholine (2 mg/kg) than adults (1 mg/kg) despite the lower plasma cholinesterase activity in infants under 6 months of age. The higher dose requirement is due to the distribution of the drug throughout the relatively large ECF compartment. Recovery is similar to that in the adult, as the cholinesterase activity, though lower, is quite adequate to metabolize the drug.

Cardiac arrhythmias are common after IV succinylcholine; brady-cardia is particularly common after a second dose but may occur with the first dose in pediatric patients. This bradycardia can be prevented by prior administration of an adequate dose of atropine (0.02 mg/kg IV). The IM administration of succinylcholine (4 mg/kg) causes little change in heart rate or rhythm even in unatropinized anaesthetized children.

Though myoglobinemia and myoglobinuria occur more commonly following succinylcholine in children than in adults (especially if halothane is being administered), the incidence of strong fasciculations and muscle pains is less. However, older children who are ambulant should receive pretreatment with *d*-tubocurarine (0.05 mg/kg) to prevent muscle pains. Serious rhabdomyolysis, severe myoglobinuria, and cardiac arrest may occur in children with Duchenne's muscular dystrophy (*see* page 352).

Masseter spasm has been reported to occur as frequently as 1 in 100 cases if IV succinylcholine is given following induction of anesthesia with halothane. The significance of this and its relationship to malignant hyperthermia (MH) is unclear; all reports indicate that the MH trait is much less common. It has been known for many years that succinylcholine interacts with halothane and results in increased skeletal muscle damage. Masseter spasm is extremely rare following induction with thiopental and succinylcholine and if it occurs must be considered a significant warning sign of the MH trait. It is probably wisest to avoid the routine use of a halothane-succinylcholine induction sequence. Thiopental, on the other hand, may "tame" succinylcholine, decreasing the incidence of both muscle effects and arrhythmias.

Succinylcholine causes less rise in intragastric pressure in infants and young children than in older children and adults. Therefore, pretreatment with *d*-tubocurarine is unnecessary for the former group prior to "crash induction." Intraocular pressure is increased by succinylcholine, as is the tension of the extraocular muscles. Therefore, the drug should be avoided if intraocular pressure is to be measured (i.e., in glaucoma), or if forced duction testing is planned (for strabismus surgery).

Serum potassium levels may become dangerously elevated following succinylcholine administration in children with burns, massive trauma, major neurologic disease, or renal failure.

It has been suggested that dreaming during anesthesia may be more common if repeated doses of succinylcholine are used.

d-Tubocurarine

It has been widely accepted that neonates experience a myasthenic-type response to nondepolarizing neuromuscular blocking agents. However, recent studies confirm that full relaxation of infants requires doses similar to those used in adults. This has been shown to be due to the combined effects of a larger volume of distribution and a lower plasma concentration required to achieve neuromuscular blockade in the infant. The response of individual infants to curare varies more than in adults; the use of a nerve stimulator to judge dosage is advised. Inhalation agents (especially isoflurane) potentiate curare and reduce the requirements for this drug.

In children, even small doses of curare depress the ventilatory capacity; therefore, controlled ventilation must be instituted in all those given this drug. Curare is best avoided in asthmatic patients, in whom bronchospasm secondary to histamine release may occur.

The effects of curare on the CVS are less in infants and children than in the adult. Hypotension is rare.

Pancuronium

Pancuronium, a nondepolarizing muscle relaxant, is five times as potent as *d*-tubocurarine, and the duration of its action may be slightly longer. Supplementary doses should be given carefully, using a nerve stimulator for guidance; each should be only 10–20% of the initial paralyzing dose.

Pancuronium causes less histamine release than *d*-tubocurarine and therefore does not cause bronchospasm; hence, it is the relaxant of choice for asthmatics. Pancuronium causes an increase in heart rate and BP. These effects are more pronounced in younger patients and may be partially concealed if atropine is administered. In preterm infants, pancuronium causes a sustained tachycardia and hypertension and an increase in plasma epinephrine level. Pancuronium is principally excreted via the kidney and should not be given to patients whose renal function is impaired (prolonged neuromuscular block may occur).

Metocurine

Metocurine is dimethyl *d*-tubocurarine; it is approximately twice as potent as *d*-tubocurarine and has a similar duration of action. There is, however, marked variation in the response of infants to the neuromuscular blocking effects of metocurine. The drug causes very little change in BP, though a slight increase in heart rate may occur. Metocurine is reported to cause less histamine release than *d*-tubocurarine.

Atracurium

Atracurium is a nondepolarizing neuromuscular blocking agent with a shorter duration of action (± 30 minutes) than *d*-tubocurarine or pancuronium. It decomposes at physiologic pH to inactive compounds (Hofmann elimination) and hence has a predictable rate of elimination even in the presence of severe hepatic or renal disease. The shorter duration of action and constant rate of metabolism make this drug ideal for administration by continuous infusion. In children, an initial bolus of 0.3 mg/kg followed by an infusion of 6 µg/kg/hr results in satisfactory relaxation during halothane or isoflurane anesthesia. Slightly higher doses are required if narcotics are substituted for volatile agents. Atracurium usually has little effect on the CVS. It does release histamine, especially if large doses are given rapidly, and should not be given to patients with asthma (bronchospasm has been described following administration of the drug in adults and children). A rash is common, but significant hypotension is rare. Very uncommonly, precipitous severe hypotension has followed the use of atracurium, especially when it has been given in a large dose (>0.4 mg/kg) and preceded by thiopental. An anaphylactoid reaction has been described in an infant following induction with thiopental and atracurium. In pediatric practice, atracurium is especially useful in the short case (e.g., pyloric stenosis) and in the patient with hepatic or renal impairment.

Vecuronium

Vecuronium is an intermediate-acting nondepolarizing neuromuscular blocking agent. It has a duration of action that is 35–45 minutes in children but may be longer (70 minutes plus) in small infants. The effective dose (ED_{95}) of vecuronium is higher in children 2–10 years old (81 µg/kg) than in infants (47 μg/kg) or adolescents (55 μg/kg). It is a highly specific drug causing virtually no cardiovascular effects and no significant histamine release. The duration of action of vecuronium is increased in patients with some forms of liver disease and in those with impaired renal function. Because vecuronium has no vagal blocking effect, bradycardia may occur if vagotonic drugs (e.g., fentanyl, halothane) are given concurrently; hence, atropine may be required. Vecuronium may be used as an infusion; infants require a considerably lower rate (± 60 μg/kg/hr) than older children (± 150 μg/kg/hr).

Mivacurium

Mivacurium is a new synthetic nondepolarizing neuromuscular blocking agent with a short duration of action; it is hydrolyzed by plasma cholinesterase. A dose of 0.1–0.2 mg/kg produced a profound degree of block in under 2 minutes, but the onset of block is not as rapid as that which follows succinylcholine. The duration of action is approximately 50% of that of vecuronium. The cardiovascular effects of the drug are minimal. The short duration of action of the drug suggests that it may prove useful for intubation for minor procedures and possibly for use as an infusion. As the recovery time has been shown to relate to plasma cholinesterase activity, prolonged effects may be expected in those with abnormality of the plasma cholinesterases.

REVERSAL OF NEUROMUSCULAR BLOCK

Nondepolarizing neuromuscular blocking agents should always be reversed at the end of the procedure unless it is planned to provide postoperative controlled ventilation. Reversal may uncertain in patients who are hypothermic ($<35°C$); therefore, controlled ventilation should be continued. Antibiotics very rarely cause problems with reversal in infants or children, but this possibility must be considered, especially in those receiving aminoglycoside derivatives (e.g., neomycin, gentamicin, tobramycin).

The adequacy of reversal of relaxants can be difficult to judge, especially in infants. The train of four should demonstrate four equal contractions. Muscle tone can be examined and is often best judged by the flexion of the arms and lifting of the legs. The ability to generate an inspiratory pressure of 25 cm H_2O has been suggested as a useful index. When any doubt whatsoever exists about the adequacy of reversal, continue with controlled ventilation and reevaluate the situation.

Commonly used regimens to reverse nondepolarizing muscle relaxants in infants and children are as follows:

Neostigmine mixed with atropine is effective and results in few and insignificant cardiac arrhythmias even in those with congenital heart disease. Glycopyrrolate does not have any advantage over atropine during reversal and may increase arrhythmias.

Edrophonium has a more rapid onset of action than neostigmine, but its vagotonic effects are also seen more rapidly. Hence, atropine should be given first and its effect observed before giving edrophonium.

Suggested Additional Reading

Inhalation Agents

Brandom BW, RB Brandom, and DR Cook: Uptake and distribution of halothane in infants: in vivo measurements and computer simulations. Anesth Analg 62:404, 1983.

Cameron CB, S Robinson and GA Gregory: The minimum anesthetic concentration of isoflurane in children. Anesth Analg 63:418–420, 1984.

Fisher DM, S Robinson, CM Brett, G Perin and GA Gregory: Comparison of enflurane, halothane, and isoflurane for diagnostic and therapeutic procedures in children with malignancies. Anesthesiology 63:647–650, 1985.

Friesen RH, and JL Lichtor: Cardiovascular effects of inhalation induction with isoflurane in infants. Anesthe Analg 62:411, 1983.

Kenna JG, J Neuberger, G Mieli-Vergani, A Mowat and R Williams: Halothane hepatitis in children. Br Med J 294:1209–1211, 1987.

Lerman J, MM Willis, GA Gregory, and EI Eger: The effect of age on the solubility of volatile anesthetics in blood. Anesthesiology 59A:30, 1983.

Lerman J, S Robinson, MM Willis, and GA Gregory: Anesthetic requirements for halothane in young children 0–1 month and 1–6 months of age. Anesthesiology 59A:446, 1983.

Lindahl SGE, MG Hulse and DJ Hatch: Ventilation and gas exchange during anaesthesia and surgery in spontaneously breathing infants and children. Br J Anaesth 56:121–129, 1984.

Lindahl SGE, AP Yates, and DJ Hatch: Respiratory depression in children at different end tidal halothane concentrations. Anaesthesia 42:1267–1275, 1987.

Phillips AJ, JR Brimacombe and DL Simpson: Anaesthetic induction with isoflurane or halothane: oxygen saturation during induction with isoflurane or halothane. Anaesthesia 43:927–929, 1988.

Salintre E, and H Rackow: The pulmonary exchange of nitrous oxide and halothane in infants and children. Anesthesiology 30:388, 1969.

Walton B: Halothane hepatitis in children. Anaesthesia 41:575–578, 1986.

Wark J: Postoperative jaundice in children—the influence of halothane. Anaesthesia 38:237, 1983.

Watcha MF, JE Forestner, MT Connor, et al: Minimum alveolar concentration of halothane for tracheal intubation in children. Anesthesiology 69:412–416, 1988.

Whitburn RH, and E Sumner: Halothane hepatitis in an 11 month old child. Anaesthesia 41:611–613, 1986.

Wolf WJ, MB Neal and MD Peterson: The hemodynamic and cardiovascular effects of isoflurane and halothane anesthesia in children. Anesthesiology 64:328–333, 1986.

Intravenous Agents

Baskett PJF, J Hyland, M Deane, and G Wray: Analgesia for burns dressing in children: a dose-finding study for phenoperidine and droperidol with and without 50 percent nitrous oxide and oxygen. Br J Anaesth 41:684, 1969.

Brummitt WM, and JS Whalen: Pediatric experience with ketamine hydrochloride (Ketalar). *In*: Ketalar. Montreal, Parke, Davis & Co., 1971, p. 85.

Cole WHJ: Midazolam in paediatric anaesthesia. Anaesth Intensive Care 10:36–39, 1982.

Hollister GR, and JMB Burn: Side effects of ketamine in pediatric anesthesia. Anesth Analg 53:264, 1974.

Jonmarker C, P Westrin, S Larsson, and O Werner: Thiopental requirements for induction of anesthesia in children. Anesthesiology 67:104–107, 1987.

Kay B: Neuroleptanesthesia for neonates and infants. Anesth Analg 52:970, 1973.

Lockhart CH, and WL Nelson: The relationship of ketamine requirement to age in pediatric patients. Anesthesiology 40:507, 1974.

Meursing AEE, B Bell, R Lobatto, and W Erdmann: A comparison of Propofol with thiopentone for induction of anesthesia in unpremedicated children. Anesthesiology 69A:741, 1988.

Patel DK, PA Keeling, GB Newman, and P Radford: Induction dose of Propofol in children. Anaesthesia 43:949–952, 1988.

Silvasi DL, DA Rosen, and KR Rosen: Continuous intravenous midazolam infusion for sedation in the pediatric intensive care unit. Anesth Analg 67:286–288, 1988.

Sorbo S, RJ Hudson, and JC Loomis: The pharmacokinetics of thiopental in pediatric surgical patients. Anesthesiology 61:666-670, 1984.

Yeung ML, and RSH Lin: Laryngeal reflexes in children under ketamine anaesthesia. Br J Anaesth 44:1089, 1972.

Rectal Drugs

Goresky GV, and DJ Steward: Rectal methohexitone for induction of anaesthesia in children. Can Anaesth Soc J 26:213, 1979.

Forbes RB, DJ Murray, JB Dillman, DL Dull, KL Croskey, and K Murphey: Pharmacokinetics of 2% rectal methohexital in children. Anesthesiology 69A:757, 1988.

Liu LMP, P Gaudrealt, PA Friedman, NG Goudsouzian, and PL Liu: Pharmacodynamics of rectal methohexital in children. Anesthesiology 59A:450, 1983.

Narcotic Analgesic Drugs

Davis PJ, KA Robinson, RL Stiller, and DR Cook: Sufentanil kinetics in infants and children. Anesthesiology 63A:472, 1985.

Davis PJ, A Killian, RL Stiller, DR Cook, and RD Guthrie: Alfentanil pharmacodynamics in premature infants and older children. Anesthesiology 69A:758, 1988.

Greeley WJ, NP de Bruijn, and DP Davis: Pharmacokinetics of sufentanil in pediatric patients. Anesthesiology 65A:442, 1986.

Greeley WJ, and NP deBruijn: Changes in sufentanil pharmacokinetics within the neonatal period. Anesth Analg 67:86–90, 1988.

Goresky GV, G Koren, MA Sabourin, JP Sale, and L Strunin: The pharmacokinetics of alfentanil in children. Anesthesiology 67:654–659, 1987.

Hertzka RE, IS Gauntlett, DM Fisher, and MJ Spellman: Fentanyl induced ventilatory depression: effects of age. Anesthesiology 70:213–218, 1989.

Johnson KL, JP Erickson, FO Holley, and JC Scott: Fentanyl pharmacokinetics in the pediatric population. Anesthesiology 61A:441, 1984.

Koehntop dE, JH Rodman, DM Brundage, MG Hegland, and JJ Buckley: Pharmacokinetics of fentanyl in neonates. Anesth Analg 65:227–232, 1986.

Purcell-Jones G, F Dorman, and E Sumner: The use of opioids in neonates. A retrospective study of 933 cases. Anaesthesia 42:1316–1320, 1987.

Singleton MA, JI Rosen, and DM Fisher: Pharmacokinetics of fentanyl for infants and adults. Anesthesiology 61A:440, 1984.

Way WL, EC Costley, and EL Way: Respiratory sensitivity of the newborn infant to meperidine and morphine. Clin Pharmacol Ther 6:454, 1965.

Yaster M: The dose response of fentanyl in neonatal anesthesia. Anesthesiology 66:433–435, 1987.

Youngberg JA, C Subaiya, GB Graybar, et al: Alfentanil for day stay surgery in children: an evaluation. Anesth Analg 63:284, 1984.

Muscle Relaxants

Bennett EJ, S Ramamurthy, FY Dalal, and ME Salem: Pancuronium and the neonate. Br J Anaesth 47:75, 1975.

Brandom BW, DR Cook, SK Woelfel, GD Rudd, B Fehr, and CG Lineberry: Atracurium infusion requirements in children during halothane, isoflurane, and narcotic anesthesia. Anesth Analg 64:471–476, 1985.

Bush GH, and AL Stead: The use of d-tubocurarine in neonatal anaesthesia. Br J Anaesth 34:721, 1962.

Cook DR: Muscle relaxants in infants and children. Anesth Analg 60:335, 1981.

Cook DR, BW Brandom, RL Stiller, S Woefel, A Lai, and J Slater: Pharmacokinetics of atracurium in normal and liver failure patients. Anesthesiology 61A:433, 1984.

Cook DR, and CG Fischer: Neuromuscular blocking effects of succinylcholine in infants and children. Anesthesiology 42:662, 1975.

Craythorne NWB, H Turndorf, and RD Dripps: Changes in pulse rate and rhythm associated with the use of succinylcholine in anesthetized children. Anesthesiology 21:465, 1960.

Fisher DM, C O'Keefe, DR Stanski, R Cronnelly, GA Gregory, and RD Miller: Phramacokinetics and dynamics of d-tubocurarine in infants, children, and adults. Anesthesiology 55A:391, 1981.

Goudsouzian NG: Atracurium in infants and children. Br J Anaesth 58 (Suppl 1):23S–28S, 1986.

Goudsouzian NG: The physiology and pharmacology of neuromuscular transmission in infants and children. In: Some Aspects of Paediatric Anaesthesia (DJ Steward, ed). Amsterdam, Excerpta Medica, 1982, p. 59–77.

*Goudsouzian NG. Maturation of neuromuscular transmission in the infant. Br J Anaesth 52:205–213, 1980.

Goudsouzian NG, JK Alifimoff, C Eberly et al: Neuromuscular and cardiovascular effects of mivacurium in children. Anesthesiology 70:237–242, 1989.

Goudsouzian NG, JV Donlon, JJ Savarese, and JF Ryan: Reevaluation of dosage and duration of action of d-tubocurarine in the pediatric age group. Anesthesiology 43:416, 1975.

Goudsouzian NG, LM Liv, and JJ Savarese: Metocurine in infants and children: neuromuscular and clinical effects. Anesthesiology 49:266, 1978.

Goudsouzian NG, JF Ryan, and JJ Savarese: The neuromuscular effects of pancuronium in infants and children. Anesthesiology 41:95, 1974.

Goudsouzian NG, JJA Martyn, LMP Liu and M Gionfriddo: Safety and efficacy of vecuronium in adolescents and children. Anesth Analg 62:1083–1088, 1983.

Hobbs AJ, GH Bush and DY Downham: Perioperative dreaming and awareness in children. Anaesthesia 43:560–562, 1988.

Hannalah RS, TH Oh, WA McGill and BS Epstein: Changes in heart rate and rhythm after intramuscular succinylcholine with or without atropine in anesthetised children. Anesth Analg 65:1329–1332, 1986.

Meretoja OA: Vecuronium infusion requirements in pediatric patients during fentanyl-N_2O-O_2 anesthesia. Anesth Analg 68:20–24, 1989.

---

* Key article

Meretoja OA, K Wirtavuori and PJ Neuvonen: Age dependence of the dose-response curve of vecuronium in pediatric patients during balanced anesthesia. Anesth Analg 67:21–26, 1988.

Montgomery CJ, and DJ Steward: A comparative study of intubating doses of atracurium, *d*-tubocurarine, pancuronium, and vecuronium in children. Can J Anaesth 35:31–35, 1988.

Nightingale DA: Use of atracurium in neonatal anaesthesia. Br J Anaesth 58(Suppl 1):32S–36S, 1986.

Nightingale DA, and GH Bush: A clinical comparison between tubocurarine and pancuronium in children. Br J Anaesth 45:63, 1973.

Ryan JF, LK Kagen, and Al Hyman: Myoglobinemia after a single dose of succinylcholine. N Engl J Med 285:824, 1971.

Salem MR, AY Wong, and YH Lin: The effect of suxamethonium on the intragastric pressure in infants and children. Br J Anaesth 44:166, 1972.

Salem MR, T Toyama, AY Wong, HK Jacobs, and EJ Bennett: Haemodynamic responses to antagonism of tubocurarine block with atropine-neostigmine mixture in chidlren. Br J Anaesth 49:901, 1977.

Woods I, P Morris and G Meakin: Severe bronchospam following the use of atracurium in children. Anaesthesia 40:208–209, 1985.

Zsigmond ED, and JR Downs: Plasma cholinesterase activity in newborns and infants. Can Anaesth Soc J 18:278, 1971.

Reversal of Muscle Relaxants

Fisher DM, R Cronnelly, M Sharma and RD Miller: Clinical pharmacology of edrophonium in infants and children. Anesthesiology 61:428–433, 1984.

Fisher DM, R Cronnelly, RD Miller and M Sharma: The neuromuscular pharmacology of neostigmine in infants and children. Anesthesiology 59:220–225, 1983.

Mason LJ, and EK Betts: Leg lift and maximum inspiratory force, clinical signs of neuromuscular blockade reversal in neonates and infants. Anesthesiology 52:441–442, 1980.

Salem MR, LB Ylagan, JJ Angel, VS Vedam and VJ Collins: Reversal of curarization with atropine-neostigmine mixture in patients with congenital heart disease. Br J Anaesth 42:991–998, 1970.

Wong AY, MR Salem, M Mani, E Padillo and AB Mehta: Glycopyrrolate as a substitute for atropine in the reversal of curarization in pediatric cardiac patients. Anesth Analg 53:412–418, 1974.

ROUTINE PREPARATION FOR SURGERY

A careful physical examination must be made at the time of the preoperative visit. Look particularly for special problems that may complicate anesthesia. Upper respiratory tract infection (URI) is common, and if present, the decision to proceed must be made with due consideration of the urgency of the operation. Provided the temperature is normal and there are no abnormal physical findings in the chest, perioperative complications following minor surgery do not seem to occur more often in patients with mild coryza. Major procedures demand more careful consideration of existing or recent (within 2 weeks) URI.

PREOPERATIVE FEEDING ORDERS

Infants and children must not be subjected to unnecessarily prolonged preoperative fasting. The higher rate of fluid turnover in these patients dictates that fluid restriction will lead quite rapidly to hypovolemia and dehydration. In addition, fasting, if excessive, may precipitate hypoglycemia and/or metabolic acidosis.

Infants who are breast fed should have the last feeding completed by 4 hours preoperatively.

For children under 2 years, regular formula feedings are given up to 6 hours preoperatively; for the last feed (timed to be completed by 4 hours preoperatively), clear fluid must be given.

Children over 2 years of age should have no food for 8 hours before surgery or on the day of surgery but may be offered drinks of clear fluids up to 4 hours preoperatively (water, ginger ale, apple juice, etc., are considered clear fluids; milk and orange juice are *not*).

These rules must, of course, be modified in special cases (e.g., diabetics). Patients for whom any period of fluid deprivation might pose a risk (e.g., the patient with polycythemia associated with congenital heart disease) should have an IV infusion established at the commencement of the period of restricted oral intake (*see* page 129).

The above rules probably err very much on the side of safety; studies have shown that clear fluids are absorbed from the stomach within 2 hours in healthy infants and children. Indeed, it has been reported that a small drink of apple juice 2 hours before anesthesia will reduce gastric contents at induction (possibly by speeding gastric emptying) and in addition will reduce hunger and thirst. It is anticipated that fluids will, in the future, be offered to infants and small children up to 2 hours before surgery.

BASIC LABORATORY TESTS

Preoperative urinalysis and hemoglobin (Hb) results must be recorded on the chart; these must be recent and reflect the patient's current status. The value of routine Hb screening of healthy children is presently under debate; however, in many regions this is a legislated requirement. A Hb or hematocrit (Hct) should certainly be obtained on all infants and any children who are other than completely healthy. In addition, a sickle cell test is necessary for all patients at risk; if this is positive, an Hb electrophoresis should be ordered (*see* page 116).

PREMEDICATION

Drugs are given preoperatively to block unwanted autonomic reflex (vagal) responses, produce prepoperative sedation and tranquillity, and reduce the amount of general anesthetic requirement to supplement balanced anesthetic techniques.

Vagal Blocking Drugs (Atropine, Scopolamine, Glycopyrrolate)

Despite a trend to omit routine administration of vagal blocking drugs to adult patients, most authorities believe that they are indicated for infants and children. Bradycardia caused by cholinergic drugs (succinylcholine, halothane) or during instrumentation of the airway is common in young patients and may lead to serious hypotension or more dangerous arrhythmias. Therefore, I advise that every patient be given an anticholinergic agent unless it is specifically contraindicated (rare).

Atropine is the preferred anticholinergic agent. It is more effective in blocking the cardiac vagus and causes less drying of secretions than scopolamine or glycopyrrolate. Respiratory tract secretions are not a serious problem with current potent agents, for example, halothane, enflurane, isoflurane. Atropine (0.02 mg/kg; maximum 0.6 mg) may be given IV at induction mixed with thiopental. This is the preferred method; it ensures effective drug action and spares the child a possibly painful IM injection and subsequent dry mouth. If successful venipuncture is in doubt, the same dose of atropine should be given IM 30 minutes preoperatively, ensuring a peak effect at the time of induction. Atropine may also be given rectally if rectal barbiturate is used for induction of anesthesia (*see* page 48). In an emergency, the usual dose of atropine diluted in 1 ml of saline is very effective by the intratracheal route.

Sedatives and Tranquilizers

There are a voluminous literature and many divergent opinions concerning sedative premedication for children. In practice, there is no ideal drug for this purpose. Sedatives, narcotics, or tranquilizers do not ensure calm cooperation at the time of induction but do significantly increase the likelihood of postoperative depression, delirium, or vomiting. Psychological preparation is more important in the management of the child and may be more effective, both at the time of induction and in preventing lasting psychological sequelae.

Narcotics

Narcotics are rarely indicated for the premedication of healthy children. Dizziness, nausea, and vomiting are common after their use. Morphine causes severe respiratory depression in infants and should not be given to patients under 1 year of age. Morphine has been advocated in the premedication of patients with cyanotic congenital heart disease (*see* page 264). Meperidine is a poor sedative and may cause vomiting. Thus, its use as a premedicant in pediatric patients makes little sense. Narcotics all have the disadvantage of necessitating an IM injection, which children find unpleasant.

Barbiturates

Barbiturates may be given by the oral (PO), rectal (PR), or IM route. Pentobarbital, 2–4 mg/kg PO or PR, usually produces sedation and hypnosis, but some children, especially if in pain, become restless and irrational. Barbiturates should not be given to young infants (<6 months) except in much smaller doses because infants metabolize these drugs more slowly than do older children or adults.

Tranquilizers

Several tranquilizers have been used as premedicants, but the response of individual children is quite unpredictable unless very large doses are used; such doses may delay postoperative recovery.

Diazepam suspension may be given PO (up to 0.5 mg/kg 1.5 hours preoperatively) to older children, but the degree of sedation achieved varies considerably. Diazepam should not be ordered for IM injection, as this may cause severe pain. Diazepam displaces protein-bound bilirubin (*see* page 31).

Lorazepam has been successfully used for premedication of adult patients and produces a significant degree of amnesia. Unfortunately, in pediatric patients, doses that produce sedation and amnesia also result in an unacceptable incidence of side effects.

Midazolam by IM injection has been used for premedication; it is reported to allay anxiety, facilitate induction, and produce some retrograde amnesia.

SPECIAL CONSIDERATIONS

1. Neurosurgical patients must not receive any premedication except atropine, which is usually given IV at induction (*see also* page 147).
2. Atropine should not be given IM to children with pyrexia, as it may exacerbate the fever by abolishing sweating. It may be given IV at the time of induction.
3. Children over 10 kg who have congenital heart disease are usually given morphine preoperatively (*see* Cardiac Surgery and Cardiologic Procedures, page 264).
4. Most patients undergoing strabismus correction are assessed by the ophthalmologist immediately before the operation and should not be heavily sedated. They should receive atropine (0.02 mg/kg IV) at induction to block the oculocardiac reflex (*see* page 166).

Suggested Additional Reading

Dawkins MJR: Biochemical aspects of developing function in new-born mammalian liver. Br Med Bull 22:27, 1966.

*Done AK: Developmental pharmacology. Clin Pharmacol Ther 5:432, 1964.

*Eger EI II: Atropine, scopolamine, and related compounds. Anesthesiology 23:365, 1962.

Peters CG, and JT Brunton: Comparative study of lorazepam and trimeprazine for oral premedication in paediatric anaesthesia. Br J Anaesth 54:623, 1982.

Sandhar BK, G Goresky, EA Shaffer, and L Strunin: Preoperative fasting in children: how long is enough? Can J Anaesth 35S:141, 1988.

Splinter WM, JA Stewart and JG Muir: The effect of preoperative apple juice on gastric contents, thirst, and hunger in children. Can J Anaesth 36:55–58, 1989.

Steward DJ: Psychological preparation and premedication. *In*: Pediatric Anesthesia (GA Gregory, ed). New York, Churchill Livingstone, 1983, p 423–436.

Taylor MB, PR Vine, and DJ Hatch: Intramuscular midazolam premedication in small children. Anaesthesia 41:21, 1986.

Thomas DKM: Hypoglycemia in children before operation: its incidence and prevention. Br J Anaesth 46:66, 1974.

Watson BG: Blood glucose levels in children during surgery. Br J Anaesth 44:712, 1972.

---

* Key article

MANAGEMENT OF THE AIRWAY

MASK ANESTHESIA

1. During mask anesthesia, have equipment for endotracheal intubation immediately at hand:
   (a) Selection of suitably sized tubes with connectors in place (Table 3-1).
   (b) Laryngoscope with suitable blade.
   (c) Syringe loaded with succinylcholine.
2. Select a mask to fit the contours of the face and minimize the dead space. The Rendell Baker mask is preferred for infants and small children.
3. The relatively large tongue in infants and adenoidal hypertrophy in older children may cause obstruction. If this occurs, insert an oropharyngeal airway of suitable size.
4. Infants have soft laryngeal cartilages and tracheal rings. Therefore, the anesthesiologist's finger may compress the airway during mask anesthesia.

TABLE 3-1. APPROXIMATE SIZE AND LENGTH OF PEDIATRIC ENDOTRACHEAL TUBES[a]

Approximate Age of Patient (yr)	Internal Diameter (mm)[b]	Length (cm)	
		Oral	Nasal
Premature	2.5–3.0	11	13.5
Newborn	3.5	12	14
1	4.0	13	15
2	4.5	14	16
4	5.0	15	17
6	5.5	17	19
8	6.0	19	21
10	6.5	20	22
12	7.0	21	22
14	7.5	22	23
16	8.0	23	24

[a] Thin-walled, uncuffed tubes of clear PVC.

[b] Formula: $\dfrac{\text{age of patient (yr)}}{4} + 4.0$ size of tube (ID).

The tube diameters listed are given only as a guide. Always prepare a selection of tubes, and use the one with the best fit (*see above*).

ENDOTRACHEAL INTUBATION

LARYNGOSCOPY

1. Ensure that the head is correctly positioned in the "sniffing" position and supported in a low head ring.
2. Examine the teeth carefully—many children have loose deciduous teeth. The teeth must be kept in view throughout laryngoscopy; retract the lip with your thumb and exert no pressure on the teeth during intubation.
3. In children, the epiglottis may obscure one's view of the glottis unless it is elevated with the tip of the blade; therefore, use a straight blade (a curved blade is not a reliable method for visualizing the glottis in infants and small children).
4. Insufflation of oxygen into the pharynx during laryngoscopy (especially in infants or those with difficult airways) will improve oxygenation during attempts at intubation. Specially designed blades with an oxygen port are available (Mil-Port*), or a suction catheter can be taped to any blade and supplied with 4 L/min of oxygen.

INTUBATION

1. The optimal size of the tube is the largest that passes easily through the glottis and subglottic region. There should be a slight leak around the tube when 20 cm H_2O positive pressure is applied to the circuit.
2. Clear, thin-walled polyvinyl chloride (PVC) tubes (Z79 approved) are preferred. The "Murphy eye" type tube is not recommended, as the additional side hole encourages accumulation of secretions and accelerates tube blockage. Do not use cuffed tubes of less than 5.5 mm inside diameter (ID); the cuff is unnecessary, and such tubes have a smaller ID. The use of Coles tubes is not recommended: they displace easily, and the "shoulder" of the tube may dilate and damage the glottis.
3. Endotracheal connectors must have a lumen at least equal to the ID of the tube and must be firmly inserted.
4. Tubes must be firmly taped in place, preferably near the middle of the mouth, and they must be supported by a bite block to prevent kinking.
5. Pressure by anesthetic hoses, etc., on the patient's face or head must be prevented by suitable padding (e.g., Dalzofoam).
6. Ventilation must be checked in all areas of both lungs after intubation. The anesthetic circuit and tube must be carefully positioned and supported to prevent any traction on the tube that might cause it to kink.

---

* Anesthesia Medical Specialties, Santa Fe Springs, CA.

Pediatric endotracheal tubes kink very easily, and this is still a potential cause of disastrous accidents.

7. Remember that extension of the neck moves the tip of the tube proximally in the trachea (and flexion advances the tip); 1–3 cm of movement may occur between full flexion and full extension in infants. Position the tube carefully and consider the effects of changing the head position.

"DIFFICULT INTUBATION"

General physical examination detects those patients who may be difficult to intubate. Some problems may be obvious, for example, the large cystic hygroma, but other times the ease of laryngoscopy will be more difficult to assess. Therefore always:

1. Check ability to open the mouth wide; check for loose teeth.
2. Assess the length and mobility of the neck.
3. Check the mandible—is the distance between the genu and the hyoid bone normal (one fingerbreadth in infants, three in adolescents)?
4. When the patient has the mouth wide open, can you see the uvula and the palatoglossal arch completely? If these structures are partly hidden by the tongue, intubation may be difficult.

If there are any indications from the history or from your examination that intubation may be difficult.

1. Do not give IV barbiturates or muscle relaxant drugs.
2. Prepare a variety of laryngoscope blades, endotracheal tubes (ETTs), and stylets, and oropharyngeal airways.
3. Induce anesthesia with halothane and nitrous oxide and deepen anesthesia with halothane in oxygen. Establish an IV infusion and administer atropine, 0.02 mg/kg.
4. Maintain spontaneous ventilation.
5. When the patient is adequately anesthetized, give lidocaine, 1 mg/kg IV, wait 3 minutes and then perform laryngoscopy and attempt to visualize the glottis. Lidocaine IV greatly diminishes the possibility of breath-holding and laryngospasm during attempts to visualize the glottis.
6. Remember that it may be easier to push the glottis into view by external manipulation of the larynx than to visualize it by movement of the laryngoscope blade. Therefore, have an assistant present to hold the larynx in a good position during intubation.

FIBEROPTIC LARYNGOSCOPE

The use of fiberoptic laryngoscopes in pediatric patients is limited by the fact that many models cannot pass through small-size ETTs. Alternative methods for their use in pediatric patients have been suggested, for example, to visualize the glottis and pass through a stylet over which the ETT can be threaded. Fiberoptic laryngoscopy is often hampered by blood or saliva in the pharynx.

LIGHT WAND INTUBATION

The use of a malleable lighted stylet* that can be passed blindly into the trachea has been described. As the light passes into the trachea, the anterior neck can be seen to transilluminate. An ETT can be advanced over the stylet into the trachea. This method requires practice but may be successful in many patients.

BLIND NASOENDOTRACHEAL INTUBATION

Blind nasoendotracheal intubation is necessary if one cannot visualize the patient's glottis (see **Note** after item 7).

1. Inspect the nares for size and patency; use the larger one. The success rate is usually higher if the left nostril is used as the bevel of most tubes is on the left. (Special tubes are made, with the bevel on the right, for the right nostril.)
2. Prepare and lubricate suitable tubes (ID 0.5 mm, smaller than for oral intubation).
3. Use an inhalation induction, for example, $N_2O + O_2 +$ halothane; 5% CO_2 may be added to increase the tidal volume prior to intubation attempts. *Do not use barbiturates or muscle relaxants.*
4. When the patient is deeply anesthetized, position the head slightly extended as in the sniffing position.
5. Insert the tube through the nostril and advance it. It goes in one of five directions:
   (a) Larynx: desired location.
   (b) Right of larynx: withdraw the tube slightly; turn it to the left and turn the patient's head to the right.
   (c) Left of larynx: withdraw the tube slightly; turn it to the right and turn the patient's head to the left.

---

* Flexi-Lum, Concept Inc., Clearwater, FL.

(d) Esophagus: withdraw the tube slightly and extend the head maximally before readvancing the tube.

(e) Anterior to epiglottis: withdraw the tube slightly and flex the head.

6. If unsuccessful, repeat using the other nostril.

7. Other useful maneuvers include:

(a) Listening at the end of the tube for maximal gas exchange.

(b) Passage of a second tube through the other nostril to block the esophagus.

(c) External pressure to the neck to direct the glottis toward the tip of the tube.

(d) Use of a smaller size tube for initial intubation. The tube can then be changed up in size by passing a flexible stylet and leaving this in place to guide the larger tube.*

Extubation

1. Children are very prone to laryngeal spasm on extubation, especially after halothane or if extubated during a light plane of anesthesia. Therefore:

(a) Before extubation, ensure that all facilities are available to ventilate with O_2 and to reintubate if necessary.

(b) Extubate when the child is fully awake (or, if indicated, deeply anesthetized).

(c) Extubation when child is coughing or is straining on the tube must be avoided.

2. The following patients must be fully awake before extubation:

(a) All those in whom intubation was difficult.

(b) All those having emergency surgery: these patients may vomit gastric contents during emergence from anesthesia.

(c) All infants.

3. Some patients should not be allowed to cough and strain on the tube, for example, after neurosurgery or intraocular surgery. This may be achieved with a planned ''deep'' extubation, preceded by careful suctioning of the stomach and pharynx. Lidocaine, 1–2 mg/kg IV, prior to extubation will decrease the risk of coughing and breathholding.

---

* **Note.** The technique of blind intubation requires considerable skill that can be acquired only by extensive practice. If the anesthesiologist is not sufficiently experienced and has no such skilled assistance at hand, some other technique (e.g., awake intubation) may be preferable.

Suggested Additional Reading

Bosman YK, and PA Foster: Endotracheal intubation and the head posture in infants. S Afr Med J 59:71, 1977.

Brandstater B: Dilation of the larynx with Cole tubes. Anesthesiology 31:378, 1969.

Cave P, and G Flectcher: Resistance of nasotracheal tubes used in infants. Anesthesiology 29:588, 1968.

Eckenhoff JE: Some anatomic considerations of the infant larynx influencing endotracheal intubation. Anesthesiology 12:401, 1951.

Koka BV, IS Jeon, JM Andre, I MacKay, and RM Smith: Postintubation croup in children. Anesth Analg 56:501, 1977.

Lane GA, NRT Pashly, RA Fishman: Tracheal and cricoid diameters in the preterm infant. Anesthesiology 53S:326, 1980.

Ledbetter JL, DK Rasch, TG Pollard et al: Reducing the risks of laryngoscopy in anaesthetised infants. Anaesthesia 43:151–153, 1988.

Morgan GAR, and DJ Steward: Linear airway dimensions in children: including those with cleft palate. Can Anaesth Soc J 29:1, 1982.

Rayburn RL: Light wand intubation. Anaesthesia 34:677, 1979.

Ring WH, JC Adair, and RA Elwyn: A new endotracheal tube. Anesth Analg 54:273, 1975.

PEDIATRIC ANESTHETIC CIRCUITS

The ideal pediatric anesthetic circuit should be lightweight, with low resistance and dead space, adaptable to spontaneous, assisted, or controlled ventilation, and readily humidified and scavenged. These conditions are most nearly met by the T-piece systems.

T-PIECE

The T-piece, originally described by Ayre in 1973, was modified by Jackson Rees to provide artificial ventilation. We use the modified T-piece for all children under 20 kg in weight and for some older patients. The T-piece relies on continuous flow from the fresh gas limb to flush the expiratory limb and so remove expired gas. The performance of the T-piece therefore depends on the rate of fresh gas flow and the ventilation of the patient. A fresh gas flow at least 2.5 times the minute volume eliminates the possibility of significant rebreathing, whatever the pattern of ventilation. During spontaneous ventilation, the minute ventilation can be estimated by counting the respiratory frequency and multiplying this by 5 ml for each kilogram of body weight. This volume multiplied by 2.5 should be provided as the fresh gas flow (Table 3-2). The volume of the expiratory

TABLE 3-2.   FRESH GAS FLOW REQUIRED TO PREVENT
REBREATHING[a] IN A T-PIECE SYSTEM (INCLUDING COAXIAL
CIRCUITS)

Patient's Body Weight (kg)	Flow Rate (L)[b]	
	Mask Anesthesia	Endotracheal Anesthesia
5	8	6.0
10	8	6.0
15	10	7.5
20	12	9.0

[a] *Important.* The flow rates cited are those required to prevent rebreathing in the T-piece. Lower fresh gas flow (FGF) rates, as recommended by some authors result in a degree of rebreathing; this can be compensated for only if the patient can increase ventilation. I believe that during spontaneous ventilation the safest course is to eliminate rebreathing completely.

[b] These flow rates should be used during spontaneous ventilation. They are calculated from the following formulas, which were derived by Rose et al. as an extension of theoretical work by Seeley et al. (*see* page 74). Patients under 30 kg: Mask anesthesia: FGF = 4 × [1,000 + (100 × kg body wt)]. Intubated patients: FGF = 3 × [1,000 + (100 × kg body wt)]. Patients over 30 kg: Mask anesthesia: FGF = 4 × [2,000 + (50 × kg body wt)]. Intubated patients: FGF = 3 × [2,000 + (50 × kg body wt)].

The safety of these flow rates has been confirmed clinically.

limb should exceed 75% of the predicted V$_T$. (**N.B.** MIE* extension tubes are approximately 40 ml in volume; the bag holds 500 or 750 ml.) The dead space of the MIE metal T-piece is 3 ml. The NESI mask angle with a central fesh gas inlet has virtually no dead space. Because the T-piece has no valves, it cannot malfunction and has a very low resistance. Because it is also lightweight and convenient and has minimal dead space, it is considered the ideal circuit for infants and young children. However, the relatively high fresh gas flow required is a potential source of atmospheric pollution. (Whenever a T-piece is used, an exhaust system should—and can easily—be added to the expiratory limb or ventilator to remove waste anesthetic gases and vapors.)

CIRCLE ABSORBER SEMICLOSED SYSTEM

The adult circle absorber semiclosed system can be used for older children. Pediatric circle systems are available and are routinely used in some centers. The circle system is economical and provides limited hum-

---

* Medical & Industrial Equipment (Canada), Niagara Falls, Ontario, Canada.

idification of inspired gases, but the higher circuit resistance and possibility of valve malfunction led us to prefer the T-piece system for infants and small children.

HUMIDIFICATION OF ANESTHETIC GASES

Humidification of inspired gases during anesthesia is recommended:

1. To prevent damage to the respiratory tract by dry gases.
2. To minimize heat loss via the respiratory tract and thus assist in maintaining normothermia.

Dry gases inhibit ciliary activity and lead to accumulation of inspissated secretions that may, in the extreme, progress to obstruct the ETT. Degenerative changes in cells exfoliated from the trachea following exposure to dry gas have been described, but an increased incidence of postoperative morbidity from pulmonary complications remains unproved.

Humidified anesthetic gases significantly reduce heat loss during the operation (*see* page 35). This is valuable in managing the newborn infant, especially those who are preterm or small for gestational age (SGA). The use of a heated humidifier with heated fresh gas delivery tube to the T-piece system is preferred for small infants. The temperature of inspired gases should be 35–36°C and must be monitored with a thermistor probe. When using a heated humidifier, extreme care should be taken to ensure that this does not run dry.

An alternative means of humidification for older children is the use of a heat and moisture exchanger (HME) at the point of connection of the ETT to the circuit. The HME conserves approximately 50% of the water normally lost via the respiratory tract and hence prevents a corresponding heat loss. Studies have demonstrated that the inspired gases entering the trachea have a water content of approximately 24 mg/L when an HME is used.

The use of a circle system provides some humidification of inspired gases, but if a dry fresh gas is delivered into the inspiratory limb, the actual humidity is dictated by the ratio of fresh gas flow to minute ventilation. The temperature of the gases in the inspiratory limb does not usually exceed room temperature, and this limits the water content of the inspired gases. Thus, the circle system is less effective than the other methods described.

CONTROLLED VENTILATION DURING ANESTHESIA

During anesthesia, ventilation may be controlled by manual or mechanical means.

Manual ventilation is used during many operative procedures in neonates. It enables the anesthesiologist to monitor compliance continuously and to compensate rapidly for changes. Rapid ventilation with small V_{TS} provides optimal results in the newborn, as this pattern of ventilation tends to maintain the FRC and prevent airway closure. However, hyperventilation (and consequent respiratory alkalosis) should be avoided. Manual ventilation should also be used whenever there is any doubt about the adequacy of ventilation or in the event of sudden deterioration in the patient's vital signs.

Mechanical ventilators can be used in conjunction with the T-piece; connection of the ventilator to the expiratory limb of the T-piece produces intermittent inflation of the lungs. Most standard types of adult ventilator can be used for this purpose, but low inspiratory flow rates must be set on the ventilator controls (the gas flow from the ventilator is complemented by the fresh gas flow into the T-piece during inspiration). Therefore, set flow and pressure at their lower limits. When the ventilator is attached to the patient circuit, gradually increase these settings to produce a satisfactory pattern of ventilation as judged by auscultation of the lungs and observation of expansion of the thorax. During major surgery the level of ventilation should be confirmed by blood gas analysis and/or measurement of end-tidal CO_2. When using a mechanical ventilator with the T-piece, (1) incorporate a pressure-relief valve (set to release at 40 cm H_2O) into the anesthetic circuit to prevent barotrauma to the lungs if the equipment malfunctions; and (2) attach a low-pressure alarm to warn of accidental disconnection of the ventilator.

During controlled ventilation, avoid excessive hyperventilation and maintain the $PaCO_2$ at near physiologic levels. When using the T-piece, it is possible to regulate the $PaCO_2$ quite accurately by limiting the fresh gas flow while slightly hyperventilating the patient. This introduces a controlled degree of rebreathing to compensate for overventilation. The following fresh gas flow* will result in a $PaCO_2$ of 35–40 mmHg:

Patients 10–30 kg: 1,000 ml + 100 ml/kg
Patients over 30 kg: 2,000 ml + 50 ml/kg

---

* Higher rates of fresh gas flow are required if there is a large leak around the ETT. Remember that flowmeters are only accurate to $\pm 10\%$; therefore, check the $PaCO_2$ for all major procedures.

Minute ventilation should be set at double the rate of fresh gas flow.

During spontaneous ventilation, the fresh gas flow rate must never fall below 2.5 times the predicted minute ventilation.

Suggested Additional Reading

Ayre P: Anaesthesia for intracranial operation: new technique. Lancet 1:561, 1937.

Ayre P: Endotracheal anesthesia for babies, with special reference to harelip and cleft-palate operations. Anesth Analg 16:330, 1937.

*Ayre P: The T-piece technique. Br J Anaesth 28:520, 1956.

*Boys JE, and TH Howells: Humidification in anesthesia: a review of the present situation. Br J Anaesth 44:879, 1972.

Brown ES, and RF Hustead: Resistance of pediatric breathing systems. Anesth Analg 48:842, 1969.

*Harrison GA: Ayre's T-piece: a review of its modifications. Br J Anaesth 36:115, 1964.

*Harrison GA: The effect of the respiratory flow pattern on rebreathing in a T-piece system. Br J Anaesth 36:206, 1964.

Inkster JS: The T-piece technique in anaesthesia: an investigation into the inspired gas concentrations. Br J Anaesth 28:512, 1956.

MacKuanying N, and J Chalon: Humidification of anaesthetic gases for children. Anesth Analg 53:387, 1974.

*Mapleson WW: The elimination of rebreathing in various semi-closed anaesthetic systems. Br J Anaesth 26:323, 1954.

Mapleson WW: Theoretical considerations of the effects of rebreathing in two semiclosed anaesthetic systems. Br Med Bull 14:64, 1958.

Ramanthan S, J Chalon, and H Turndorf: A safety valve for the pediatric Rees system. Anesth Analg 55:741, 1967.

Rashad KF, and DW Benson: Role of humidity in prevention of hypothermia in infants and children. Anesth Analg 46:712, 1967.

Rees GJ: Neonatal anaesthesia. Br Med Bull 14:38, 1958.

*Rose DK, RJ Byrick, and AB Froese: Carbon dioxide elimination during spontaneous ventilation with a modified Mapleson D system: studies in a lung model. Can Anaesth Soc J 25:353, 1978.

Seeley HF, PK Barnes, and CM Conway: Controlled ventilation with the Mapleson D system: a theoretical and experimental study. Br J Anaesth 49:107, 1977.

Steward DJ: A disposable condensor humidifier for use during anesthesia. Anesthesiology 54:337, 1981.

Weeks DB: Evaluation of a disposable humidifier for use during anesthesia. Anesthesiology 54:337, 1981.

---

* Key article

MONITORING DURING ANESTHESIA

ROUTINE MONITORS

Routinely, monitoring during anesthesia must include the following:

1. Stethoscope, precordial or esophageal: heart and breath sounds must be monitored continuously throughout anesthesia.
2. Blood pressure cuff of suitable width.* Use of a Doppler flowmeter† is indicated in most cases. This permits accurate determination of systolic BP and also provides for continuous audible monitoring of pulsatile flow at the radial artery. An automatic BP cuff (e.g., Dinamap) may be used, but this has the disadvantage of only providing an update at set intervals.
3. Pulse oximeter should be applied before induction and remain in place until the patient leaves the operating room. The light source and sensor must be positioned to transilluminate part of the body (ear lobe, finger, or palm of hand, depending on the size of the patient). The sensor should be covered to prevent outside light from interfering with the reading. The absorption of light by the arterial blood is analyzed to derive the percent saturation of the hemoglobin. This equipment requires no calibration, very rarely causes skin burns, and provides readings even when superficial skin blood flow is reduced (e.g., during hypotension). Accurate readings of saturation can be made through pigmented skin, but methemoglobin or carboxyhemoglobin if present will affect the accuracy of readings. Arterial saturation of 80–95% has been demonstrated to indicate a PaO_2 of 40–80 mmHg in most patients: a safe range for the preterm infant. This monitor functions more reliably during anesthesia and surgery than does the transcutaneous PO_2 ($TCPO_2$) monitor. If considered necessary, an arterial sample can be obtained to confirm which level of saturation is appropriate in terms of PaO_2 for each patient. This level of saturation can then be maintained by varying the FiO_2.
4. Electrocardiogram (ECG) (use adhesive electrodes).
5. Thermistor probe (axillary, esophageal, or rectal).

In many cases the following additional monitors may be indicated:

---

* The cuff should occupy two-thirds of the upper arm. If the cuff is too narrow, the BP readings will be falsely high, and if it is too wide, they will be falsely low. A width of 4 cm is recommended for use on term neonates.

† We prefer the Parks Electronics model 811, Parks Electronics, Beaverton, OR.

6. End-tidal CO_2. This measurement provides a useful noninvasive means to measure the adequacy of ventilation. It also provides a most reliable indicator of successful endotracheal intubation. Unfortunately the method is not as easy to apply in infants and small children owing to the small size of the V_T. When a partial rebreathing circuit is used (e.g., a T-piece plus ventilator), end-tidal sampling must be obtained from the distal tip of the endotracheal tube for all small patients (<12 kg) if useful numbers are to be obtained. If a nonrebreathing circuit is used (e.g., circle, Siemen's ventilator, or Sechrist infant ventilator), proximal sampling at the endotracheal connector will give valid results even for small patients.

7. Peripheral nerve stimulator: should be used whenever practical if relaxant drugs are administered.

8. An arterial line should be inserted for direct measurement of BP and to provide for intermittent blood gas analysis when continuous access to such information is required. The radial artery is usually cannulated. Do not use the femoral artery in neonates (high incidence of perfusion-related complications) or the brachial artery (uncertain collateral flow). The left radial artery is usually preferred for arterial puncture.

   (a) Locate the artery by palpation; if this is difficult, use the Doppler flowmeter or, in small infants, transilluminate the wrist with a bright cold light.

   (b) Use careful aseptic technique and prepare the skin with Betadine (povidone-iodine) (your finger, which is used to palpate the artery, should be prepared also—arterial puncture with gloves is almost impossible).

   (c) Make a small skin incision over the artery with an 18-guage needle. This prevents damage to the tip of the cannula during skin puncture.

   (d) Perform arterial puncture; as soon as blood issues into the hub of the needle, turn the needle so that the bevel faces down.

   (e) Advance the cannula gently into the artery (Fig. 3-1).

   (f) If it will not advance, withdraw until blood flows freely and carefully insert a fine guide wire* then advance the cannula over this.

   (g) Apply antibiotic spray or ointment to skin puncture site and cover with a sterile dressing.

   (h) Secure cannula carefully with adhesive tape. All connections should be Luer-Lok or similar to prevent accidental bleeding.

---

* Arrow 0.45 mm by 25 cm no. AW 04018 duoflex spring wire guide.

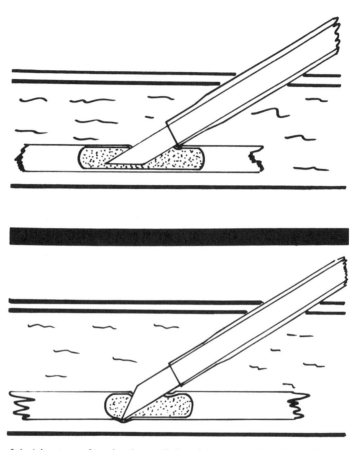

Fig. 3-1. Advantage of turning the needle bevel down when inserting an intravenous cannula into a small vein or artery. (Reproduced with permission from HC Filston and DG Johnson: Percutaneous venous cannulation in neonates and infants: a method for catheter insertion without cutdown. *Pediatrics* 48:896–901, 1971.)

Precautions with arterial lines:

(a) Insert the cannula with meticulous asepsis (*see* page 77).

(b) Secure all connections, using Luer-Lok fittings, to exclude the danger of accidental disconnection and hemorrhage. Plug sampling taps when not in use.

(c) Immobilize the forearm and wrist on a padded splint to prevent accidental decannulation.

(d) Use a continuous flush device, but beware of accidental fluid overload.
(e) Beware of embolization.
   (i) Do not reinfuse blood removed during sampling.
   (ii) Do not use high pressure to attempt to clear a blocked cannula.
   (iii) Infuse only small volumes of flush fluid after sampling. In small infants, volumes of only 0.5–1.0 ml injected into the radial artery may flow retrogradely into the cerebral vessels.
(f) Remove the arterial line as soon as it has served its purpose. Complications (especially arterial thrombosis and sepsis) increase with the duration of cannulation of the vessel.

9. Urine output: record this for all patients undergoing major surgery as well as all who have hypovolemic shock or whose renal function may be impaired.
10. Central venous pressure (CVP): recorded from a catheter inserted centrally via the external jugular vein, median cubital vein, or the internal jugular vein.* This should be monitored in patients in whom major blood loss and/or impaired cardiac performance is anticipated.

External jugular vein cannulation:

(a) Position the patient with a 15° head-down tilt and a small pillow under the shoulder.
(b) Locate the external juglar vein and prepare and drape the area.
(c) Puncture the vein and insert a 22-gauge IV catheter.
(d) Feed a J-wire through the catheter and advance it centrally, rotating as necessary. A 6-mm-diameter J-wire is most likely to pass easily. The catheter must be manipulated gently to avoid the possibility of damage.
(e) When the wire has advanced, a dilator may be gently used, but do not pass this further than into the external jugular vein or a tear at the junction of the subclavian may result.
(f) Advance the central catheter over the guide wire until it is sited at the junction of the superior vena cava (SVC) and right atrium (RA). This distance can be judged by measuring the distance from skin puncture to manubrio-sternal junction.

_____

* Internal jugular cannulation in infants and children has a higher complication rate than in adults; thus, it may be preferable to attempt central cannulation initially via the external jugular vein if this is easily visible.

(g) The position of long-dwelling CVP lines should be checked by radiography. Complications (including perforation) may occur if the line is too long.

Internal jugular cannulation (method of Dr. Michael Smith, B.C.C.H.):

(a) Position the patient—head to left, with 20° Trendelenburg, with a rolled towel under the shoulders to reduce concavity of the neck.

(b) Palpate the carotid pulse medial to the sternocleidomastoid muscle and pick this muscle up to identify its bulk at the level of the thyroid cartilage prominence.

(c) Prepare and drape, gown and glove.

(d) Make a skin stab (no. 11 blade) at the anterior border of the sternomastoid at the level of the thyroid prominence (if <15 kg) or at the level of the cricothyroid membrane (if >15 kg), avoiding the external jugular vein.

(e) Use a 22-gauge plastic cannula (e.g., Angiocath). Advance this through the skin stab medial to the sternomastoid at an angle of 30° to the skin toward the ipsilateral axilla. Aspirate intermittently to identify venous blood. If the vein is not found withdraw the cannula slowly, aspirating continuously. If still unsuccessful, repeat insertion in a more medial direction toward the ipsilateral nipple. Throughout this procedure use care to avoid the carotid pulsation.

(f) When the vein is found, advance the cannula and verify easy aspiration of blood. In cyanotic patients, is it advisable to attach the cannula to a transducer and confirm that the pressure is venous.

(g) Insert a guide wire and complete cannulation by the Seldinger technique.

(h) To position the tip of the catheter in SVC-RA junction, the length should be equal to the distance from skin penetration to a point 2 cm below the upper border of the manubrium.

OTHER FORMS OF MONITORING

TRANSCUTANEOUS O_2

Transcutaneous O_2 ($TCPO_2$) monitoring became routine practice in the neonatal intensive care unit (ICU) and may provide a very useful guide to oxygen therapy. Unfortunately, these devices do not perform well during anesthesia.

1. Any factor that decreases skin blood flow results in falsely low readings when compared with arterial values. Thus, vasoconstriction in response to surgical stimuli, hypotension, hypovolemia, etc, may cause low readings.
2. Anesthetic gases and vapors are excreted through the skin and may pass into the electrode and influence its accuracy:
   (a) Nitrous oxide may mimic oxygen in the electrode and cause a falsely high reading. The extent of this effect depends on the polarizing voltage of the electrode and is minimal with some machines.
   (b) Halothane is also reduced in the electrode and produces falsely high readings for oxygen. This halothane effect can be prevented by fitting a membrane to the electrode that is impermeable to halothane. Unfortunately, such action also impairs the sensitivity to oxygen.

In summary, $TCPO_2$ monitoring during anesthesia is an unreliable means to accurately observe the PaO_2. It may, however, provide valuable information about trends in tissue perfusion.

TRANSCUTANEOUS CO_2 TENSION

Equipment is available to measure transcutaneous CO_2 tension. Such machines may be useful to monitor changes during endoscopic procedures.

INVASIVE SYSTEMS TO MONITOR OXYGENATION

INTRAVASCULAR OXYGEN ELECTRODE

Small-gauge catheters with an O_2 electrode at the tip that can be inserted via the umbilical artery are available. These are expensive to use and may fail, but they are not subject to the errors caused by changes in skin blood flow that affect the performance of the $TCPO_2$ electrode.

INTRAVASCULAR SATURATION MONITOR

A fiberoptic catheter system enables Hb saturation to be measured in the lumen of a major artery or vein. The introduction of the transcutaneous arterial saturation monitor decreases the need for invasive monitoring. However, the use of a pulmonary artery saturation probe may provide useful information when treating patients in shock.

BLOOD GLUCOSE

Preterm infants are very prone to hypoglycemia. Blood sugar levels should be checked frequently and hypoglycemia (<40 mg/dl) corrected by infusions of glucose (6 mg/kg/min). Avoid excessive glucose administration, however, as it may result in hyperglycemia, glycosuria, and dehydration (*see* page 32) and may increase the risk of cerebral damage should a hypoxic episode occur. A compact Glucometer* should be available in the OR.

FLUID ADMINISTRATION

The IV administration of fluids must be very carefully monitored to avoid overload. Syringe pumps or controlled IV infusion lines (e.g., IVAC) should always be used. Determine the total of all fluids given, including those given with drugs. The use of a low-volume remote injection site (Portex Industries Ltd.) or an injection cap at the IV site minimizes the need for flushing fluid. Small (tuberculin) syringes should be used to measure small doses accurately.

ANESTHESIA CHART

The anesthesia chart is an important monitor and, if well kept, permits the anesthesiologist to detect important trends in the progress of the patient.

Suggested Additional Reading

Badgwell JM, ME Mcleod, J Lerman and RE Creighton: End-tidal PCO_2 monitoring in infants and children during ventilation with the Air Shields Ventimeter ventilator. Anesthesiology 65A:418, 1986.

Badgwell JM, JE Heavner, WS May, JF Goldthorn, and J Lerman: End tidal PCO_2 monitoring in infants and children ventilated with either a partial rebreathing or a non-rebreathing circuit. Anesthesiology 66:405–410, 1987.

Badgwell JM, ME Mcleod, J Lerman and RE Creighton: End-tidal PCO_2 measurements in infants and children ventilated with the Sechrist ventilator. Anesthesiology 67A:511, 1987.

Berry FA: Monitoring in pediatric anesthesia. *In*: Some Aspects of Pediatric Anesthesia (DJ Steward, ed). Amsterdam, Elsevier/North Holland Biomedical Press, 1982, p. 137–163.

Cote CJ, EA Goldstein, MA Cote, et al: A single blind study of pulse oximetry in children. Anesthesiology 68:184–188, 1988.

---

* Miles Canada Inc., Etobicoke, Ontario, Canada.

Damen J: Positive bacterial cultures and related risk factors associated with percutaneous internal jugular vein catherisation in pediatric cardiac patients. Anesthesiology 66:558–562, 1987.

Deckhart R, and DJ Steward: Continuous transcutaneous arterial oxygen saturation measurement. II. Arterial hemoglobin saturation versus oxygen tension monitoring in the preterm infant. Crit Care Med 12:935–939, 1984.

Eberhard P, and W Mindt: Interference of anesthetic gases at oxygen sensors. Birth Defects 15:65, 1979.

Glenski JA, FM Beynen and J Brady: A prospective evaluation of femoral artery monitoring in pediatric patients. Anesthesiology 66:227–229, 1987.

Gothgen I, and E Jacobsen: Transcutaneous oxygen measurement. II. The influence of halothane and hypotension. Acta Anaesthesiol Scand [Suppl] 67:71, 1978.

Hansen TN, and WH Tooley: Skin surface carbon dioxide tension in sick infants. Pediatrics 64:942, 1979.

Hill GE, and RH Machin: Doppler determined blood pressure recordings: the effect of varying cuff sizes in children. Can Anaesth Soc J 23:323, 1976.

Lowenstein E, JW Little, and HH Lo: Prevention of cerebral embolization from flushing radial artery cannulas. N Engl J Med 285:1414, 1971.

Lum LG, and MD Jones: The effect of cuff width on systolic blood pressure measurements in neonates. J Pediatr 91:963, 1977.

Miyasaka K, JF Edmonds, and AW Conn: Complications of radial artery lines in the paediatric patient. Can Anaesth Soc J 23:9, 1976.

Nordstrom L, and R Fletcher: A comparison of two different J-wires for central venous cannulation via the external jugular vein. Anesth Analg 62:365, 1983.

Severinghaus JW, RB Weiskopf, M Nishimura, et al: Oxygen electrode errors due to polarographic reduction of halothane. J Appl Physiol 31:640, 1971.

Todres ID, MC Rogers, DC Shannon, FMB Moylan, and JF Ryan: Percutaneous catheterization of the radial artery in the critically ill neonate. J Pediatr 87:273, 1975.

Tremper KK and SJ Barker: Pulse oximetry. Anesthesiology 70:98–108, 1989.

Versmold HT, O Lindekamp, M Holzmann, I Strohhacker, and K Riegel: Transcutaneous monitoring of pO_2 in newborn infants. Where are the limits? Influence of blood pressure, blood volume, blood flow, viscosity and acid base state. Birth Defects 15:285, 1979.

Waltemath CL, and DD Preuss: Determination of blood pressure in low-flow states by the Doppler techniques. Anesthesiology 34:77, 1971.

Wilkinson AR, RH Phibbs, and GA Gregory: Continuous in vivo oxygen saturation in newborn infants with pulmonary disease: a new fiberoptic catheter oximeter. Crit Care Med 7:232, 1979.

MANAGEMENT OF BODY TEMPERATURE

MONITORING

Continuous body temperature monitoring with a thermistor probe is essential for all patients undergoing general anesthesia. In larger children having minor surgery, the temperature is usually recorded from the axilla. This reflects body core temperature accurately, provided the tip of the probe is close to the axillary artery and the patient's arm is adducted. In smaller children and infants, and for major surgery, the temperature should be monitored in the esophagus or the rectum. Esophageal temperatures should be recorded in the lower third of the esophagus to avoid falsely low readings caused by gas flow in the trachea. When using an esophageal stethoscope, attach a thermistor probe (or use a combined stethoscope-thermistor); when the heart sounds are best heard, these monitors are optimally placed behind the left atrium.

CONSERVATION OF BODY HEAT IN NEONATES

The objective of body heat conservation is to prevent cold stress and avoid hypothermia (which prolongs recovery from anesthetic drugs, impairs myocardial efficiency, and may depress ventilation).

Preoperatively. Adjust the operating room (OR) ambient temperature to 24°C (75°F) or higher. Ensure that a heating blanket set at 40°C and covered by two layers of flannelette is in place on the OR table. Keep the patient in the transport incubator until you are ready to induce anesthesia.

Perioperatively. Position an infrared heating lamp at the correct distance over the patient during induction and preparation for surgery. Keep a woolen cap on the infant's head whenever possible. Use warmed IV solutions and heated humidified anesthetic gases (at 36°C). Warmed (40°C) skin preparation solution should be used and any excess dried from the skin to prevent cooling by evaporation.

Postoperatively. Use the infrared heater during extubation and other procedures at the end of anesthesia. Place the infant in a warmed incubator and return the infant promptly to the postanesthesia room (PAR), ICU, or neonatal unit.

HYPERTHERMIA DURING SURGERY

Hyperthermia sometimes develops during surgery if all the above heat-conserving procedures are followed. If this occurs, the temperature of the inspired gases should be reduced or the heating blanket switched off.

Other causes for hyperthermia during surgery include pyrexial reactions (e.g., as a result of manipulation of an infected organ or a blood transfusion reaction); very rarely, it may be caused by the malignant hyperpyrexia syndrome (*see* page 133).

Suggested Additional Reading

Bennett EJ, KP Patel, and EM Grundy: Neonatal temperature and surgery. Anesthesiology 46:303, 1977.

Engelman DR, and CH Lockhart: Comparisons between temperature effects of ketamine and halothane anesthesia in children. Anesth Analg 51:98, 1972.

Goudsouzian NG, RH Morris, and JF Ryan: The effects of a warming blanket on the maintenance of body temperatures in anesthetized infants and children. Anesthesiology 39:351, 1973.

Meyers MB, and TH Oh: Prevention of hypothermia during cystoscopy in neonates. Anesth Analg 55:592, 1976.

Rashad KF, and DW Benson: Role of humidity in prevention of hypothermia in infants and children. Anesth Analg 46:712, 1967.

INTRAVENOUS THERAPY

1. For all children under 20 kg, insert a Buretrol or similar graduated reservoir between the IV bag and the administration set; this prevents accidental fluid overload and allows for a check of infused volumes.
2. Use an infusion pump (e.g., IVAC) whenever possible. This allows accurate control of the rate of infusion and easy monitoring of volumes adminsitered.
3. Percutaneous insertion of a plastic cannula into a vein is considered optimal. Use a 22-guage cannula or larger if blood transfusion may be required. Observe strict asepsis when performing cannulation; use Betadine skin preparation and cover the puncture site with a sterile dressing. Insertion of a plastic cannula into a small vein can be facilitated by turning the bevel of the needle down and injecting a small volume of fluid. Label the IV with the size of the cannula and the date of insertion.

4. For major abdominal surgery, the IV lines must be placed in the upper limbs.
5. Before surgery is begun, ensure that the IV line is working well.

VENIPUNCTURE AND INSERTION OF INTRAVENOUS CANNULAS

The ability to perform a venipuncture painlessly and to cannulate small veins successfully is essential for the pediatric anesthesiologist. Some tips that may help are

1. For venipuncture:
    (a) Make sure that you have a skilled assistant who can distract the child, who is gently restrained. (Use EMLA* if available.)
    (b) Never use a rubber tourniquet on a young child; have your assistant grasp the arm to gently impede venous return and thus fill the veins. Do not attempt venipuncture unless the vein is obviously well filled: filling can be facilitated by having the assistant hold the hand below the patient's body level and applying gentle manual constriction to the limb.
    (c) Never inject drugs into veins of the antecubital fossa. Accidental intra-arterial injection is more common here than at any other site. The risk is higher in children because of close proximity of vessels and the possibility that the child might move during the injection.
    (d) Usually a vein on the dorsum of the hand is most suitable. Look and palpate across the back of the hand opposite the fourth digit.
    (e) Use the smallest size needle and syringe possible, and keep the equipment from the child's view at all times.
    (f) Hold needle and syringe firmly and avoid accidentally touching the skin with the needle until ready to puncture the vein.
    (g) When ready, puncture the skin and vein firmly with one rapid movement and then hold the needle firmly in place until the injection is completed.
2. To cannulate a vein: usually this is performed after induction of anesthesia; otherwise, use a local analgesic (1% lidocaine).
    (a) Select a suitable vein; the best sites usually are
        (i) Dorsum of hand.
        (ii) Medial aspect of ankle.
        (iii) Lateral aspect of foot.
        (iv) Scalp vein (in infants).
        (v) Lateral aspect of wrist (older children).
            (Remember, some patients must have an IV line in the upper

---

* Astra Pharmaceuticals Inc., Missisauga, Ontario, Canada.

limb, for example, those with abdominal trauma or tumor, etc.)
(b) Use careful aseptic technique and prepare the skin with Betadine solution.
(c) Make sure the vein selected is well filled and make a small incision over it with an 18-gauge needle.
(d) Note direction of the bevel on the cannula needle. After the initial venous puncture is made, turn the bevel face down before attempting to advance the cannula into the vein. This ensures that the point of the needle is unlikely to be in the distal wall of a small vein and that the cannula will advance unimpeded into the vein (Fig. 3-1).
(e) When the cannula is in place, apply antibiotic spray or ointment to the puncture site and cover this with a sterile dressing. Tape the cannula firmly in place and immobilize the limb on a splint.

PREOPERATIVE FLUID REPLACEMENT

Preoperative dehydration can be classified by the size of the deficit as mild, moderate, or severe:

Mild	50 ml/kg (5% body weight loss)
Moderate	100 ml/kg (10% body weight loss)
Severe	150 ml/kg (15% body weight loss)

Replacement of water and electrolytes should proceed in three phases:

1. *Treatment of overt or impending shock* (severe dehydration and hypovolemia): Order an initial infusion of whole blood (10 ml/kg); if this is not available, give plasma or 5% albumin (20 ml/kg).
2. *Replacement of extracellular water and sodium:* Half the estimated fluid deficit can be replaced over the initial 6–8 hours as 0.3N saline. If the deficit is severe, give an initial infusion of 0.9N saline (20 ml/kg). The degree of success of this therapy can be gauged from the clinical signs (heart rate, arterial and venous pressures, and urine output). The following formula is useful in correcting sodium deficiency:

$$Na^+ \text{ deficit (mEq)} = \text{normal } Na^+ \text{ (mEq)} - \text{measured } Na^+ \text{ (mEq)} \times 0.6 \times \text{weight (kg)}$$

where 0.6 = diffusion constant.

Metabolic acidosis should be treated simultaneously, using the formula:

$$\text{Dose required (mEq of HCO}_3^-) = \text{base deficit} \times \text{weight (kg)}$$
$$\times 0.3 \ (0.4 \text{ for infants})$$

Give half the calculated requirement; then reassess the acid-base status.

3. *Replacement of K^+:* Potassium replacement should be initiated when a good urinary output has been established, according to the following:
   (a) Replace a maximum of 3 mEq of K/kg/24 hr.
   (b) Rate of administration should not exceed 0.5 mEq/kg/hr.
   (c) Complete correction of severe K deficiency should take 4–5 days.

Remember. These figures are only a guide and must be adjusted for changes in metabolic activity, clinical conditions, and extrarenal losses (e.g., gastric suction).

Note. A neonate's insensible water loss decreases by 30–35% when the infant is nursed in a high-humidity atmosphere or ventilated with humidified gases. Insensible water loss is increased by crying, sweating, hyperventilation, and the use of radiant heater or "bili" lights. Pyrexia increases water loss by 12%/1°C.

PERIOPERATIVE FLUID MANAGEMENT

Calculation of the volume and type of fluid required must take into consideration:

1. Dehydration present *before* preoperative fasting.
2. Fluid deficit incurred *during* preoperative fasting.
3. Maintenance fluid requirement during surgery.
4. Estimated ECF loss resulting from surgical trauma.
5. Alterations in body temperature.

For short surgical procedures (under 1 hour) in otherwise healthy children, fluid is usually not given IV perioperatively if the preoperative deficit was small and blood loss or tissue trauma is minimal, provided oral intake is likely to be reestablished early in the postoperative period, for example, hernia and hydrocele repair, circumcision, minor plastic and orthopedic procedures.

For surgical procedures of longer duration, when reestablishment of oral intake may be delayed:

1. An IV infusion is established.
2. Fluid is administered perioperatively and postoperatively until oral intake is reestablished.

TABLE 3-3. DAILY
MAINTENANCE
REQUIREMENTS

Weight (kg)	Maintenance Fluid Requirement (ml/kg/hr)
Newborn	3
4–10	4
11–20	3
21–40	2.5–3.0
41 +	2.0–2.5

3. 5% dextrose in lactated Ringer solution is usually given for simple procedures.
4. For extensive surgery, especially in infants, it is advantageous to separate the administration of dextrose from other fluid therapy. Thus, an infusion of 5 or 10% dextrose can be established at a rate that will deliver 4–6 mg/kg/min. Blood glucose levels should be checked periodically. Other fluids given to replace losses should be free of dextrose.

The hourly rate of infusion is based on daily maintenance requirements (Table 3-3). Adjust the hourly rate if (1) factors affecting insensible fluid loss are present (e.g., increased body temperature) or (2) there are extrarenal losses (e.g., gastrointestinal).

Sufficient fluid should be given to compensate for preoperative fasting. The total volume to be administered during surgery is calculated by multiplying the number of hours (fasting plus surgery) by the hourly maintenance requirement; for example, for a 10-kg child fasting for 4 hours and then undergoing an estimated 4-hour operative procedure, replacement and maintenance requirements would total $160 + 160 = 320$ ml (i.e., 8 ml/kg/hr).

ADDITIONAL FLUIDS

For surgical procedures causing significant tissue trauma and/or blood loss, give additional fluids to replace ECF loss in blood or sequestered into damaged tissue. This deficiency should be replaced with a multiple-electrolyte solution, for example, lactated Ringer solution in which the electrolyte concentrations are similar to those in ECF (Table 3-4).

The adequacy of fluid replacement is best judged by monitoring the cardiovascular indices and urine output.

TABLE 3-4. COMPOSITION OF ELECTROLYTE SOLUTIONS

Solution	Conc. (mEq/L)					Conc. HCO_3^- (mEq/L)		
	Na^+	K^+	Mg^{2+}	Ca^{2+}	Cl^-	Acetate	Gluconate	Lactate
Normal saline (0.9%)	154	—	—	—	154	—	—	—
0.3N saline in D_5W	51	—	—	—	51	—	—	—
0.2N saline in D_5W	34	—	—	—	34	—	—	—
Normosol-M	40	13	3	—	40	16	—	—
Normosol-R	140	5	3	—	98	27	23	—
Lactated Ringer solution	130	4	—	3	109	—	—	28

Magnesium sulfate (2 ml amp., 50% w/v): 4.0 mEq Mg^{2+}/ml
Sodium bicarbonate (50 ml amp., 7.5% w/v): 0.9 mEq HCO_3^-/ml
Calcium gluconate (10 ml amp., 10% w/v): 0.447 mEq Ca^{2+}/ml
Calcium chloride (10 ml amp., 10% w/v): 1.36 mEq Ca^{2+}/ml

Suggested Additional Reading

*Bennett EJ: Fluids for Anesthesia and Surgery in the Newborn and Infant. Springfield, IL, Charles C Thomas, 1975.

Bennett EJ, MJ Daughety, and MT Jenkins: Some controversial aspects of fluids for the anesthetized neonate. Anesth Analg 49:478, 1970.

Berry FA: Practical aspects of fluid and electrolyte therapy. *In*: Anesthetic Management of Difficult and Routine Pediatric Patients (FA Berry, ed). New York, Churchill Livingstone, 1986.

Bush GH: Intravenous fluid therapy in paediatrics. Ann R Coll Surg Engl 49:92, 1971.

Filston HC, and DG Johnson: Percutaneous venous cannulation in neonates and infants: a method for catheter insertion without cutdown. Pediatrics 48:896, 1971.

Hall SC, HJ Przybylo, and AJ Roth: 5% and 10% dextrose intravenous solutions during neonatal surgery. Anesthesiology 69A:738, 1988.

Rickham PP, J Lister, and IM Irving (eds): Neonatal Surgery, 2nd ed. London, Butterworth, 1978, p. 41–47.

Shepard FM, LM Arango, and FA Berry: Acid-base response of the newborn to major surgery. Anesth Analg 50:31, 1971.

The Hospital for Sick Children: Residents' Handbook, 5th ed (rev). Toronto, 1978.

Wellborn LG, RS Hannalah, WA McGill, UE Ruttimann, and JM Hicks: Glucose concentrations for routine intravenous infusion in pediatric outpatient surgery. Anesthesiology 67:427–430, 1987.

BLOOD REPLACEMENT

PREOPERATIVE ASSESSMENT

A normal Hb level (above 10 g/dl or 14 g/dl in neonates) is desirable in every case of elective surgery (Table 3-5); below this, the risk of anesthesia may be increased and the decision whether to proceed must take into account all relevant factors in relation to the individual patient. In some patients, elective surgery can be delayed until the anemia has been investigated and treated. In some anemic patients, surgery may be more urgent, and anesthesia for these patients must be with a technique that is compatible with their anemia (*see* page 114). When surgery cannot be delayed despite a very low Hb value, packed cells should be infused preoperatively. Approximately 4 ml of packed cells/kg is required to raise the Hb level by 1 g/dl.

---

* Key article

TABLE 3-5. NORMAL Hb LEVELS

Age	Normal Hb Values[a] (g/dl)
1st day of life	20 (18–22)
2nd week	17
3 months	10–11
2 years	11
3–5 years	12.5–13.0
5–10 years	13.0–13.5
10+ years	14.5

[a] The Hb concentration declines gradually to about 10–11 g/dl during the first few months of life as fetal Hb is replaced. It then gradually increases and is maximal at about 14 years.

Hb content of:

Stored whole blood = 12 g/dl
Packed cells = 24 g/dl
Buffy-coat-poor washed cells = 28 g/dl

When blood loss of 10% of the estimated blood volume (EBV) or greater is expected, the patient's blood should be grouped and cross-matched for a volume depending on expected losses. Insert a CVP line preoperatively in patients who are hypovolemic and/or may require massive blood replacement during surgery.

PERIOPERATIVE MANAGEMENT

At commencement of the operation, record on the anesthesia chart the EBV and the preoperative Hb level.

ASSESSMENT OF BLOOD LOSS

Accurate estimates of blood loss must be maintained throughout the operation.

1. Monitor CVS indices; in infants, the systolic BP is the most reliable indicator of blood volume.
2. Measure blood loss from the surgical site:
   (a) All sponges must be weighed before they dry out. This is simple and accurate (assume 1 g = 1 ml of blood and subtract the known dry weight).

(b) Measure blood from suction (in graduated flasks).

(c) Estimate blood on drapes.

3. Chart the running total continually.

4. Be aware of the possibility that blood losses may accumulate in body cavities (e.g., peritoneum, pleura).

BLOOD TRANSFUSION

The decision whether to transfuse blood must be based on the pre-operative Hb level, the measured surgical blood loss, and the patient's cardiovascular response. As a rough guide, in otherwise healthy children, blood replacement is probably necessary after loss of 15% of the EBV. The need for blood transfusion can be determined more accurately from serial Hct measurements (normally, the Hct should be maintained at or above 30%).

Check each unit of blood against the patient's identity bracelet and mix it well by repeated inversion of the bag. Blood should be warmed to 37°C before administration. It should not be heated above 38°C or it may be damaged.

Calcium gluconate is rarely necessary during massive transfusion in children but may be given (0.1 ml/kg of a 10% solution) if persistent hypotension follows apparently adequate volume replacement in infants.

In severely shocked patients who require rapid massive transfusion, be prepared to give sodium bicarbonate if indicated by serial acid-base determinations.

If it becomes apparent that massive blood transfusion will be required (i.e., >75% of the EBV), institute monitoring of coagulation indices. Platelet counts, prothrombin time, and partial thromboplastin time together with tests for fibrinolysis (determination of fibrin split products) should be repeated at least after every 50% blood volume replacement. It is helpful to have a preoperative platelet count if massive transfusion is a possibility. A low initial count will indicate the need for early platelet transfusion. Platelet counts of under 65,000 will increase clinical bleeding and should be corrected. In practice, if platelets are being monitored during a continuing massive replacement, this means that platelets should be ordered as the count goes down through 100,000. Infusion of 1 unit of platelet concentrate per 5 kg will increase the platelet count by 30,000–40,000/mm^3. Platelets must be stored at room temperature and not refrigerated. Other deficiencies that become apparent should be dealt with by appropriate therapy (e.g., fresh frozen plasma or appropriate blood component therapy).

Suggested Additional Reading

*Ballinger CM (ed): Blood transfusion. Int Anesthesiol Clin 5:871, 1967.

Bourke DL, and TC Smith: Estimating allowable hemodilution. Anesthesiology 41:609, 1974.

Cote CJ, LMP Liu, SK Szyfelbein, et al: Changes in serial platelet counts following massive blood transfusions in pediatric patients. Anesthesiology 62:197–201, 1985.

Consensus Conference: Perioperative red blood cell transfusion. JAMA 260:2700–2703, 1988.

*Davenport HT, and MN Barr: Blood loss during pediatric operations. Can Med Assoc J 89:1309, 1963.

Furman EB, DG Roman, LAS Lemmer, J Hairabet, M Jasinska, and MB Laver: Specific therapy in water, electrolyte and blood-volume replacement during pediatric surgery. Anesthesiology 42:187, 1975.

Jacobs RG, WS Howland, and AH Goulet: Serial microhematocrit determinations in evaluating blood replacement. Anesthesiology 22:342, 1961.

SPECIAL PROVISIONS FOR THE NEWBORN

The following measures are important for all infants but are especially vital for the low-birth-weight and/or premature neonate.

PROPHYLAXIS AGAINST HEMORRHAGE

Ensure that the infant has been given vitamin K_1 to prevent hemorrhage resulting from lack of vitamin K-dependent factors. Aqueous vitamin K_1, 1 mg IM, corrects such deficiency within a few hours and therefore should be given as early as possible.

TEMPERATURE

Avoid cold stress and decreases in body temperature.

1. A heated transport incubator should be used to transfer the neonate to and from the OR.
2. The OR must be warmed to at least 75°F (24°C).
3. Leave the infant in the incubator until all preparations are complete

---

* Key article

and return the infant to a warm environment as soon as possible after surgery.

4. Use heating pads and blankets (set at 40°C).
5. Use an overhead infrared lamp to maintain skin temperature at 36°C.
6. Humidify anesthetic gases with a heated humidifier. Monitor the temperature of inspired gases, which should be 36°C.
7. Ensure that warmed skin preparation solutions (40°C) are used and that excess solutions are dried from the skin (to prevent heat loss by evaporation).
8. Ensure that the incubator is kept operating and warm during surgery.
9. Cover the head with a woolen cap to prevent heat loss from the scalp.

AIRWAY

1. In some instances it may be preferable to intubate the neonate awake.*
2. Use a tube that passes the glottis early and allows a slight lead during positive-pressure ventilation.
3. Use sterile ETTs and do not handle the tracheal portion or allow it to come into contact with other materials before insertion.
4. Position the tip of the tube carefully. Remember that in a term newborn the trachea is only 4–5 cm long; therefore, pass the tube 2–3 cm below the vocal cords for optimal positioning.
5. Check the air entry to all areas of the lung fields.
6. Tape the ETT firmly in place, preferably in the center of the mouth to avoid kinking, and support it with a soft rubber bite block.

ANESTHESIA CIRCUIT

1. The Jackson Rees modification of the T-piece is most suitable for the newborn. For prematures, the NESI angle can be incorporated to reduce apparatus dead space further.
2. Manual control of ventilation is preferable for thoracoabdominal surgery, as subtle changes in compliance can be detected rapidly and adjustments made to maintain ventilation. Mechanical ventilation is pre-

---

* However, this awake intubation has been demonstrated to cause a rise in ICP and might, in the preterm infant, add to the risk of intraventricular hemorrhage (IVH). The rise in ICP is diminished if the patient is anesthetized or if relaxants are used. The risks of these measures must be weighed against the uncertain consequences of ICP fluctuations associated with intubation. There is some evidence that the hemodynamic responses to endotracheal intubation (tachycardia and hypertension) may be less in the neonate than in the older infant. There does not appear to be any evidence that the anesthetic period is one of high risk for IVH.

ferred for cardiac surgery (so that the PCO_2 can be held more constant and respiratory alkalosis can be avoided).

ADDITIONAL CONSIDERATIONS FOR THE PRETERM INFANT

1. **Size.** Anesthetic management of the preterm infant is complicated by the very small size of the patient. Before starting any anesthetic, ensure that suitable miniature equipment is available. Prepackaged sterile trays containing all necessary items for the preterm infant should be available for immediate use.

2. **Apneic spells.** Apneic spells are common in preterm infants (*see* page 16), who must be monitored very closely at all times and especially during and after anesthesia. Postoperatively, an apnea alarm should be ordered for all preterm infants of less than 45 weeks postconceptual age. Perioperative apnea is more common in infants of low postconceptual age and those with residual pulmonary disease. In very small infants, the risk of apnea may extend as long as 72 hours into the postoperative period. Apnea may be less common following surgery performed under spinal analgesia, but it still may occur, so the patient must be monitored. Caffeine therapy (10 mg/kg IV slowly after induction) may prevent apnea, but monitoring is still advised.

3. **Temperature control.** The preterm infant is extremely vulnerable to heat loss—even more so than the term newborn. The surface area is even larger relative to body mass, and there are no insulating subcutaneous tissues. Be especially alert to prevent heat loss at all times while the infant is in your care.

4. **Oxygenation.** Oxygenation must be very carefully controlled if hypoxia is to be avoided and the risk of retrolental fibroplasia minimized. Inspired concentrations must be kept to the minimum that will allow safe conduct of general anesthesia. Monitor with the pulse oximeter and attempt to keep the saturation between 90 and 95%.
   (a) Ascertain the FiO_2 required preoperatively to achieve satisfactory oxygenation. During nonthoracic surgery with controlled ventilation, continue with this FiO_2 and check saturation.
   (b) Whenever N_2O is contraindicated, use an air-O_2 mixture to achieve the desired FiO_2 and saturation.
   (c) During intrathoracic surgery it is essential to increase the FiO_2, but monitor saturation and limit the O_2 concentration as far as possible while avoiding the possibility of inducing hypoxemia.

5. **Hypoglycemia and hyperglycemia.** Preterm infants are very prone to hypoglycemia. Blood sugar levels should be checked frequently and hypoglycemia (<40 mg/dl) corrected by infusions of glucose. The preterm infant is also subject to hyperglycemia, which is usually iatrogenic but may also be due to poor insulin response and continued glycolysis. Hyperglycemia leads to glycosuria, osmotic diuresis, and dehydration and should be avoided by frequent blood sugar determinations and limited IV glucose administration.

6. **Fluid administration.** Avoid fluid overload by very careful control of IV fluids. Determine the total of IV fluids given, including those given with drugs. Use tuberculin syringes to accurately measure small volumes of drugs. Syringe pumps and controlled infusion lines are essential.

7. **Coagulation.** The preterm infant is subject to coagulopathy associated with shock and sepsis. Thrombocytopenia is common. Perform coagulation studies on all seriously ill preterm infants. Platelet concentrates, fresh frozen plasma, or exchange transfusion may be required.

Suggested Additional Reading

Betts EK, JJ Downes, DB Schaffer, and R Johns: Retrolental fibroplasia and oxygen administration during general anesthesia. Anesthesiology 47:518, 1977.

Bush GH: Neonatal anaesthesia. *In*: General Anaesthesia, 3rd ed. (TC Gray and JF Nunn, eds). London, Butterworth, 1971, vol. 2, p. 410.

Charlton AJ, and SG Greenhough: Blood pressure response of neonates to tracheal intubation. Anesthesia 43:744–746, 1988.

Friesen RH, AT Honda, and RE Thieme: Perianesthetic intracranial hemorrhage in preterm neonates. Anesthesiology 67:814–816, 1987.

Gross SJ, and MJ Stuart: Hemostasis in the premature infant. Clin Perinatol 4:259, 1977.

Hatch DJ, and E Sumner: Neonatal Anaesthesia. London, Arnold, 1981.

Maze A, and SI Samuels: Hypoglycemia-induced seizures is an infant during anesthesia. Anesthesiology 52:77, 1980.

Mayhew JF, DL Bourke, and WS Guinee: Evaluation of the premature infant at risk for postoperative complications. Can J Anaesth 34:627–631, 1987.

Phibbs RH: Oxygen therapy: a continuing hazard to the premature infant. Anesthesiology 47:486, 1977.

Sarasohn C: Care of the very small premature infant. Pediatr Clin North Am 24:619, 1977.

Smith PC, and NT Smith: The special considerations of the premature infant. *In*: Some Aspects of Pediatric Anesthesia (DJ Steward, ed). Amsterdam, Elsevier/North Holland Biomedical Press, 1982, p. 273–329.

Steward DJ: Preterm infants are more prone to perioperative complications following minor surgery than are term infants. Anesthesiology 56:304, 1982.

Stow PJ, ME Mcleod, and FA Burrows: Anterior fontanel pressure response to endotracheal intubation in neonates and young infants. Anesth Analg 66S:169, 1987.

Welborn LG, RS Hannalah, R Fink, and JM Hicks: The role of caffeine in the prevention of postoperative apnea in former premature infants; if some is goood, is more better? Anesthesiology 69A:753, 1988.

POSTANESTHESIA ROOM

GENERAL MANAGEMENT

All patients must be placed in a lateral position for transport to the postanesthesia room (PAR); the anesthesiologist walks behind the cart or bed, in a good position to continuously observe the child. The time of transfer of the patient to the PAR is a danger time for respiratory obstruction, so be alert to this possibility. All patients, other than the absolutely healthy child having minor surgery, should have oxygen administered during transport. There is evidence from monitoring O_2 saturation during transport that many children show a fall in saturation at this time. A clear airway and good ventilation must be ensured. In the PAR, the anesthesiologist (1) transfers the patient to the care of the nurses (see below) and explains the operative procedure plus any complications of surgery or anesthesia: (2) finishes the anesthesia record; and (3) writes postoperative orders, including those for analgesics, IV therapy, and respiratory therapy.

In the PAR, every patient is given humidified oxygen via a face mask. An anesthesiologist should not hand over care of the patient until satisfied that the patient no longer needs an oropharyngeal airway. *If a patient still requires an orpharyngeal airway, the patient still needs an anesthesiologist.*

Postoperative stridor may occur, especially after endoscopy, in patients with Down syndrome or following unwise use of too large an ETT. Use of humidified oxygen and administration of dexamethasone (Decadron) IV may reduce subglottic edema. If stridor persists, administer racemic epinephrine by intermittent positive-pressure breathing for 15 min; this is usually efficacious.

Laryngospasm may occur. It should be managed by ventilation with O_2 via a face mask and a Jackson Rees T-piece, maintaining positive pressure on the bag. Be ready to reintubate if necessary and do not delay this too long if cyanosis occurs.

Remember that small infants (under 3 months) are obligate nose-breathers and therefore *ventilation may become obstructed* if the nasal passages are blocked (e.g., following cleft lip repair). If this occurs, insertion of an orpharyngeal airway or orogastric tube permits ventilation until the nasal airway is clear.

Shivering and rigidity are common during recovery from anesthesia, greatly increasing the metabolic rate and O_2 requirements. They are more severe after halothane, and if they cause concern (e.g., in an orthopedic patient with a recently reduced fracture), they can be abolished by IV injection of Ritalin (methylphenidate HCI, 0.15–0.4 mg/kg).

After *ketamine anesthesia*, recovery should take place in a quiet area with minimal tactile and auditory stimulation. If hallucinations develop, give diazepam (0.2–0.4 mg/kg IV).

DURATION OF STAY IN THE POSTANESTHESIA ROOM

Patients are kept in the PAR until they are fully awake and have recovered from the effects of anesthesia. Be alert for significant likely postoperative complications (e.g., stridor after surgery of or near the airway or after endoscopy; bleeding after a kidney or liver biopsy) and specify a longer stay in the PAR for such patients.

Patients staying longer than 1 hour must have deep breathing and coughing exercises and be turned hourly. Each patient must be signed out of the PAR by an anesthesiologist.

POSTOPERATIVE ANALGESIA

The provision of optimal postoperative analgesia for every infant and child should be the objective; postoperative pain hurts and may have adverse physiologic and psychological effects. Good pain relief will minimize the metabolic rate for oxygen, reduce cardiorespiratory demands, and speed recovery; postoperative emotional disturbance may be reduced. There are now a variety of means to combat postoperative pain, and most of these can be applied to appropriate pediatric patients.

Regional Nerve Block or Local Infiltration

The pain following many pediatric procedures can be very effectively treated by local or regional analgesic techniques. Frequently, no other medication will be required. Thus, the side effects of narcotics are avoided and the child rapidly returns to full activity after minor surgery.

Following more major surgery, appropriate regional blocks (e.g., intercostal nerve block) may permit reduction of narcotic dosage and earlier mobilization of the patient.

Bupivacaine to a maximum of 2.5 mg/kg may be used.

The following blocks are suggested. For details of technique, the reader is referred to the articles listed at the end of this section.

1. For thoracotomy or flank incisions (e.g., renal), a block of appropriate intercostal nerves with 1–2 ml of 0.25% bupivacaine should be performed. The use of equal volumes of dextran 40 and 0.5% bupivacaine will produce a more prolonged block. In infants and small children, the needle should be introduced at an angle oblique to rather than vertical to the rib.
2. For inguinal surgery, block the ilioinguinal and iliohypogastric nerves with 1–2 ml of 0.25% bupivacaine. This block has been shown to be as effective as a caudal block for such procedures.
3. For umbilical surgery, block the 10th intercostal nerve bilaterally below the lowest part of the 10th rib in the midaxillary line with 1–2 ml of 0.25% bupivacaine.
4. For circumcision, perform a dorsal nerve block of the penis. Use 0.25% bupivacaine without epinephrine, 0.5 ml in an infant and up to 4 ml in an adolescent. Topical lidocaine gel may also be effective.
5. For extensive penile or perineal surgery, perform a caudal block with 0.125% bupivacaine in a dose of 0.75 ml/kg.
6. Local infiltration of the wound with 0.125% bupivacaine may provide pain relief when there is no suitable nerve to block.

Regional anesthesia in children should be performed by the same methods and taking the same precautions as for adults, but with special attention to the total drug dose, as it is very easy to approach toxic levels of local analgesics in children.

Systemic Analgesic Drugs

Following minor procedures, when no regional or local analgesia regimen is possible, the use of a systemic analgesic is indicated. Dosages in common use are

Acetaminophen 10 mg/kg PO
Codeine 1–1.5 mg/kg IM or PO q4h
Meperidine 1 mg/kg IM q4h *or* 0.2 mg/kg IV q2h
Morphine 0.1–0.2 mg/kg IM q4h

The appropriate drug should be chosen for the magnitude of the pain, and a satisfactory effect should be confirmed. It is often preferable to administer the first parenteral dose of analgesia before the patient emerges from general anesthesia, for example for tonsillectomy, give 1.5 mg/kg of meperidine IM.

Continuous Narcotic Infusion

Morphine by continuous infusion with a dilute solution and a syringe pump provides for more even levels of analgesia and is appropriate for many patients after major surgery. The patient must have close nursing supervision when this technique is used. A loading dose of 0.1 mg/kg should be given, and an infusion commenced to deliver 10–30 μg/kg/hr. An infusion can be prepared by adding 1 mg of morphine for each kilogram of body weight to 100 ml of fluid. This infused at 1 ml/hr will equal 10 μg/kg/hr. For some patients, the loading dose may have to be repeated to establish an initially satisfactory level of analgesia.

Patient-Controlled Analgesia

Pediatric patients of over 5 years of age have been shown to be able to manage a patient-controlled analgesia (PCA) system and so to obtain good pain relief. It is important that a safe regimen be established, and the child and parents should be reassured that the system has an appropriate lock-out time and total dosage safeguards. The combination of a loading dose, a slow continuous infusion, and PCA supplements may give the best results.

Epidural Narcotics

Epidural morphine by the lumbar or the caudal route has been shown to be effective following major cardiac, general, urologic, or orthopedic surgery in children. The complications seen are similar to those in adults, with pruritis, urinary retention, and nausea being the most common. Ventilatory depression may occur, and the ventilatory response to CO_2 is depressed for up to 24 hours; the patient should receive appropriate nursing observation. A dose of 0.05–0.1 mg/kg of preservative-free morphine in 5 ml of preservative-free saline has been suggested. When the caudal route is used, 0.1 mg/kg of morphine in a dilution of 0.5 mg/ml has been recommended.

Continuous Epidural Analgesia

Continuous epidural analgesia has been used to provide pain relief following abdominal, perineal, and lower limb surgery. Bupivacaine may be delivered by continuous infusion via an epidural catheter or by intermittant top-up doses. A loading dose of 0.5 ml/kg of 0.25% bupivacaine and an infusion rate of 0.08 ml/kg/hr of 0.25% bupivacaine is reported to provide good analgesia with safe plasma bupivacaine levels. The patients must be provided with constant nursing observation.

Patients must remain in the PAR for at least 30 minutes after receiving an analgesic. Exercise great care when ordering drugs for infants weighing less than 5 kg and do not give morphine.

Cryopexy

Cryopexy of the intercostal nerves is a useful method to provide prolonged analgesia following thoracotomy. This may be especially useful in patients with chronic lung disease, for example, cystic fibrosis. The nerve must be exposed and treated with two 30-second freezy cycles from a $-60°C$ cryoprobe. Recovery of sensation is usually complete by 30 days.

Suggested Additional Reading
Review Article

Yaster M, and LG Maxwell: Pediatric regional anesthesia. Anesthesiology 70:324–338, 1989.

Other References

Anand KJS, and PR Hickey: Pain and its effects on the human neonate and fetus. N Engl J Med 317:1321–1329, 1987.

Blasie G, and WL Roy: Postoperative pain relief after hypospadius repair in pediatric patients: regional analgesia versus systemic analgesics. Anesthesiology 65:84–86, 1986.

Dalens B, A Tanguy, and JP Haberer: Lumbar epidural anesthesia for operative and postoperative pain relief in infants and young children. Anesth Analg 65:1069–1073, 1986.

Dalens B, and A Hasnaoui: Caudal anesthesia in pediatric surgery: success rate and adverse effects in 750 consecutive patients. Anesth Analg 68:83–89, 1989.

Desparmet J, C Meistelamn, J Barre, and C Saint-Maurice: Continuous epidural infusion of bupivacaine for postoperative pain relief in children. Anesthesiology 67:108–110, 1987.

Evelyn R, and DJ Steward: Oxygen consumption in infants in the early postoperative period: effect of analgesic therapy and subsequent activity. Can J Anaesth 34:S95–S96, 1987.

Katz J, W Nelson, R Forest, and DI Bruce: Cryoanalgesia for post-thoracotomy pain. Lancet 1:512, 1980.

Krane EJ, LE Jacobson, AM Lynn, C Parrot, and DC Tylor: Caudal morphine for postoperative analgesia in children. Anesth Analg 66:647–653, 1987.

Lunn JN: Postoperative analgesia after circumcision. Anaesthesia 34:552–554, 1979.

Lynn AM, KE Opheim, and DC Tyler: Morphine infusion after pediatric cardiac surgery. Crit Care Med 12:863–866, 1984.

Rosen K, D Rosen, and E Bank: Caudal morphine for post-op pain control in children undergoing cardiac procedures. Anesthesiology 67A:510, 1987.

Shapiro LA, RJ Jedeikin, D Shalev, and S Hoffman: Epidural morphine analgesia in children. Anesthesiology 61:210–212, 1984.

Tree-Trakarn T, and S Pirayavaraporn: Postoperative pain relief for circumcision in children: comparison among morphine, nerve block, and topical analgesia. Anesthesiology 62:519–522, 1985.

Wolf A, RD Valley, DW Fear, WL Roy, and J Lerman: The minimum effective concentration of bupivacaine for caudal analgesia after surgery in pediatrics. Anesthesiology 67A:509, 1987.

REGIONAL ANALGESIA TECHNIQUES FOR SURGERY

Regional analgesia techniques are of limited value for pediatric surgical procedures (except as outlined above for the management of postoperative pain, where they are invaluable). The overall nonacceptance and lack of cooperation in the young results in the need for such large doses of sedatives that general anesthesia usually becomes preferable. However, spinal anesthesia is useful for small infants, especially the expreterm infant with a hernia and residual lung disease. Epidural analgesia may be a suitable alternative to general anesthesia in some older children (e.g., those with cystic fibrosis) and may be continued into the postoperative period. In addition, some older children (5 years and over) can be charmed into cooperation and have their upper limb fractures reduced under a regional block. The possibility of using regional analgesia should also be considered for any minor procedure in a high-risk patient (e.g., skeletal muscle biopsy in a child with cardiomyopathy).

Rarely, regional blocks are also indicated for chronic pain therapy and/or diagnostic purposes.

Basic rules for regional analgesia:

1. Calculate the allowable dose of the local analgesic agent for each child and do not exceed this.
2. Do use as much of this allowable dose of the agent as is necessary to ensure a good block.

3. Use careful aseptic technique; beware of intravascular injection: test by aspirating frequently.
4. Allow plenty of time for the block to become established before allowing the surgeon to approach the patient.

Suggested maximum doses for epidural or peripheral nerve blocks.

Lidocaine 5 mg/kg (8 mg/kg with 1:200,000 epinephrine)
Bupivacaine 2.5 mg/kg

Useful blocks include the following:

Brachial plexus block. The axillary approach is recommended because of its simplicity and lack of complications; it is easy to perform if the patient can place a hand behind the head. It is useful for forearm fractures, plastic procedures, and insertion of shunts for dialysis. For the older child, 10 ml of 1% lidocaine with 1:200,000 epinephrine added is adequate.

Femoral nerve block. This is useful for fractures of the shaft of the femur and for muscle biopsy in patients suspected of myopathy. For the latter procedure, a lateral femoral cutaneous nerve block should also be performed.

Intravenous regional analgesia (the Bier block). This may be useful in older children having excision of lesions on the limbs (e.g., ganglion). Use a reliable double tourniquet and do not exceed 5 mg/kg of 0.25% lidocaine. In general, the success of the block varies with the degree of limb exsanguination that can be achieved prior to injection of the local analgesic. Intravenous blocks are not suitable for fractures as it is difficult to apply an optimally tight cast to an ischemic limb.

SPINAL ANESTHESIA IN INFANTS

Spiral anesthesia is most commonly indicated for surgery at or below the umbilicus in small infants with a history of respiratory disease. It avoids the necessity to intubate and ventilate the patient and hence the risk of further airway damage or ventilator dependence. Little change in CVS parameters occurs in infants during spinal block. Postoperative apnea may be less common but has been reported after a spinal block. Remember that the spinal cord ends at L3 in the infant (vs. L2 in the adult), so perform lumbar puncture below L3.

Contraindications:

1. Sepsis or infected lumbar puncture site.

2. Coagulopathy.
3. Lack of enthusiastic parental consent.

Anesthetic Management

Preoperative
1. The patient should receive nothing by mouth for 4 hours.
2. No premedication is necessary.

Perioperative
1. Observe all special precautions for infants and preterm infants. Prepare anesthesia machine, ETTs, etc.
2. Brandy and sugar soother is often useful to settle the infant.
3. Establish a reliable IV infusion with local analgesia.
4. Scrub, gown, and glove.
5. Gently but firmly restrain the patient in a lateral position, avoiding neck flexion, which may compromise the airway.
6. Prepare and drape; infiltrate interspaces below L3 with 1% lidocaine.
7. Use a neonatal spinal needle (e.g., 22 gauge by 1 inch [26 mm]).
8. Insert at L4–L5 until cerebrospinal fluid is obtained.
9. Slowly inject 1% tetracaine, 0.4–0.6 mg/kg (higher dose for smaller infants). Add an equal volume of 10% dextrose. Use a tuberculin syringe.
10. Add extra volume for dead space of needle (= 0.2 ml).
11. Turn to supine. Motor function in lower limbs usually ceases immediately.
12. Duration of anesthesia is approximately 1.5 hours.

Postoperative
1. Continue to nurse the patient in a horizontal position, until motor function in legs returns.

Suggested Additional Reading

Abajian JC, P Mellish, AF Browne, et al: Spinal anaesthesia for surgery in the high risk infant. Anesth Analg 63:359–362, 1984.
Harnick E, GR Hoy, S Potolicchio, DR Stewart, and RE Siegelman: Spinal anesthesia in premature infants recovering from respiratory distress syndrome. Anesthesiology 64:95–99, 1986.
Yaster M, and LG Maxwell: Pediatric regional anesthesia. Anesthesiology 70:324–338, 1989.

ANESTHESIA FOR OUTPATIENT SURGERY

ADVANTAGES OF OUTPATIENT SURGERY

1. Psychological upset of the child is minimized.
2. Less risk of hospital-acquired infection.
3. Reduced cost of care; availability of hospital beds for others.

SELECTION OF CASES

1. The child must be healthy or have chronic disease under good control.
2. The child's parents must be reliable and willing to follow instructions concerning preoperative and postoperative care.
3. The operation must be short with minor physiologic upset.
4. Infants who were full-term and are still under 3 months' postnatal age or less than 45 weeks' postconceptual age should be admitted to the hospital. There is a higher incidence of perioperative complications in these patients (especially apnea).

PREOPERATIVE PREPARATION

Preoperative preparation is as for inpatient surgery (*see* page 62).

The parents should be given written instructions concerning preoperative fasting and methods to prepare their child for the visit to the hospital (*see* page 3). They should also be given a questionnaire to complete and bring with them to facilitate obtaining a medical history for the child (Fig. 3-2).

On the day of operation, the child is brought to the outpatient department surgical unit. Urinalysis is performed and the Hb determined; if indicated, a sickle cell preparation is obtained. The parent's or legal guardian's consent for operation must be obtained. The parent is encouraged to stay with the child, to remove the child's clothes and gown the child for the OR, and to await the child's return from the recovery room.

The anesthesiologist makes a preoperative assessment by taking the history, examining the patient, and noting hematology and urinalysis data.

SELECTION OF ANESTHETIC TECHNIQUES

Premedication is not routinely given to outpatients, so that the recovery phase is not prolonged. Most children attending for outpatient surgery with their parents are not very upset, and "pharmacologic crutches"

AMBULATORY SERVICES
OUT-PATIENT SURGERY

INSTRUCTIONS:
— CHECK ONE ANSWER TO EACH QUESTION
— PLEASE COMPLETE THIS SIDE ONLY
— PLEASE BRING THIS FORM WITH YOU ON THE DAY OF SURGERY

	YES	NO	DON'T KNOW
1. HAS YOUR CHILD EVER BEEN IN HOSPITAL?	☐	☐	☐
2. HAS HE BEEN IN THIS HOSPITAL BEFORE?	☐	☐	☐
3. HAS YOUR CHILD EVER HAD AN ANAESTHETIC?	☐	☐	☐
4. DID YOUR CHILD HAVE ANY PROBLEMS WITH THE ANAESTHETIC?	☐	☐	☐
5. DOES YOUR CHILD HAVE ANY ALLERGIES?	☐	☐	☐
6. WAS THE ALLERGY DUE TO:			
a) A DRUG OR MEDICINE?	☐	☐	☐
b) ANY TYPE OF FOOD?	☐	☐	☐
c) OTHER THINGS?	☐	☐	☐
7. IF HE HAD AN ALLERGY, DID HE HAVE:			
a) A SKIN RASH OR HIVES?	☐	☐	☐
b) WHEEZING OR TROUBLE BREATHING?	☐	☐	☐
c) HAY FEVER OR A RUNNY NOSE?	☐	☐	☐
d) A HIGH FEVER?	☐	☐	☐
8. HAS THIS CHILD HAD A HEAD COLD OR COUGH WITHIN THE PAST WEEK?	☐	☐	☐
9. DOES YOUR CHILD WEAR A DENTAL PLATE OR BRIDGE?	☐	☐	☐
10. HAS YOUR CHILD HAD A CORTISONE TYPE DRUG WITHIN THE PAST TWO YEARS?	☐	☐	☐
11. IS YOUR CHILD RECEIVING ANY MEDICINE JUST NOW?	☐	☐	☐

	YES	NO	DON'T KNOW
12. IS THERE ANYONE IN THE FAMILY WITH A BLEEDING PROBLEM?	☐	☐	☐
13. HAS THE PATIENT HAD ANY MINOR INJURIES, OPERATIONS, OR TOOTH EXTRACTION FOLLOWED BY AN UNUSUAL AMOUNT OF BLEEDING?	☐	☐	☐
14. DOES THE CHILD BRUISE EASILY ON BODY AREAS OTHER THAN THE LEGS?	☐	☐	☐
15. HAS YOUR CHILD BEEN EXPOSED TO ANY INFECTIOUS DISEASE WITHIN THE PAST MONTH?	☐	☐	☐
16. HAS YOUR CHILD EVER HAD:			
DIABETES	☐	☐	☐
ASTHMA	☐	☐	☐
CYSTIC FIBROSIS	☐	☐	☐
TUBERCULOSIS	☐	☐	☐
RHEUMATIC FEVER	☐	☐	☐
RHEUMATISM	☐	☐	☐
HEART DISEASE	☐	☐	☐
LIVER DISEASE	☐	☐	☐
ANEMIA	☐	☐	☐
CONVULSIONS OR FITS	☐	☐	☐
GLAUCOMA	☐	☐	☐
JAUNDICE	☐	☐	☐
17. IS THERE ANY PROBLEM ABOUT YOUR CHILD NOT MENTIONED SO FAR?	☐	☐	☐
18. HAS ANYONE IN YOUR FAMILY EVER HAD A PROBLEM WITH AN ANAESTHETIC?	☐	☐	☐

IF ANY QUESTIONS ABOVE RECEIVED A "YES" ANSWER GIVE DETAILS BELOW:

DATE COMPLETED:_____ SIGNATURE OF PARENT:_____

Fig. 3-2. Questionnaire for outpatients.

are usually unnecessary. In the (rare) event that the child is very nervous, the mother should be instructed to give an appropriate dose of diazepam orally before leaving home. However, all patients are given atropine, 0.02 mg/kg, preferably IV, at induction.

Use simple general anesthetic techniques likely to result in rapid recovery and do not give drugs that might increase morbidity postoperatively. In general, volatile agents are preferred to IV drugs: halothane is the agent of first choice. For some limb procedures in older children, an IV infusion block may be more appropriate.

Induction may be by inhalation (N_2O with halothane), IV (thiopental), or rectally (methohexital). If succinylcholine is to be used for intubation, precede it with a small dose (0.05 mg/kg) of curare IV to prevent postoperative muscle pain. Intubation should be used if indicated. Postintubation complications can be avoided by gentle laryngoscopy and use of a tube that passes easily through the glottis. A nasotracheal tube is used for dental surgery; at the end of the procedure, perform laryngoscopy, suction the pharynx well, and ensure that all throat packs, etc., have been removed.

Maintain anesthesia with mixtures of N_2O and halothane. Avoid ketamine and neuroleptanalgesics because of prolonged recovery time. Enflurane, although widely advocated for outpatient anesthesia, has no advantage over halothane in pediatric patients. Isoflurane may result in a marginally more rapid recovery than halothane, but the incidence of coughing and laryngospasm is higher.

Tonsillectomy is sometimes performed in the day care unit. It is important that these patients are well hydrated during and after the operation as a return to adequate oral fluid intake may be delayed. I suggest that IV fluids be given to fully replace the preoperative deficit and to "load" the patient slightly before discharge home. Careful surgical technique and follow-up for bleeding is an obvious requirement.

POSTOPERATIVE CARE

Many patients require no analgesics postoperatively, especially if a regional block has been performed (for hernia, etc.; *see* page 100). If required, codeine can be given IM in the usual dosage. More potent analgesics are only very rarely indicated for outpatients.

Patients should be taking and retaining oral fluids well before discharge. Those who have had tonsillectomy or adenoidectomy are offered Popsicles* ad lib.

---

* Popsicle Industries Canada, Burlington, Ontario, Canada.

Every patient must be examined and signed out by an anesthesiologist. Infants can be taken home when they are obviously fully recovered. Children should be tested for street fitness and should be able to walk out; if dizzy or nauseated, they must stay longer. If the anesthesiologist considers a patient unfit for discharge within 4 hours, overnight admission is recommended.

Children must be accompanied home by an adult. Warn the parents that their child must not ride a bicycle or engage in dangerous activities for 24 hours. A follow-up service should be provided and the parents encouraged to seek advice from the hospital if problems develop during the postoperative period.

Complications following pediatric outpatient surgery are rare. It is also very seldom (<1%) that a child needs to be admitted overnight following a planned day care procedure; the most common reasons are protracted vomiting or complicated surgery. Complications that may occur at home include vomiting, cough, sleepiness, sore throat, and hoarseness. If the parents are well prepared, these can usually be treated effectively in the home.

Suggested Additional Reading

Ahlgren EW, EJ Bennett, and CR Stephen: Outpatient pediatric anesthesiology: a case series. Anesth Analg 50:402, 1971.

Booker PD, and DH Chapman: Premedication in children undergoing day-care surgery. Br J Anaesth 51:1083, 1979.

Cloud DT, WA Reed, JL Ford, LM Linkner, DS Trump, and GW Dorman: The surgicenter: a fresh concept in outpatient pediatric surgery. J Pediatr Surg 7:206, 1972.

Cox JMR: Intravenous regional anaesthesia. Can Anaesth Soc J 11:503, 1964.

Davenport HT, CP Shah, and GC Robinson: Day surgery for children. Can Med Assoc J 105:498, 1971.

Fleming SA, JA Veiga-Pires, RM McCutcheon, and CI Emanuel: A demonstration of the site of action of intravenous lignocaine. Can Anaesth Soc J 13:21, 1966.

Morse TS: Pediatric outpatient surgery. J Pediatr Surg 7:283, 1972.

Shah CP, GC Robinson, C Kinnis, and Davenport HT: Day care surgery for children: a controlled study of medical complications and parental attitudes. Med Care 10:437, 1972.

Patel RI, and RS Hannallah: Anesthetic complications following pediatric ambulatory surgery. Anesthesiology 69:1009–1012, 1988.

Shandling B, and DJ Steward: Regional analgesia for post-operative pain in pediatric outpatient surgery. J Pediatr Surg 15:477, 1980.

Smith BL, and MLM Manford: Postoperative vomiting after paediatric adenotonsillectomy: a survey of incidence following differing pre- and post-operative drugs. Br J Anaesth 46:373, 1974.

Smith RM, JB Stetson, and A Sanchez-Salazar: Postoperative distress in children [abstract]. Anesthesiology 22:145, 1961.

Steward DJ: Anaesthesia for day care surgery; a symposium. IV Anaesthesia for paediatric outpatients. Can Anaesth Soc J 27:412, 1980.

Steward DJ: A simplified scoring system for the post-operative recovery room. Can Anaesth Soc J 22:111, 1975.

* Steward DJ: Outpatient pediatric anesthesia. Anesthesiology 43:268, 1975.

---

* Key article. *See also* Appendix II.

4

Miscellaneous Disorders with Significant Implications for Anesthesia

MALIGNANT HYPERPYREXIA
Detection of susceptibility
Clinical manifestations
Therapeutic regimen
Anesthesia regimen
Cases at risk
Preoperative investigation
Preoperative preparation
Suggested additional reading

CYSTIC FIBROSIS
Suggested additional reading

THE CHILD WITH AN UPPER RESPIRATORY TRACT INFECTION

Pediatric patients often have, or are recovering from, a runny nose or other manifestations of upper respiratory tract infection (URI) when they are seen for evaluation prior to general anesthesia. Some children seem to have a runny nose most of the time. There are several causes for a runny nose in children, including viral or bacterial infections and allergies.

Several studies have suggested that patients with uncomplicated URI who are otherwise well do not have a higher incidence of perioperative problems during *minor* surgery performed under general anesthesia. There is even one report that suggests that halothane anesthesia may favourably influence the course of a URI. However, infants under 1 year with URI may show an increased incidence of complications during induction of anesthesia. Pulmonary complications in patients having *major* surgery may be more common if there is a recent (within 2 weeks) history of URI. This may be due to the fact that virus infections alter the reactivity of the airway for such a period.

The following plan of action is suggested:

1. Patients who need emergency or urgent surgery must be accepted for general anesthesia for the needed procedure. No special modifications to the anesthesia technique should be made (e.g., endotracheal intubation should be performed for the usual indications, but make sure that gases are warmed and humidified.
2. Patients for elective surgery should be carefully assessed:
   (a) A history of their URI should be obtained along with a detailed history of any other illnesses.
   (b) A careful physical examination should be performed, looking particularly for any evidence of lower respiratory tract disease.
3. Patients without pyrexia or any other evidence of disease may be accepted for minor surgical procedures knowing that studies indicate no increased risk of complications (exception—infants under 1 year of age should be deferred if possible).
4. Patients with URI who have pyrexia, evidence of lower respiratory tract or other disease, and those having major surgery should be deferred for 3–4 weeks if possible.
5. Patients who are in the recovery phase from a URI, especially if there was also lower respiratory tract involvement (e.g., cough, wheezing), should have major surgery deferred for 2–3 weeks if possible.

Suggested Additional Reading

Liu LMP, JF Ryan, CJ Cote, and NG Goudsouzian: Influence of upper respiratory infections on critical incidents in children during anesthesia. Abstracts of the 9th World Congress of Anaesthesia. A0786, 1988.

McGill WA, LA Coveler, and BS Epstein: Subacute upper respiratory infection in small children. Anesth Analg 58:331–333, 1979.

Mcleod ME, and L Roy: Anaesthesia and upper respiratory tract infection in the paediatric patient. Can Anaesth Soc J 30:586, 1983.

Tait AR, TR Ketcham, MJ Klein, and PR Knight: Perioperative respiratory complications in patients with upper respiratory tract infections. Anesthesiology 59A:433, 1983.

Tait AR, and PR Knight: Anesthesia and upper respiratory viral infections: a prospective cohort study. Anesthesiology 63A:526, 1985.

Tait AR, BS McLear, and PR Knight: Anesthesia and the common cold: why not sleep on it? Anesthesiology 65A:492, 1986.

HEMATOLOGIC DISORDERS

ANEMIA

Children requiring surgery may be anemic. Remember that the hemoglobin (Hb) level, normally 18–20 g/dl at birth, falls to a low of about 10–11 g/dl by 3 months of age and thereafter climbs gradually to 14 g/dl by 6 years of age. In the preterm infant, the Hb often falls to lower levels, owing to a low red blood cell (RBC) mass at birth, short survival of fetal RBCs, and poor erythropoietin response. Frequent blood sampling compounds this anemia. In children, Hb levels below normal for age are most frequently due to poor diet. Anemia discovered before elective surgery should be fully investigated and adequately treated before scheduling the operation. Usually elective surgery is postponed if the Hb is less than 10 g/dl, but in each case the whole clinical situation must be fully considered before the decision is made. Remember that in patients with anemia:

1. O_2 transport to the tissues can be maintained only by increased cardiac output or increased O_2 extraction from the blood. The major compensation is the increase in the cardiac output; shift of the Hb/O_2 dissociation curve caused by increased 2,3-diphosphoglycerate contributes relatively little. Below a Hb level of about 8 g/dl the cardiac output must increase to compensate for the decreased oxygen-carrying capacity in the blood.

2. Coronary sinus blood is normally very desaturated; therefore, in anemia, O_2 transport to the heart muscle can be maintained only by in-

creased coronary blood flow. At Hb levels below 5 g/dl the ability of the myocardium to meet its own needs is compromised and congestive cardiac failure may occur.

3. Anemic patients are suggested to be at increased risk of cardiac arrest during anesthesia. The factual data to support this are scant, but the concept seems reasonable.
4. Patients with cardiac or serious respiratory disease require a higher Hb level than normal children: a level of 14 g/dl should be considered as the minimum acceptable, and some patients need higher levels (*see also* page 262).
5. Preterm infants who are anemic are more prone to apnea.

If surgery cannot be delayed, a decision must be made whether to proceed despite the anemic state or whether to transfuse packed cells to correct the anemia.

If blood transfusion is contraindicated, unwarranted, or refused, use techniques that are optimal in the anemic state:

1. Avoid excessive preoperative sedation.
2. Oxygenate the patient before induction.
3. Use high inspired O_2 concentrations during anesthesia.
4. Always use an endotracheal tube.
5. Use controlled ventilation to a normal carbon dioxide tension.
6. Be cautious with myocardial depressant drugs, although halothane has been suggested to be advantageous as it decreases myocardial oxygen demand.
7. Carefully replace fluids to maintain the intravascular volume; hypovolemia must be avoided if the cardiac output is to be maintained.
8. Do not extubate the patient until the child is fully awake.
9. Give additional O_2 continuously during transportation to and in the postanesthesia room (PAR).
10. Keep the patient warm throughout.

Suggested Additional Reading

Allen JB, and RB Allen: The minimum acceptable level of hemoglobin. Int Anesthesiol Clin 20:1–22, 1982.

Barrera M, DJ Miletich, RF Albrecht, and WE Hoffman: Hemodynamic consequences of halothane anesthesia during chronic anemia. Anesthesiology 61:36–42, 1984.

Blanchette VS, and A Zipursky: Assessment of anemia in newborn infants. Clin Perinatol 11:489–510, 1984.

Cropp G: Cardiovascular function in children with severe anemia. Circulation 39:775, 1969.

Gillies IDS: Anaemia and anaesthesia. Br J Anaesth 46:589, 1974.

Howells TH: Anaesthesia and blood diseases. *In*: Recent Advances in Anaesthesia and Analgesia, No. 12 (CL Hewer and RS Atkinson, eds). Edinburgh, Churchill Livingstone, 1976, p. 120–130.

Wardrup CAJ, BN Holland, KE Anne Veal, JG Jones, and OP Gray: Nonphysiological anaemia of prematurity. Arch Dis Child 53:855–860, 1978.

SICKLE CELL STATES

In sickle cell conditions an abnormal hemoglobin (HbS) is present. HbS forms a gel when deoxygenated, distorting the erythrocytes; these then occlude vessels, causing infarction. In addition, erythrocyte life span is reduced and there is increased hemolysis with consequent anemia and increased bilirubin level. The course of the disease is one of many crises: sickling, hemolytic, or aplastic. Sickling crises result in ischemic pain; hemolytic crises result in further anemia; aplastic crises may cause death. The disease is almost entirely confined to the black races and may become evident during infancy when HbS replaces fetal hemoglobin (HbF) (Table 4-1).

The severity of the disease depends on the percentage of HbS and the presence or absence of other abnormal forms of Hb.

1. Sickle cell trait (mild form): low concentration of HbS (<50%). This is unlikely to give rise to serious problems during anesthesia.
2. Sickle cell disease (severe form): high concentration of HbS (>75%). This may cause serious complications during anesthesia and surgery.

   Note: The incidence of sickle cell trait is ±8%. Sickle cell disease may occur in 0.16–1.3% of a black population.
3. If another abnormal Hb is present it may modify the disease; for example, HbC if present may result in a greater tendency to sickling. On the other hand, HbF if present (e.g., thallasemia) may protect by re-

TABLE 4-1. INCIDENCE OF SICKLE CELL STATES

	Incidence (% of Black Population)	
State	Africa	North America
Trait	1–40 (regional variation)	9
Disease	?	0.5–1.0

ducing hemolysis and sickling. It is therefore most important to know the results of Hb electrophoresis.

4. Neonates who have a high percentage of HbF are not usually anemic or usually considered at risk of sickling. However, sickle cell crises have been reported in severely stressed neonates. Usually, the clinical signs appear by the time the child is a few months old.
5. Splenic function is impaired, serious infections may occur, and prophylactic antibiotics are indicated. Later, autosplenectomy may occur owing to vaso-occlusive events.
6. In later life, pulmonary infarction leads to pulmonary hypertension and cor pulmonale.

Special Anesthetic Problems

1. A sickling crisis may be precipitated by general or local hypoxemia.
2. Sickling is more likely if the patient is anemic, acidotic, hypotensive, dehydrated, and/or hypothermic or if the blood contains other abnormal Hb as well.
3. If the patient has sickle cell disease, previous vascular occlusive crises may have permanently impaired cardiac, hepatic, and/or renal function.
4. Serum cholinesterase activity may be low.

Anesthetic Management

The management of the sickle cell diseases is evolving as we gain more experience with these conditions. The assistance of a hematologist may be helpful in deciding which measures are appropriate for each patient. Do not be surprised if some previously held concepts change.

Preoperative

1. Screening: All black patients who require anesthesia must be screened for sickle cells:
   (a) Sickle cell preparation (microscopy for "sickled" cells) takes 2 hours to complete.
   (b) Sickledex test results are available in 5 minutes.
   (c) Screening is unreliable in infants under 6 months of age, but electrophoresis will provide accurate diagnosis.
   (d) Some authorities recommend that all patients at risk should have Hb electrophoresis to establish the exact diagnosis.
2. If screening tests are positive, the severity of the condition should be determined by Hb electrophoresis. In general, a severe form of the disease is unlikely if anemia is absent, but Hb electrophoresis is essential to exclude other abnormal Hb. For example, patients with HbSC disease may have a normal Hb level but be at increased risk of sickling.

3. If the patient has sickle cell trait (<50% HbS):
   (a) Avoid preoperative dehydration—start intravenous (IV) fluids during the fasting period.
   (b) Avoid excessive preoperative sedation.
4. If the patient has sickle cell disease (70–90% HbS):
   (a) Assess the patient carefully, particularly for sequelae of previous sickling crises (cardiac or renal infarction, etc.).
   (b) Preoperative transfusions of packed cells over several days are necessary; this suppresses erythropoiesis as evidenced by a fall in reticulocyte count. It is desirable to reduce the HbS level to below 40% for most operations. Those patients who require cardiopulmonary bypass with hypothermia should have packed cell infusions or exchange transfusion to reduce the HbS level to below 5%.
   (c) In an emergency, exchange transfusion should be performed.
   (d) Treat as outlined above for sickle cell trait.

Perioperative

1. Use high inspired O_2 concentrations (at least 50%) to maintain 100% saturation and control the ventilation.
2. Monitor the acid-base status carefully and avoid acidosis.
3. Ensure maintenance of body temperature.
4. Beware of regional ischemia:
   (a) Do not use a tourniquet unless essential. If so, exsanguinate the limb well and use for the minimal time.
   (b) Check blood pressure (BP) cuff, etc., frequently to see that no locally constricting effects are produced.
5. Maintain blood volume and hydration.

Postoperative

1. Patient must be awake before extubation.
2. Give additional O_2 continuously during transport to and in the PAR.
3. Hydration and warmth must be maintained.
4. Be alert for the possibility of pulmonary complications—these are common in patients with sickle cell disease.

Suggested Additional Reading

Bentley PG, and ER Howard: Surgery in children with homozygous sickle-cell anemia. Ann R Coll Surg Engl 61:55, 1979.

Browne RA: Anaesthesia in patients with sickle-cell anaemia. Br J Anaesth 37:181, 1965.

Burrington JD, and MD Smith: Elective and emergency surgery in children with sickle cell disease. Surg Clin North Am 56:55, 1976.

Esseltine DW, MRN Baxter, and JC Bevan: Sickle cell states and the anaesthetist. Can J Anaesth 35:385–403, 1988.

Homi J: General anaesthesia in sickle-cell disease. Br Med J 2:739, 1979.

Riethmuller R, EM Grundy, and R Radley-Smith: Open heart surgery in a patient with homozygous sickle-cell states: a review. Anaesthesia 37:324, 1982.

Searle JF: Anaesthesia in sickle cell states: a review. Anaesthesia 28:48, 1973.

Vichinsky EP, and BH Lubin: Sickle cell anemia and related hemoglobinopathies. Pediatr Clin North Am 27:429, 1980.

THALASSEMIA

Thalassemia, which occurs in two forms (major and minor), may affect any race but is commonest in individuals from the Mediterranean countries and Southeast Asia. The primary defect is a slow rate of Hb synthesis. (A high percentage of HbF is present.)

1. *Thalassemia minor* (heterozygous condition): Hb level is usually 9–12 g/dl. No special treatment is required, and there are usually no anesthesia problems.
2. *Thalassemia major* (homozygous form), also called Cooley's anemia: low Hb levels may necessitate repeated transfusion, which may result in hemosiderosis.

Special Anesthetic Problems (Thalassemia Major)

1. Anemia may be severe (5–7 g/dl).
2. Hemosiderosis may have developed and may impair myocardial and hepatic function.
3. Facial deformity (overgrowth of the maxillary region) may make intubation difficult.

Anesthetic Management

Preoperative

1. Packed cells should be transfused to elevate the Hb level to 10 g/dl. A chelating agent (e.g., deferoxamine) may be given with the blood.
2. Assess the patient carefully and anticipate any difficulty with intubation.

Perioperative

1. If intubation is considered likely to be difficult:
   (a) Do not use IV induction agents.

   (b) Perform inhalation induction and proceed as suggested for difficult intubation (*see* page 68).
2. Use caution when infusing fluids IV. (The plasma volume may be high and circulatory overload may occur.)

Postoperative
1. No special treatment is required.

Suggested Additional Reading

Oduntan SA, and WA Isaacs: Anaesthesia in patients with abnormal haemoglobin syndromes: a preliminary report. Br J Anaesth 43:1159, 1972.

Ohene-Frempong K, and E Schartz: Clinical features of thalassemia. Pediatr Clin North Am 27:403, 1980.

Orr D: Difficult intubation: a hazard in thalassemia; a case report. Br J Anaesth 39:585, 1967.

IDIOPATHIC THROMBOCYTOPENIC PURPURA

In idiopathic thrombocytopenic purpura (ITP), an antiplatelet factor is present that results in the excessive destruction of platelets by the spleen, with consequent thrombocytopenia and bleeding. The disease may be acute or chronic; the incidence is highest at about 7 years of age. The acute form, which lasts about 1 month before spontaneous remission, may be complicated by severe intracranial bleeding or exsanguinating gastrointestinal (GI) hemorrhage, but the overall death rate is under 2%. Steroid hormones may be of some value during the acute episodes.

Surgical Therapy

Splenectomy results in improvement in almost all patients with acute ITP and many of those with the chronic condition.

Special Anesthetic Problems
1. Platelet counts may be very low and cannot be improved by infusions until the spleen is removed. Therefore, infusing platelets preoperatively is useless.
2. Many patients will have been treated with steroid hormones.

Anesthetic Management

Preoperative
1. Order steroid therapy as necessary.
2. Order blood and platelet concentrates (to be transfused if necessary after the spleen has been removed).

3. Do not order intramuscular injections.

Perioperative
1. Intubate the patient gently; avoid trauma to the mucosa that might cause bleeding. Use a well-lubricated tube.
2. Surgical bleeding is not usually a problem, but if it is, give platelets after the spleen has been removed.

Postoperative
1. The platelet count usually rises rapidly within hours after removal of the spleen.
2. Prophylactic antibiotic therapy is not necessary. (Children who have undergone splenectomy for ITP do not seem to be as prone to overwhelming infection as those whose spleens have been removed for other indications.

Suggested Additional Reading
Baldini MG: Idiopathic thrombocytopenic purpura and the ITP syndrome. Med Clin North Am 56:47, 1972.

HEMOPHILIA

FACTOR VIII DEFICIENCY (CLASSIC HEMOPHILIA TYPE A)
Classic hemophilia is characterized by episodes of bleeding, either spontaneous or after minimal injury. The presenting sign may be bleeding from the umbilical cord in neonates or after circumcision in infants. During childhood many sites may be involved, hemarthrosis is common, and retroperitoneal bleeding may occur. Hemophilic children require special care during any operation, including (most frequently) dental extractions.

Surgical Management
Patients with hemophilia should undergo elective surgery only in hospitals with full facilities to care for this condition. Team care by hematologist, surgeon, and anesthesiologist is essential.

If an emergency operation is absolutely essential but the facilities of a hematology department are not available, give fresh frozen plasma (20 mg/kg) preoperatively.

Preoperative Measures
1. If there is any doubt about the diagnosis, the patient's blood must be

tested. Investigation should include screening for factor VIII inhibitors. (which rarely complicate hemophilia; *see* Postoperative Measures).
2. One hour before surgery, an infusion of cryoprecipitate (3 ml/kg) should be given followed by an assay for plasma factor VIII activity. Surgery can proceed if factor VIII activity is over 50% (or preferably 75% for major surgery).

Perioperative Measures
1. Exercise great care during instrumentation of the airway. Avoid trauma that might provoke submucosal hemorrhage.

Postoperative Measures
1. Depending on the nature of the surgery, the factor VIII levels in the blood should be maintained at 50% for several days. This is achieved by giving infusions of cryoprecipitate, as dictated by repeated assay for factor VIII.
2. After dental extraction, ϵ-aminocaproic acid (Amicar) may help to inhibit fibrinolysis of formed blood clot.

Note. When factor VIII inhibitors are present (rarely), cryoprecipitate cannot be used and treatment presents a grave problem. At present, our patients are given factor IX infusions.

FACTOR IX DEFICIENCY (CHRISTMAS DISEASE, HEMOPHILIA TYPE B)

Patients with factor IX deficiency are treated as for factor XIII deficiency, except that factor IX levels are assayed and factor IX infusions are given.

Suggested Additional Reading

Abildgaard CF, M Britton, and J Harrison: Prothrombin complex concentrate (Konyne) in the treatment of hemophilic patients with factor VIII inhibitors. J Pediatr 88:200, 1976.
Buchanan GR: Hemophilia. Pediatr Clin North Am 27:309, 1980.
Davies RM, and JG Scott: Anaesthesia for major oral and maxillofacial surgery. Br J Anaesth 40:202, 1968.
Needleman HL, LB Kaban, and SV Kevy: The use of epsilon-aminocaproic acid for the management of hemophilia in dental and oral surgery patients. J Am Dent Assoc 93:586, 1976.
Rizza CR: Clinical management of haemophilia. Br Med Bull 33:225, 1977.

ATYPICAL PLASMA CHOLINESTERASES

The genetically determined abnormal cholinesterases may result in prolonged apnea after the administration of succinylcholine. In the homozygous state (about 1 in 2,500 children), recovery of muscle power may be delayed for hours; in the heterozygous state, the delay is usually 15–25 minutes (Table 4-2).

MANAGEMENT OF PROLONGED APNEA

If muscle activity fails to recover after administration of succinylcholine:

1. Continue to ventilate the patient and continue anesthesia.
2. Confirm persistence of the neuromuscular block by using a nerve stimulator.
3. Allow the child to recover completely before you discontinue ventilation (this may take 3–6 hours).

   Note. Prolonged apnea after succinylcholine owing to an atypical cholinesterase is not serious provided the above steps are followed. Do not attempt to modify the neuromuscular block by giving drugs or infusing fresh blood, etc., as further complications may arise. Ventilate the child well, and be patient.

TABLE 4-2.   PLASMA CHOLINESTERASES: VARIATION IN RESPONSE TO SUCCINYLCHOLINE

Genotype	Incidence	Response to Succinylcholine	Dibucaine No.	Fluoride No.
Homozygous				
$E_1^u E_1^u$		Normal	70	50
$E_1^a E_1^a$	1:2,800	Grossly prolonged	15–25	20–25
$E_1^s E_1^s$	1:140,000	Grossly prolonged	—	—
$E_1^f E_1^f$	1:300,000	Moderately prolonged	60–70	30–40
Heterozygous				
$E_1^u E_1^a$	1:25	Almost normal	50–70	40–50
$E_1^u E_1^f$	1:280	Almost normal	70–80	50–55
$E_1^u E_1^c$	1:190	Almost normal	70	50
$E_1^a E_1^f$	1:29,000	Grossly prolonged	45–50	30–40
$E_1^a E_1^s$	1:20,000	Grossly prolonged	15–25	20–25
$E_1^f E_1^s$	1:200,000	Grossly prolonged	60–70	30–35

4. Obtain blood samples for cholinesterase studies:
   (a) Cholinesterase activity (normal range is 60–200 units but varies with the individual laboratory).
   (b) Dibucaine number (DN; normal range 75–85).
   (c) Fluoride number (FN; normal range 55–65) (Table 4-2).

   Characteristically, patients with the atypical enzyme have a low DN (0–20) and FN (15–25). Those heterozygous for the condition have intermediate values (DN 40–60; FN 40–50). The results of these tests may not be available for some days and hence are of no value in the immediate management of the patient.

Postoperative Measures
1. When the diagnosis is confirmed, the patient's family should have blood tests and be informed of their status. Those having homozygous atypical states should be advised to carry a warning card or wear a "medic-alert" bracelet.

Suggested Additional Reading

Ernst EA: Genetic defects. Int Anesthesiol Clin 6:269, 1968.
Goedde HW, and K Altland: Suxamethonium sensitivity. Ann NY Acad Sci 179:695, 1971.
Horne JA, TD Watson III, AH Giesecke Jr, PP Raj, and EW Ahlgren: Prolonged apnea in an infant following the use of succinylcholine. Anesthesiology 39:545, 1973.
McLaren RG, and EA Moffitt: Case history number 92: prolonged apnea after succinylcholine in a dental outpatient. Anesth Analg 55:737, 1976.

DIABETES MELLITUS

In children, the onset of type 1 diabetes mellitus may be very abrupt, often manifesting with dehydration and metabolic acidosis. All of these patients require insulin, and control may be difficult. However, vascular complications seldom occur in diabetic children. As childhood diabetes is often unstable, the anesthesiologist should cooperate closely with the pediatrician in planning the management of these patients.

Anesthetic Management

Anesthetic management must be designed to avoid hypoglycemia or severe hyperglycemia. Mild hyperglycemia and some degree of glycosuria are not dangerous and must be expected during the operative period.

Preoperative
1. Diabetic children should be admitted several days before elective surgery for stabilization of the diabetes. If possible, defer emergency surgery until diabetic ketoacidosis is corrected.
2. Severe hyperglycemia and ketosis should be treated with appropriate insulin adjustments before surgery is scheduled.
3. *Short procedures* (less than 1 hour):
   (a) Schedule as early as possible in the morning.
   (b) Determine preoperative blood glucose level.
   (c) Give one-half to two-thirds the usual dose of insulin as intermediate acting insulin only (NPH or Lente). No short-acting insulin should be given.
   (d) Start an IV infusion of glucose-containing solutions, and infuse at a slow rate unless the blood glucose is less than 5.5 mmol/L (<100 mg/dl).
   (e) Determine blood glucose immediately after the procedure. Use capillary blood with one of the available strip methods for measuring blood glucose, for example, Chemstrip BG. Verify results with the laboratory.
4. *Long procedures* (greater than 1 hour):
   (a) An insulin infusion can be used to give insulin for longer procedures. Add 50 units of regular insulin to 500 ml of isotonic saline (each milliliter contains 0.1 unit of regular insulin). Saturate the insulin-binding sites of the IV tubing by allowing 50–100 ml of the solution to run through.
   (b) Use a Y-tube or piggyback into the maintenance IV line and control the rate with an infusion pump.
   (c) Infuse 0.1 units of insulin/kg/hr (1 ml/kg/hr).
   (d) Blood glucose levels should be determined every 0.5 hour during the surgery. Maintain blood glucose at 8.5–14 mmol/L (150–250 mg/dl) by infusing IV glucose solution.
   (e) Postoperatively, the insulin infusion can be continued as long as is necessary depending on the circumstances. The child's pediatrician should control the rate and amount of the infusion based on the blood glucose levels.

Perioperative
1. The usual anesthetic agents and techniques appropriate to the surgery may be employed.
2. Check blood glucose readings every 0.5 hour during surgery. (The level usually rises during surgery.)

Postoperative

1. *Short procedures:*
   (a) If the patient is receiving subcutaneous insulin, give appropriate doses of short-acting insulin as required based on blood glucose levels. Continue the IV until the child is taking fluids orally.
   (b) Usual insulin regimen can be resumed the next day if the patient is able to tolerate fluids or food.
2. *Long procedures:*
   (a) Change to subcutaneous insulin when the child's condition allows, for example, when the child is taking fluids orally and the IV is discontinued.
   (b) Pediatricians should observe and manage the patient's diabetes.

Suggested Additional Reading

Drash A: Diabetes mellitus in childhood: a review. J Pediatr 78:919, 1971.
Ehrlich RM: Diabetes mellitus in childhood. Pediatr Clin North Am 21:871, 1974.
Holvey SM: Surgery in the child with diabetes. Pediatr Clin North Am 16:671, 1969.

MALIGNANT DISEASES

The anesthesiologist frequently has to care for children with malignant disease. Special problems may arise depending on the site and type of the disease, but all of these children require special attention to their emotional status. Extreme care must be taken to ensure a minimum of discomfort and upset for the child and parents.

Special Anesthetic Problems

1. Abnormal anatomy, including the airway. (Beware of the child with enlarged hilar lymph nodes [*see* page 240]).
2. Myocardiopathy may follow total body irradiation and cyclophosphamide therapy or the use of Adriamycin or daunomycin (*see* below).
3. Increased susceptibility to infection: care in asepsis is vital to these children.
4. A history of long-term steroid therapy necessitates preoperative corticosteroids.
5. Nausea and vomiting may complicate radiotherapy and/or drug therapy and lead to dehydration and electrolyte disturbance: check the biochemistry levels.

6. Hypercalcemia may accompany malignant tumors of bone.
7. Hematologic disease may reuslt in anemia, coagulopathy, and immune deficiency. Check laboratory results.
8. Nephropathy may lead to impaired renal function.
9. Raised intracranial pressure may occur with involvement of the central nervous system (CNS).
10. Peripheral neuropathy may occur.
11. Muscle weakness and hypotonia occur in advanced malignant disease.
12. Toxic effects of chemotherapy (*see below*).

Adverse Effects of Commonly Used Drugs

All antineoplasic drugs may cause:

1. Leukopenia, anemia, and thrombocytopenia.
2. Anorexia, nausea, and vomiting.
3. Stomatitis and alopecia.
4. Decreased resistance to infection.

In addition, specific drugs have special effects of importance to anesthesiologists.

1. Daunomycin—used in leukemia therapy. Adriamycin—used in therapy of solid tumors and leukemias. Both drugs affect the heart:
   (a) Nonspecific electrocardiographic (ECG) changes may occur with any dose.
   (b) Disturbances of conduction: supraventricular tachycardia, atrial and ventricular extrasystoles, and ventricular fibrillation may occur.
   (c) Drug-induced cardiomyopathy occurs in 1–2% of patients and leads to congestive heart failure.
   (d) The cardiac effects of Adriamycin are dose related. A total cumulative dose of 250 mg/m^2 or 150 mg/m^2 if combined with mediastinal radiation must alert the anesthesiologist and is indication for a full cardiologic assessment. Patients with a history of congestive heart failure are particularly likely to suffer perioperative complications.
   (e) Myocardial depressant drugs (e.g., halothane) should be avoided, and cardiac parameters should be closely monitored.
2. Bleomycin—used in therapy of testicular tumors and Hodgkin's disease. This drug causes pulmonary fibrosis in approximately 10% of patients and may result in death (1%). The effects on the lung are accelerated by hyperoxia, and O_2 therapy should be carefully controlled at all times. Fluid overload may further compromise lung function.

3. Cyclophosphamide—used for lymphomas, Hodgkin's disease, leukemias, and various other tumors.
   (a) This drug inhibits serum cholinesterase, and prolonged apnea with succinylcholine may occur.
   (b) Pulmonary fibrosis may occur and be accelerated by hyperoxia.

Suggested Additional Reading

Azizkhan RG, DL Dudgeon, JR Buck, and PM Colombani, et al: Life-threatening airway obstruction as a complication to the management of mediastinal masses in children. J Pediatr Surg 20:816–822, 1985.

Burrows FA, PR Hickey, and S Kolin: Complications of anesthesia in Adriamycin treated pediatric patients. Anesthesiology 59A:434, 1983.

Keon TP: Death on induction of anesthesia for cervical node biopsy. Anesthesiology 55:471–472, 1981.

Klein DS, and PR Wilds: Pulmonary toxicity of antineoplastic agents: anaesthetic and postoperative implications. Can Anaesth Soc J 30:399, 1983.

McQuillan PJ, BA Morgan, and J Ramwell: Adriamycin cardiomyopathy. Anaesthesia 43:301–304, 1988.

ANESTHESIA FOR NONCARDIAC SURGERY IN CHILDREN WITH CONGENITAL HEART DISEASE

Children with congenital heart disease (CHD) sometimes require anesthesia for noncardiac procedures (e.g., dental surgery). Many of the potential problems are identical to those associated with cardiac surgery (*see* page 258 et seq.). Anesthesia must be carefully planned to minimize the possibility of adversely affecting the cardiovascular status of these patients. The anesthesiologist must understand the pathophysiology of the patient's disease and carefully assess the current hemodynamic status.

Anesthetic Management

Preoperative

1. Assess the patient carefully. Consider:
   (a) Type of cardiovascular anomaly and its present status.
   (b) Possibility of disease in other systems (e.g., respiratory infections) that may have implications for general anesthesia.
2. Elective surgery: ensure that the patient is in optimal condition; otherwise, surgery should be delayed.

3. Ensure that suitable antibiotic prophylaxis is ordered.

Antibiotic Routine for Patients with Cardiac Disease.

1. Dental procedures, oropharyngeal surgery, instrumentation of the respiratory tract (including nasotracheal intubation):
   (a) Standard regimen for children tolerant of penicillin:
      (i) Penicillin V, 2.0 g orally (PO) 60 minutes preoperatively (1 g for children <27 kg) followed by penicillin V, 1.0 g PO 6 hours later (500 mg for children <27 kg).
   Or if unable to take oral medications:
      (ii) Aqueous penicillin G, 50,000 units/kg intramuscularly (IM) or IV 30–60 minutes preoperatively followed by penicillin G, 25,000 units/kg IM or IV 6 hours later.
   (b) Regimen for patients at high risk of endocarditis (or with prosthetic valves):
      (i) Ampicillin, 50 mg/kg, plus gentamicin, 2 mg/kg, IV or IM 30 minutes preoperatively and repeat this 8 hours later.
   (c) Children allergic to penicillin or receiving continuous penicillin prophylaxis for rheumatic fever:
      (i) Erythromycin, 20 mg/kg PO 60–90 minutes preoperatively followed by 10 mg/kg PO 6 hours later.
   Or for high-risk patients (e.g., with prosthetic valves) allergic to penicillin:
      (ii) Vancomycin, 20 mg/kg, by slow IV infusion 30–60 min preoperatively.
2. Gastrointestinal or genitourinary procedures or instrumentation:
   (a) Children tolerant of penicillin: Ampicillin, 50 mg/kg IV, plus gentamicin, 2 mg/kg IV, 30–60 minutes preoperatively with the same doses repeated 8 hours later.
   (b) Children allergic to penicillen: Vancomycin, 20 mg/kg (maximum 1.0 g) IV, plus gentamicin, 2.0 mg/kg IV, 30–60 minutes preoperatively. Repeat the same doses 8 hours later.
   (c) Children with prosthetic valves: Vancomycin plus gentamicin as in (b) above.
4. If the hematocrit (Hct) is above 45%, order fluids to be given IV during the preoperative fasting period (to avoid hemoconcentration and therefore the risk of cerebral thrombosis).
5. Order appropriate preoperative sedation but avoid producing respiratory depression. Order atropine to be given IM.
6. Ensure that equipment for cardiopulmonary resuscitation (e.g., defibrillator) is available.

7. Check coagulation status in those with cyanotic heat disease. Coagulopathy is a common complication of polycythemia.

Perioperative
1. Attach monitors (including ECG).
2. Establish a reliable IV route.
3. Give 100% O_2 by mask.
4. Induce anesthesia with thiopental IV; use a small dose (3–4 mg/kg) injected slowly.
5. Intubate the patient for all but the most minor procedure (e.g., myringotomy). Give succinylcholine IV; if circulation time is prolonged, increase the dose by 50%.
6. Children with less severe disease will tolerate volatile agents well; for minor procedures, maintain anesthesia with N_2O and low concentrations of halothane or isoflurane with spontaneous ventilation. Patients with more severe disease and any history of congestive cardiac failure are managed with a high-dose narcotic and relaxant (vecuronium) technique, with controlled ventilation.
7. Maintain a high concentration of O_2 (at least 50%) and monitor the oxygen saturation carefully.
8. For major noncardiac surgery, insert arterial lines, etc., and monitor the patient as you would for cardiac surgery.

Postoperative
1. Continue to monitor the patient (including ECG and oxymeter) until fully recovered from all effects of anesthesia.
2. Give O_2 by mask until recovery is complete.
3. Provide good pain relief.
4. Give maintenance fluids IV until oral intake is adequate, but avoid inducing a fluid overload.

Suggested Additional Reading
Hickey PR: Anesthesia for Children with Heart Disease. International Anesthesia Research Society Review Course Lectures, 1988, p. 86–90.
Moore RA: Anesthesia for the pediatric congenital heart patient for noncardiac surgery. Anesth Rev 8:23–29, 1981.
Shulman ST, DP Amren, AL Bisno, et al: Special report: prevention of bacterial endocarditis. Circulation 70:1123A–1127A, 1984.

DOWN SYNDROME

Down syndrome (trisomy 21; T21) is common (1.5 in 1,000 live births). Mental retardation is invariably present but varies in severity from patient to patient.

Associated Conditions

1. Congenital heart disease occurs in up to 60% of patients, particularly atrioventricular canal, ventricular septal defect, patent ductus arteriosus, and tetralogy of Fallot.
2. Respiratory infections are common. This may be related to the genetic anomaly, an immune deficiency, and/or the social and institutional implications of the syndrome.
3. Atlantoaxial joint instability occurs in 12% of patients and may lead to cervical spinal cord injury. The neck is particularly unstable in the flexed position.
4. Duodenal atresia of the newborn is common in patients with Down syndrome.
5. Congenital subglottic stenosis is common. Ensure that the endotracheal tube selected is not too large.
6. Polycythemia is a frequent finding in neonates and may require phlebotomy to relieve circulatory failure.
7. Thyroid hypofunction is common as the child grows older.
8. Sleep apnea is common.

Special Anesthetic Problems

1. Airway: The large tongue and small nasopharynx predispose to respiratory obstruction, particularly during mask anesthesia and recovery stages. Congenital subglottic stenosis predisposes to postoperative stridor.
2. Lungs: Is there any acute infection present that requires therapy prior to surgery?
3. Problems of associated cardiac disease, and need for antibiotic prophylaxis against subacute bacterial endocarditis (SBE).
4. Atlantoaxial joint instability may predispose to injury during intubation. Excessive neck movement should be avoided (especially flexion).
5. Retarded children are more difficult to manage during induction of anesthesia. Often the parents can be of great help.

Note. Children with Down syndrome have been reported to be especially sensitive to the effects of atropine. This is not true and, in practice, we have used the same dosage schedule for these patients as for other patients without any problems.

Anesthetic Management

Preoperative

1. Do not order heavy sedation because of the risk of airway obstruction.
2. Order appropriate antibiotics if cardiac disease is present (*see* page 129).

3. Assess pulmonary status carefully.
4. Screening for atlantoaxial subluxation should be obtained whenever possible in all children over 4 years of age.

Perioperative

1. For older children, it may be advantageous to have a parent present for the initial stages of induction, if possible.
2. Be very cautious when selecting the correct size of endotracheal tube (i.e., not too big).
3. Avoid unnecessarily excessive neck movements during laryngoscopy.
4. Use techniques appropriate for the planned operation and the associated diseases.

Postoperative

1. Be alert to the possibility of airway problems during recovery.
2. Use care with narcotic analgesics. There is a danger of airway obstruction, and analgesics may predispose to sleep apnea. If heavy narcotic sedation is essential, the patient must be very closely supervised.
3. Postoperative stridor is more common and may require therapy (*see* page 98).
4. Following cardiac surgery, there may be a higher incidence of pulmonary complications and a need for more prolonged ventilatory support.

Suggsted Additional Reading

Beilin B, A Kadari, Y Shapira, D Shulman, and JT Davidson. Anaesthetic considerations in facial reconstruction in Down's syndrome. J R Soc Med 81:23–26, 1988.

Clark RW, HS Schmidt, and DE Schuller: Sleep induced ventilatory dysfunction in Down's syndrome. Arch Intern Med 140:45, 1980.

Greenwood RD, and AS Nadas: The clinical course of cardiac disease in Down's syndrome. Pediatrics 58:893, 1976.

Kobel M, RE Creighton, and DJ Steward: Anaesthetic considerations in Down's syndrome: experience with 100 patients and a review of the literature. Can Anaesth Soc J 29:593, 1982.

Morray JP, R MacGillivray, and G Duker: Increased perioperative risk following repair of congenital heart disease in Down's syndrome. Anesthesiology 65:221–224, 1986.

Moore RA, KW McNicholas, and SP Warran: Atlantoaxial subluxation with symptomatic spinal cord compression in a child with Down's syndrome. Anesth Analg 66:89–90, 1987.

Whaley WJ, and WD Gray: Atlantoaxial dislocation and Down's syndrome. Can Med Assoc J 123:35, 1980.

Williams JP, GM Somerville, ME Miner, and D Reilly: Atlanto-axial sub-luxation and trisomy-21: another perioperative complication. Anesthesiology 67:253–254, 1987.

MALIGNANT HYPERPYREXIA

Malignant hyperpyrexia (MH), a potentially fatal abnormal response to anesthetic agents, is genetically determined. It is characterized by a rapid rise in body temperature and profound biochemical changes usually accompanied by generalized muscular rigidity. Almost any anesthetic agent or muscle relaxant may trigger the condition, but two drugs (halothane and succinylcholine) are most frequently implicated.

Malignant hyperpyrexia is a rare condition, probably occurring in less than 1 in 100,000 cases in which general anesthetics are given. Children and young adults are most frequently affected, and it has been reported in a patient as young as 2 months of age. Increased awareness of MH, leading to earlier diagnosis and prompt institution of therapy, has reduced the mortality rate from over 70% to less than 40% of cases.

The exact pathogenesis of MH is unknown. The manifestations of the acute syndrome are due to uncontrolled acceleration of metabolic processes (particularly of skeletal muscle cells), accompanied by large increases in O_2 consumption and CO_2 production. If the acute condition persists, cellular energy substrates become depleted and failure of cellular function results.

DETECTION OF SUSCEPTIBILITY

There are no simple reliable screening tests to identify the MH-susceptible individual preoperatively. Creatine phosphokinase (CPK) levels are usually elevated, but this test is nonspecific and many other causes of an elevated CPK level exist.

At present, MH-susceptible patients can be identified with reasonable certainty only by in vitro study of muscle tissue obtained at biopsy. Caffeine- or halothane-induced contracture of the living biopsy specimen is usually diagnostic. Unfortunately, up to the present a large biopsy specimen has been required. Thus, the test is not suitable for small children (<10 years). Recently, progress has been made with smaller samples (skinned single fibers). Also, investigations of the metabolic activity of leukocytes in patients with MH may promise the possibility of a new approach to diagnosis of the trait.

Many of the affected patients have local or general muscular disease; however, the majority of patients with muscle disease are not MH susceptible. Furthermore, although a positive family anesthetic history is the most reliable clue, its absence does not guarantee an individual's non-susceptibility to appropriate triggering agents, and uneventual anesthesia does not preclude an MH crisis during administration of a subsequent anesthetic.

CLINICAL MANIFESTATIONS

1. Nonspecific early signs are unexplained tachycardia, tachypnea, sweating, cyanosis, and overheating of the soda lime.
2. Hypertonus of the skeletal muscle may occur.
   (a) Immediately after the administration of succinylcholine.
      (i) Failure of skeletal muscle to relax is an indication to postpone surgery and reevaluate.
      (ii) Abnormally severe muscle fasciculations or masseter spasm should arouse suspicion.
   (b) Later during anesthesia, after the use of potent agents, commonly halothane.
3. A rapid rise in body temperature ($>1°C$) may be a late sign. The prognosis is more favorable if the syndrome is recognized before a severe pyrexic reaction develops.

THERAPEUTIC REGIMEN

1. Discontinue all inhalational agents and relaxants, and **STOP THE SURGERY AT ONCE. SEND FOR HELP!**
2. Hyperventilate with 100% O_2 using a high flow.
3. Change to a vapor-free anesthetic machine and a vapor-free circuit (e.g., disposable plastic circuit) as soon as possible.
4. Establish a good IV line; insert a cannula with as wide a bore as practicable. Send an arterial sample for blood gas analysis.
5. Give:
   (a) Dantrolene: infuse IV at 1 mg/kg/min (up to 10 mg/kg) until the heart rate begins to slow and become regular, decreased muscle tone becomes evident, and the patient's temperature starts to fall. Then withhold the dantrolene and observe the heart rate, muscle tone, and temperature. If these regress, the infusion can be repeated at intervals of not less than 15 minutes until clinical improvement is apparent.

(b) If an IV preparation of dantrolene is not available or if arrhythmias occur: give procainamide IV (1 mg/kg/min, up to a maximum of 15 mg/kg) and monitor this with the ECG. This may relieve muscle contracture promptly and prevent further increase in body temperature.

(c) Sodium bicarbonate (7.5%), 4 ml/kg IV *stat*; repeat in accordance with blood gas analyses.

(d) Mannitol, 2 g/kg IV: to maintain adequate urine output (>2 ml/kg/hr).

(e) Steroids: hydrocortisone sodium succinate (10 mg/kg), dexamethasone (0.2 mg/kg), and chlorpromazine (1 mg/kg). These can be given but are of uncertain value.

6. Do not give drugs that may accelerate the MH crisis, e.g.:
   (a) Calcium chloride or gluconate.
   (b) Digitalis preparations.
   (c) Adrenergics.
   (d) Amide-type local anesthetics (e.g., lidocaine).

7. Commence active cooling. Place the patient on a rubber sheet, apply ice bags and ice water, and use fans. Intragastric cooling and cold enemas may also be necessary.

8. Infuse refrigerated saline solution IV at 10 ml/kg/hr.

9. Continue monitoring the patient closely by:
   (a) Stethoscope.
   (b) BP.
   (c) ECG.
   (d) Multichannel thermometer (rectal, esophageal, skin, and muscle leads).

10. Insert an arterial cannula for sampling and take serial blood specimens (10 ml) for measurement of:
    (a) Blood gases.
    (b) Electrolytes (Na, K, Cl, Ca, P_i).
    (c) Creatine phosphokinase.
    (d) Serum enzymes: serum glutamic oxaloacetic transaminase (SGOT), lactic dehydrogenase (LDH), creatine kinase (CK), 3-hydroxybutyrate dehydrogenase (3-HBDH). Repeat blood gas and electrolyte measurements every 10 minutes.

11. Correct the electrolyte imbalance on the basis of biochemical indices. To treat hyperkalemia, give 50 units of regular insulin in 50 ml of a 15% glucose solution. If hypokalemia develops, infuse KCl solution.

12. The patient is catheterized, and a urine sample is taken for hemoglobin and myoglobin estimations. Urine output is measured.

13. Complications, particularly coagulopathy and renal failure, must be expected after correction of the hyperthermia.

ANESTHESIA REGIMEN

All who may be concerned in the care of an MH-susceptible patient in the operating room (OR) and PAR must be fully acquainted with a suitable protocol that describes the location of drugs, equipment, etc., and the procedures to be implemented if MH develops.

CASES AT RISK

1. Survivors of an MH crisis.
2. Patients with a positive muscle biopsy.
3. A first-degree relative of anyone known to be MH susceptible (i.e., one with a positive muscle biopsy or a survivor of an MH crisis).
4. MH suspected on the basis of muscle abnormalities and/or an elevated serum CPK level.

In the management of children, the clinician frequently must assume MH susceptibility on questionable evidence, for example a family history of anesthetic difficulties but no positive muscle biopsy in the family.

PREOPERATIVE INVESTIGATION

This is for patients with a positive or suggestive family or personal history.

1. Review the family and personal history carefully, noting especially muscle disease, cardiac abnormality, and drug- or anesthetic-induced reactions.
2. Order laboratory investigations: serum enzymes (SGOT, LDH, CK, 3-HBDH) and coagulation indices.
3. Order an ECG and echocardiogram.
4. If the findings indicate a strong possibility of MH susceptibility and the child is over 12 years of age, it is advisable to arrange for a muscle biopsy at a suitably equipped center. Younger children and infants must be presumed to be at risk for MH susceptibility and treated accordingly until they are old enough for testing (or until an improved, less-invasive diagnostic test becomes available).

PREOPERATIVE PREPARATION

1. The patient should be admitted to the hospital 24 hours preoperatively (bed rest helps to alleviate anxiety and reduce muscle cramps). MH-susceptible patients should not have outpatient surgery.

2. Routine dantrolene sodium pretreatment for all MH patients is not recommended. It may be advantageous to administer IV dantrolene, 2.4
mg/kg, to the very high risk MH patient and to emergency or trauma
patients.
3. If diagnostic muscle biopsy is to be performed, do not given dantrolene
(it would affect the test results).

Anesthetic Management
Preoperative
1. Order a suitable barbiturate or diazepam to be given the evening before
surgery.
2. Order oral diazepam (0.2–0.5 mg/kg) 1.5 hours preoperatively (or a
narcotic of choice if more suitable).
3. At 0.5 hour before induction of anesthesia:
   (a) Insert a wide-bore cannula into a peripheral vein under local anesthesia.
   (b) Continue infusion with 5% dextrose-0.2N saline solution (2 ml/kg/
   hr).
4. Ensure that all necessary drugs and equipment have been prepared:
   (a) Drugs for anesthesia—droperidol, fentanyl, diazepam, pancuronium.
   (b) Drugs for emergency use if MH develops—including refrigerated
   lactated Ringer solution, normal saline, 7.5% $NaHCO_3$, and
   warmed 20% mannitol and 50% glucose solutions, dantrolene, procainamide, hydrocortisone, furosemide, KCl, soluble insulin, heparin, chlorpromazine, and propranolol.
   (c) Equipment: vapor-free anesthetic machine, plastic disposable circuit and reservoir bag, ventilator, two hypothermia blankets, multichannel thermometer and probes, ECG and Doppler apparatus,
   ice bags and crushed ice, capnograph.
5. Remove all triggering agents from the room (to avoid any possibility
of accidental use).

Perioperative
"Safe" drugs to use include nitrous oxide, thiopentone, narcotics,
droperidol, diazepam, pancuronium, naloxone.
Atropine should be used in small IV doses (0.005 mg/kg) as required
to treat bradycardia.

Induction
1. Ensure that the patient is placed on a hypothermia blanket (switched
to the "off" position).

2. Apply monitors:
   (a) Temperature probes in axilla and rectum.
   (b) Precordial stethoscope.
   (c) BP cuff with Doppler flowmeter (on arm).
   (d) ECG leads.
3. Monitor and record vital signs constantly.
4. Give 100% O_2 by mask for 3–5 min.
5. Give thiopentone, followed by droperidol, 0.1 mg/kg, and fentanyl, 1–2 μg/kg IV.
6. Hyperventilate the patient with 100% O_2.
7. Give additional fentanyl in increments of 1–2 μg/kg as required.
8. For intubation:
   (a) For long operations and if muscle relaxant will be required, give pancuronium, 0.1 mg/kg.
   (b) For short procedures, spray the vocal cords with 5% cocaine HCl and then intubate.
9. For all but short procedures:
   (a) Insert arterial line for direct BP recording and arterial blood gas determinations.
   (b) Insert central venous pressure line for pressure measurements and venous sampling.
   (c) Catheterize the patient and measure urine output.

Maintenance
1. Maintain anesthesia with 70% N_2O-30% O_2.
2. Hyperventilate the patient, maintaining the arterial $PaCO_2$ at 30 mmHg.
3. Give serial doses of fentanyl, 0.003 mg/kg/hr.
4. If pancuronium is used, determine timing and dose by the patient's response to peripheral nerve stimulation.
5. Monitor the vital signs and record at 5-minute intervals. Signs: temperature, BP, pulse rate, tidal volume, respiratory rate, continuous ECG tracing, skin color, end-tidal CO_2.
6. Take arterial blood samples (for measurement of blood gases, serum electrolytes, and serum enzymes) during surgery and at end of anesthesia.
7. Continue IV fluid therapy (lactated Ringer solution, at a rate appropriate to the surgery).

Signs of an MH response include sudden onset of:

Increased end-tidal CO_2
Tachycardia
Multifocal ventricular arrhythmias

Sweating
BP instability
Rapid 1–2°C rise in temperature
Slight cyanosis

Treatment must then be as outlined on page 134.

Postoperative (Following Uneventful Anesthesia)

1. Transfer the patient to the postanesthesia room (PAR), with monitoring equipment, IV cannulas, and catheter in place.
2. Ensure that *all* PAR staff are aware of the possibility of an MH reaction and know what to do if one occurs.
3. Vital signs are recorded at 5-minute intervals.
4. Do not transfer the patient to the ward until vital signs have been stable for 4 hours and results of laboratory tests are satisfactory.
5. When the patient is returned to the ward, vital signs are recorded hourly for 4 hours and then q4h for 1 day.
6. Dantrolene should be administered to any patient who exhibits any untoward signs, for example, persistent tachycardia or dysrhythmia, temperature rise, etc.
7. Day 1: 24-hour collection of urine for myoglobin determination.
8. Days 1–4: daily serum levels of SGOT, LDH, CK, 3-HBDH.

Suggested Additional Reading

*Britt BA (ed): Malignant hyperpyrexia. Int Anesthesiol Clin Vol. 17, 1979.

Gordon RA, BA Britt, and W Kalow (eds): Malignant Hyperthermia. Springfield, IL, Charles C Thomas, 1973.

Gronert GA: Malignant hyperthermia. Anesthesiology 53:395–423, 1980.

Gronert GA: Controversies in malignant hyperthermia. Anesthesiology 59:273–274, 1983.

Harrison GG: The prophylaxis of malignant hyperthermia by oral dantrolene sodium in swine. Br J Anaesth 49:315, 1977.

Lerman J, and JES Relton: Anesthesia for malignant hyperthermia susceptible patients. *In:* Malignant Hyperthermia, (BA Britt, ed). Boston, Martinus Nijhoff 1987, p. 369–392.

Relton JES, BA Britt, and DJ Steward: Malignant hyperpyrexia. Br J Anaesth 45:269, 1973.

Relton JES, DJ Steward, RE Creighton, and BA Britt: Malignant hyperpyrexia: a therapeutic and investigative regimen. Can Anaesth Soc J 19:200, 1972.

* Key article

CYSTIC FIBROSIS

Cystic fibrosis (CF) is a heritable disorder of unknown pathogenesis. It affects many body systems, including the lungs; respiratory failure develops by the second or third decade of life. Even if they appear fairly well, all of these patients have severe pulmonary ventilation-perfusion ($\dot{V}/\dot{Q}$) inequality.

Surgery for children with this condition is most commonly for nasal polypectomy (in many cases repeated), antral lavage, and bronchoscopy for removal of retained secretions and treatment of atelectasis. Some children with advanced disease may require heart and lung transplantation. Interestingly, the transplanted lungs do not appear to be affected by this otherwise generalized disease.

Special Anesthetic Problems

1. Copious, extremely viscous secretions in the respiratory tract.
2. Because of the $\dot{V}/\dot{Q}$ disturbances:
   (a) Hypoxia may develop rapidly during anesthesia.
   (b) Induction of anesthesia with inhalational agents is prolonged.
3. Reduced lung compliance. In severe late cases, very high airway pressure may be required to provide adequate ventilation and prevent hypoxemia; therefore, use a cuffed endotracheal tube or bronchoscope whenever possible.
4. Malnutrition and underweight for age is a result of malabsorption and chronic infection. Dosage of drugs should be carefully reduced accordingly.
5. Many children with advanced CF become severely emotionally upset (naturally). All of them require especially careful and considerate handling and much reassurance.

Anesthetic Management

Preoperative

1. Assess the patient's condition carefully.
2. Do not give narcotic premedication. Give diazepam, if indicated, to counter anxiety.
3. Ensure optimal hydration—fluids must not be withheld for long periods. The patient should be offered clear fluids until 4 hours preoperatively.
4. Order chest physiotherapy for immediately before anesthesia and postoperatively and ensure that it is applied.

Perioperative

Note. Whenever possible, use local or regional analgesia.

1. Establish an IV line for hydration and emergency drug administration.
   If general anesthesia is required:
2. Give 100% O_2 by mask for at least 5 minutes; then induce anesthesia IV with thiopental, atropine, and succinylcholine.
3. Intubate the patient: use a cuffed endotracheal tube for children over 10 years of age.
4. Suction the trachea and remove secretions as often as necessary.
5. Use humidified gases with sufficient O_2 added (100% may be necessary for patients with severe disease).
6. Do not give long-acting narcotic agents; use a technique that ensures early awakening of the patient postoperatively.
   Note. For bronchoscopy in the severely ill child with retained tenacious secretions, various techniques have been tried; none is perfect. We have used the following options:
   (a) Local analgesia: probably optimal for older children.
   (b) Inhalation anesthesia (halothane) with spontaneous ventilation.
   (c) Controlled ventilation with muscle relaxants.

Postoperative

1. Fluids are given IV until the patient is drinking well.
2. The patient is nursed in a humid atmosphere (e.g., croup tent).
3. Encourage the patient to cough (e.g., pharyngeal suctioning, chest physiotherapy).
4. Do not give more than the essential narcotic analgesics, as they suppress the cough reflex. Use regional analgesia for postoperative pain whenever possible. Do provide good pain relief.

Suggested Additional Reading

*Di Sant'Agnese PA, and RC Talamo: Pathogenesis and physiopathology of cystic fibrosis of the pancreas: fibrocystic disease of the pancreas (mucoviscidosis). N Engl J Med 277:1287, 1344, 1399, 1967.

Doershuk CF, AL Reyes, AG Regan, and LW Matthews: Anesthesia and surgery in cystic fibrosis. Anesth Analg 51:413, 1972.

Robinson DA, Branthwaite MA: Pleural surgery in patients with cystic fibrosis. Anaesthesia 39:655–659, 1984.

Salanitre E, D Klonymus, and H Rackow: Anesthetic experience in children with cystic fibrosis of the pancreas. Anesthesiology 25:801, 1964.

Shwachman H, and RM Smith: Case history: cystic fibrosis—problems of management. Anesth Analg 44:140, 1965.

---

* Key article

5

Neurosurgery and Neuroradiology

GENERAL PRINCIPLES

1. Perioperative management must be planned to minimize the possibility of increasing the intracranial pressure (ICP) and to ensure optimal operating conditions for the neurosurgeon.
2. Light general anesthesia is adequate for neurosurgical operations. Additional techniques may be required to prevent or treat increased ICP. All anesthetic drugs used should be short-acting, capable of being rapidly eliminated, or completely reversible. This ensures that the patient speedily emerges from anesthesia, and that accurate continuous neurosurgical assessment is possible.
3. Postoperative pain is not severe following intracranial surgery. Potent analgesics are unnecessary and may cause ventilatory depression; they therefore should not be used. Codeine, 1–1.5 mg/kg intramuscularly (IM) is adequate for most patients.

INTRACRANIAL PHYSIOLOGY AND PATHOPHYSIOLOGY

1. Autoregulation of the caliber of the cerebral vessels ensures maintenance of constant blood flow during alterations in blood pressure (BP). This operates throughout a wide range of systemic BPs (65–180 mmHg, and even as low as 45–50 mmHg in the supine infant).
2. Cerebral blood flow (CBF) varies directly with changes in arterial CO_2 tension while the latter is between 20 and 80 mmHg.
3. Vasodilation of normal reactive cerebral vessels reduces blood flow in low-resistance vessels (e.g., arteriovenous [AV] malformations and vascular tumors) and in areas that because of infection or trauma, for example, have lost autoregulation (intracerebral steal).
4. Vasoconstriction of normal reactive cerebral vessels has the opposite effect (inverse intracerebral steal).
5. The total volume of the intracranial contents cannot alter. However, any of its three constituents—blood, cerebrospinal fluid (CSF), and brain tissue—can increase or decrease if compensated by an equal opposite change in the volumes of the others (the revised Munro-Kellie hypothesis).
6. The effect of a space-occupying lesion on ICP depends on its volume and rate of expansion. Initially, the lesion displaces CSF and/or venous blood from the skull, and ICP increases slowly if at all. As expansion continues, compensation is no longer possible and small increases in volume result in progressively larger increases in ICP. With a rapidly

expanding lesion (e.g., intracranial bleeding), of course, pressure increases rapidly from the outset.

EFFECTS OF SPECIFIC ANESTHETIC DRUGS ON INTRACRANIAL PHYSIOLOGY

1. All inhalation agents may increase CBF and ICP. Halothane increases CBF more than isoflurane. N_2O may cause a small increase in CBF but has been used successfully for neurosurgery for many years.
2. Intravenous (IV) anesthetic agents, with the exception of ketamine, either have no effect on CBF or decrease it.
3. In preterm infants during controlled ventilation, halothane, isoflurane, ketamine, and fentanyl all cause a slight fall in anterior fontanelle pressure.
4. Muscle relaxants have no direct effect on CBF. (Vasodilation resulting from histamine release caused by d-tubocurarine is a rare possible exception.)
5. If an independent vasodilator effect is absent, drugs that depress neuronal function (e.g., barbiturates) decrease CBF.
6. Drugs that enhance neuronal function increase CBF.
7. Hypocarbia tends to modify or reverse the effects of agents that increase CBF (e.g., halothane or isoflurane).
8. Hypercarbia tends to modify or reverse the effects of agents that decrease CBF (e.g., barbiturates).
9. Sodium nitroprusside (SNP) inhibits cerebral autoregulation and thus may increase ICP.
10. Dexamethsaone (0.15 mg/kg IV to a maximum of 10 mg) decreases focal cerebral edema in response to surgical trauma of brain tissue.
11. Opiate-induced muscle rigidity may increase ICP by both increasing central venous pressure (CVP) and causing hypercarbia. If opiates are used, a nondepolarizing neuromuscular blocking drug should be added and ventilation should be controlled.

INTRAVENOUS THERAPY

A reliable IV line is essential for pediatric neurosurgical patients.

Normal replacement fluid (lactated Ringer solution) is given as necessary to replace fluid deficits and maintain intravascular volume. Dextrose-containing solutions should be avoided if any brain ischemia may occur owing to retraction, etc., since increased neurologic damage might result. If there is concern that hypoglycemia might result (e.g., in infants), blood glucose determinations should be performed.

Furosemide (Lasix, 0.6 mg/kg IV) is used to decrease cerebral volume in patients undergoing craniotomy. It should be given immediately after induction of anesthesia.

Mannitol 20% (1.5–2.5 g/kg) is also used to control ICP and should be given immediately after induction of anesthesia. When combined with furosemide, this produces a greater and more prolonged decrease in cerebral volume.

After a diuretic is used, the schedule of fluid therapy depends on the urine output. When urine volume = 10% of the estimated blood volume (EBV), further urine losses are replaced (volume for volume) with lactated Ringer solution.

BLOOD REPLACEMENT

As blood loss during neurosurgery cannot be measured accurately, it must be gauged clinically from observation of the amount of bleeding and measurement of the patient's cardiovascular indices. The systolic BP must be monitored carefully; fluid replacements should maintain it at 60 mmHg in infants and 70–80 mmHg in larger children. (**Note:** The latter may lose up to 20% of EBV without a fall in BP.) When surgery is complete but before the dura is closed, enough fluid is given to return the arterial pressure to the preloss level. During closure, a fluid volume equal to 10% of the EBV is given. The decision to transfuse blood may be based on determination of the hematocrit (Hct) or on clinical judgement of the losses that are occurring in relation to the allowable blood loss.

If major blood transfusion has been necessary, particularly in small infants, serum Ca^{2+} may fall. Hypotension unresponsive to further volume replacement should be treated with calcium gluconate (*see* page 93).

HYPOTENSIVE TECHNIQUES

A safe range of systolic BP in the supine position is 50–65 mmHg up to age 10 years and 70–75 mmHg in children over 10 years. If the patient is tilted head up, position the transducer at the level of the head.

VENTILATION

Controlled ventilation should be used except in the very rare instance when spontaneous ventilation is specifically indicated, for example, as a monitor of medullary integrity. Apnea in neurosurgical patients may indicate acutely raised ICP. If this occurs, hyperventilate the patient with N_2O and O_2, and advise the surgeon so a CSF tap can be performed immediately.

Controlled hyperventilation is used to decrease brain bulk and ICP during intracranial surgery and to improve the quality of cerebral arterio-grams during neuroradiology. A $PaCO_2$ of 30 mmHg is preferred during controlled ventilation.

PATIENT MONITORING

The patient should be monitored by:

1. Esophageal stethoscope and pulse oximeter.
2. BP cuff with a Doppler flowmeter.
3. Continuous recording of body temperature (usually rectal).
4. Electrocardiogram (ECG).
5. End-tidal CO_2 monitor—for infants under 8 kg. Sampling at the tip of the endotracheal tube is necessary for accurate results. The end-tidal CO_2 monitor is useful both as guide to the adequacy of ventilation and as a means to detect air embolism.
6. For major neurosurgery, an arterial line connected to a pressure trans-ducer. (If this is not available, blood gas studies on free-flowing venous samples from the dorsum of the hand are usually adequate for assessing ventilation).
7. Measurement of urinary output via catheter—during major neurosur-gery or if diuretics may be given.
8. A precordial Doppler detector should be used for operations in the sitting or head-up position, when air embolism is a danger. In such circumstances, a central catheter may be inserted to aspirate air should embolism occur.

NEUROSURGERY

ANESTHETIC MANAGEMENT

PREMEDICATION

Do not give any drug that can depress respiration, prolong recovery, or hamper postoperative assessment. Therefore, with one exception (*see below*), do not give sedative premedication to neurosurgical patients. At induction, give atropine sulfate (0.02 mg/kg IV) to minimize vagal effects on the heart.

Exception. Patients with vascular aneurysms or AV malformations, es-pecially if there is a history of hemorrhage, should have sedative pre-medication: droperidol, 0.1 mg/kg, and fentanyl, 1 μg/kg, may be given

IV by the anesthesiologist on the ward or intensive care unit (ICU). The patient is then closely observed and this dose repeated if necessary before bringing the patient to the operating room (OR).

Management during induction of anesthesia should be planned to minimize changes in ICP resulting from hypercapnia, the effects of anesthetic drugs, or instrumentation of the airway.

Intravenous induction with thiopental, 5–6 mg/kg, followed by succinylcholine chloride to facilitate rapid intubation and ensure optimal ventilation is preferred. Lidocaine, 1–1.5 mg/kg IV, may be given prior to intubation to minimize changes in ICP associated with this procedure. (If this is done, the lidocaine should be given 3 minutes before intubation, that is, it should precede the thiopental).

Patients with vascular anomalies should be induced with thiopental, and anesthesia should be deepened with inhalation agents. *d*-Tubocurarine or vecuronium and lidocaine, 1.5 mg/kg IV, are given prior to intubation. the BP is carefully monitored during induction to watch for hypertension.

For surgery in the prone position, for small infants, and for any procedures that entail changes in position, use a nasotracheal tube (an orotracheal tube may kink in the prone patient or become dislodged if saliva loosens the adhesive tape, and a nasotracheal tube is more easily accurately fixed in the infant). For surgery on older children in the supine or lateral position, use an armored orotracheal tube. Throat packing placed in the mouth will limit the flow of saliva from the mouth.

MAINTENANCE

Volatile agents or short-acting narcotics (e.g., fentanyl) that ensure rapid postoperative recovery are preferred. All volatile anesthetic agents increase CBF; therefore they should be used in the lowest concentration compatible with adequate anesthesia.

Drugs to Induce Hypotension

1. *Isoflurane*. The inspired concentration can be increased progressively until the desired pressure is obtained. This method is easy to apply and results in very stable BP levels.
2. *SNP*. Has been widely used to induce hypotension but may result in tachyphylaxis, often results in wide swings in pressure, and in large doses may cause toxic effects. SNP interferes with cerebral autoregulation and may increase ICP. Its infusion should not be commenced until the skull is opened.

POSTOPERATIVE CONSIDERATIONS

All patients should be fully recovered from the effects of anesthetic drugs and be awake at completion of the procedure. Extubation should be smooth without coughing or bucking. This can be facilitated by giving lidocaine, 1.5 mg/kg IV. If the patient remains unresponsive or if any ventilatory depression is present, the endotracheal tube should be left in and controlled ventilation continued until the cause is determined.

Postoperative nursing care should include routine neurologic signs. The fluid status should be carefully followed as regulatory mechanisms (e.g., antidiuretic hormone) may be altered following craniotomy.

HYDROCEPHALUS

Hydrocephalus may be due to a congenital defect (e.g., Arnold-Chiari malformation, aqueduct stenosis) or acquired disease (e.g., tumor). In the newborn, hydrocephalus is most commonly secondary to the Arnold-Chiari malformation. (In many cases, it is accompanied by meningomyelocele; this combined defect is present in 1–3 of 1,000 live births).

SURGICAL PROCEDURES: CREATION OF CSF SHUNTS

For noncommunicating hydrocephalus (*see also* page 10):

1. Ventriculoperitoneal shunt (lateral ventricle to peritoneum)—most common and preferred as it allows most room for growth.
2. Ventriculoatrial shunt (lateral ventricle to right atrium)—still used occasionally, but may lead to long-term complications, especially pulmonary thromboembolism and cor pulmonale.
3. Ventriculopleural shunt (lateral ventricle to pleural cavity)—rare.
4. Fourth ventriculostomy.

For communicating hydrocephalus (*see also* page 10):

1. Lumboperitoneal shunt (lumbar subarachnoid space to peritoneum).

Special Anesthetic Problems

1. Increased ICP, sometimes severe.
2. Many patients have had repeated anesthetics for shunt revisions.
3. Patient should be fully awake at end of procedure to permit assessment.

Anesthetic Management

Preoperative

1. Exercise special care if the ICP is increased. The patient should be watched carefully until surgery can be arranged, as the condition may deteriorate suddenly, necessitating immediate ventricular tap or lumbar puncture (depending on whether the hydrocephalus is noncommunicating or communicating).
2. If the patient becomes apneic: intubate, ventilate, and arrange for an immediate ventricular tap.
3. Premedication: give atropine only, preferably IV at induction.

Perioperative

1. Exercise special care during induction of anesthesia to prevent hypoventilation, hypoxia, or systemic hypertension.
   (a) An IV induction with thiopental and succinylcholine is preferred, so that the airway can be secured rapidly and adequate ventilation ensured.
   (b) Lidocaine, 1.5 mg/kg IV, may be given to attenuate the hypertensive response to laryngoscopy and intubation.
2. During surgery, maintain anesthesia with N_2O and low concentrations of isoflurane or halothane. Addition of a nondepolarizing relaxant drug permits the use of minimal volatile agent with rapid recovery upon reversal. Controlled ventilation is preferred for all patients.
3. Pay special attention to the following situations:
   (a) Hypotension at the time of CSF tap. If the arterial BP was elevated secondary to increased ICP, and if excessive inhalation agents have been given, the BP may fall precipitously as the ICP returns to normal (at the time of CSF tap). Withdraw all anesthetic agents and ventilate with 100% O_2 until the arterial BP regains a normal level.
   (b) Bradycardia and other arrhythmias may occur following placement of the IV catheter, probably due to shifts in intracranial contents.
   (c) Ventriculoatrial (VA) shunts. Apply controlled positive-pressure ventilation to prevent air embolism while the vein is open for insertion of the cardiac end of the VA shunt. The ECG may be used as a guide for positioning the atrial end of the shunt. The shunt tubing is filled with hypertonic saline and attached by an extension wire to the left arm ECG lead. Switch the ECG to lead III. The tubing is advanced, and as the tip approaches the right atrium, the P waves grow higher; when it reaches its correct position in the atrium, they become small and biphasic (Fig. 5-1).

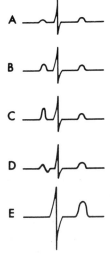

Fig. 5-1. Drawing of ECG tracings obtained as a VA shunt catheter is advanced toward the heart. A, when the catheter tip is in the SVC. P waves become larger as the tip approaches the right atrium (B,C), then smaller and biphasic as the atrium is entered (D). If the catheter is advanced too far, into the ventricle, the QRS complexes become very large (E).

4. Blood loss is usually minimal, requiring no replacement, but a reliable IV line should be placed.
5. Discontinue potent anesthetic agents before the end of surgery, so that the patient is wide awake and responding before leaving the OR.

Postoperative
1. Order routine postcraniotomy nursing care.
2. Do not give narcotic analgesics, except codeine.

CHRONIC EXTRADURAL AND SUBDURAL HEMATOMAS

Chronic extradural and subdural hematomas commonly result from birth trauma and require surgery during the first 6 months of life. Symptoms include irritability and convulsions.

Surgical Procedures
1. Burr holes.
2. Craniotomy—if membranes are present.

Special Anesthetic Problem
1. Major blood loss may occur during surgery (rare).

Anesthetic Management
See also page 147.

Preoperative
1. Check that blood is available for transfusion.
2. Premedication: give atropine only, preferably IV at induction.

Perioperative
1. An IV induction with thiopental and succinylcholine is preferred.
2. An armored orotracheal tube is essential (because of the flexed position of the head for surgery).
3. Maintain anesthesia with N_2O and isoflurane; control ventilation but avoid excessive hyperventilation. (This allows the brain to expand and fill the space occupied by the evacuated hematoma.)
4. Establish a reliable IV line and have blood ready in the OR.
5. Discontinue potent anesthetic agents before the end of surgery so that the patient is awake and responding before leaving the OR.

Postoperative
1. Order routine postcraniotomy nursing care.
2. Do not give narcotic analgesics.

CRANIOSYNOSTOSIS

Premature fusion of one suture between bones of the vault of the skull leads to deformity. Fusion of more than one suture may lead to raised ICP and later to mental retardation and possibly optic atrophy. Early surgical repair gives improved cosmetic results with less blood loss than repair at an older age.

Associated Conditions
1. Craniofacial abnormalities: for example, Crouzon's disease and Apert's syndrome.

Surgical Procedure
1. Craniectomy: division of skull along suture lines.

Special Anesthetic Problems
1. Sudden massive blood loss from damaged cerebral venous sinuses.
2. Difficult airway: in patients with craniofacial syndromes.
3. Air embolism is a potential danger.

Anesthetic Management
Preoperative
1. Check that blood is available in the OR for transfusion.
2. Premedication: give atropine only, preferably IV at induction.

Perioperative
1. An IV induction with thiopental and succinylcholine is preferred. A nasotracheal tube is preferred; otherwise, use an armored oral tube. (Choanal atresia is occasionally associated with craniosynostosis.)
2. Maintain anesthesia with N_2O-O_2 and 0.5% halothane, or N_2O-O_2 and d-tubocurarine; control ventilation.
3. Establish a reliable wide-bore IV line and have blood ready in the OR.
4. Discontinue potent anesthetic agents before the end of surgery so that the patient is wide awake and responding before leaving the OR.

Postoperative
1. Order routine postcraniotomy nursing care.
2. Do not give narcotic analgesics.

MENINGOMYELOCELE AND ENCEPHALOCELE

Meningomyelocele and encephalocele result from failure of the neural tube to fuse in the fetus. The incidence of meningomyelocele is approximately 1–4 in 1,000 live births, with a large geographic variation. Encephalocele is much less common.

Associated Conditions
Hydrocephalus, in many cases with Arnold-Chiari malformation and aqueduct stenosis, occurs in 80% of infants with meningomyelocele or encephalocele.

Surgical Procedures
Excision of the sac and repair of the defect is usually performed as soon as possible after birth to prevent infection.

Special Anesthetic Problems

1. Potential difficulty in positioning the patient for intubation.
2. Blood losses (a) are difficult to measure and (b) may be considerable.
3. Difficulty controlling heat loss during surgery.

Anesthetic Management

Preoperative

1. The lesion is kept covered with sterile dressing.
2. Ensure that cross-matched blood (250 ml) is in the OR.
3. Ensure that the OR has been warmed to at least 24°C.
4. Give atropine, 0.1 mg IV or IM.

Perioperative

1. Use warming blankets, radiant heat lamps, heated humidifier, and woolen cap on head.
2. Induce anesthesia and intubate. We prefer IV thiopental and relaxant. Laryngoscopy and intubation is easier if the patient is place left side down, with an assistant applying forward pressure at the back of the head and backward pressure on the shoulders to prevent neck extension. If intubation cannot be performed in this position, place the infant supine supported on a ring cushion to protect the defect.
3. Continue anesthesia with N_2O and isoflurane, with controlled ventilation.
4. For surgery, the patient is positioned prone on bolsters.
5. Do not give neuromuscular blocking agents until you have asked whether the surgeon wishes to use a nerve stimulator to confirm the location of nerve roots.
6. Blood loss cannot be measured accurately. Estimate the amount of bleeding and monitor the arterial systolic pressure carefully as a guide to replacement.

Postoperative

1. Return the patient to a warm incubator, to be nursed prone on a frame.
2. Instruct the nursing staff to observe closely for signs of raised ICP, especially in cases of encephalocele.
3. Do not give narcotic analgesics.
4. Check hemoglobin (Hb) and Hct on arrival in the postanesthesia room (PAR).

SPINAL CORD TUMORS AND TETHERED CORD

Spinal cord tumors are less common in children than adults but may occur at any site in the spinal cord.

Tethered cord causes bladder and bowel symptoms and weakness of one or both lower limbs. This syndrome is confirmed by myelograph and computed tomography (CT) scan, with demonstrate a low conus, a thickened filum, and a transverse orientation of nerve roots. Surgical division of the filum terminale is the treatment.

Special Anesthetic Considerations

1. Muscle relaxants should not be used, as nerve stimulation may be required intraoperatively to identify peripheral nerves. Anorectal manometry or somatosensory evoked potentials from the pudendal nerve have also been used to monitor neurologic function intraoperatively.
2. The patient must be carefully positioned on a frame or bolsters to avoid pressure on the abdomen. Such pressure diverts blood from the abdominal veins to the vertebral venous plexus and increases bleeding at the surgical site.

SELECTIVE POSTERIOR RHIZOTOMY FOR SPASTICITY

Some patients with spasticity secondary to cerebral palsy may benefit from rhizotomy of some of the fasicles of the posterior roots of L2 to S1 bilaterally. Intraoperative electromyography is used to determine which fasicles demonstrate a normal response to stimulation (brief local contraction) and which give an abnormal response (a sustained or diffuse contracture). The latter are then divided. Many children benefit significantly with a generalized reduction of spasticity and improved limb and even speech function. Sensation is not significantly affected.

Management of anesthesia should be as for tethered cord (*see above*). Nondepolarizing muscle relaxants should not be administered since neuromuscular block will compromise the interpretation of the electromyography (EMG) findings. Succinylcholine may be given for intubation if required and is safe to use in the patient with cerebral palsy.

CRANIOTOMY FOR TUMORS AND VASCULAR LESIONS

Intracerebral tumors are relatively common during childhood, with a peak incidence in the range of 5–8 years; about 60% are in the posterior fossa. Epileptogenic foci (*see* page 158) and benign vascular lesions also may be indications for craniotomy.

Surgical Procedures

1. Exploratory biopsy and/or excision of lesion.

Special Anesthetic Problems

1. Elevated ICP.
2. Anesthetic techniques must be designed to provide optimal intracranial conditions for surgery.
3. Blood losses (a) are difficult to measure and (b) may be massive.
4. Small infants with AV malformations may have associated high-output congestive heart failure. These patients have a low diastolic BP and do not tolerate further reduction in BP intraoperatively (cardiac arrest may occur).
5. Postoperatively, the patient must be free of residual effects of anesthesia to permit accurate neurologic assessment and monitoring.
6. In a few cases, it may be necessary to perform intraoperative neurophysiologic studies. During surgery for epilepsy it may be required to record the electroencephalogram (EEG) directly from the brain tissue; in such cases, it is preferable to avoid giving large doses of drugs known to suppress seizures (e.g., thiopental, diazepam). In others, it may be necessary to record cortical somatosensory evoked potentials intraoperatively. The use of 0.5% isoflurane in nitrous oxide has been demonstrated to be satisfactory during such monitoring. Higher concentrations of volatile agents may interfere with the recording.
7. In very few cases, the patient is required to be awake and cooperate during surgery (e.g., this may be necessary to map the speech area).

Anesthetic Management

See also page 147.

Preoperative

1. Assess the patient carefully. Older children: establish rapport with them and reassure them concerning the planned procedures.
2. Check that blood is available for transfusion (at least 1,000 ml for craniotomy and more for removal of vascular malformations).
3. Do not give narcotic sedative premedication except for patients with vascular lesions (*see* page 147).

Perioperative

1. Induce anesthesia IV and give a full dose of a relaxant to secure the airway rapidly and prevent hypoventilation, hypoxia, or coughing and straining.
2. Inject lidocaine, 1.5 mg/kg IV, and intubate with the largest endotracheal tube that passes the larynx easily.
3. Light general anesthesia is adequate for neurosurgery, for example, N_2O and isoflurane, 0.5–0.75%, plus a relaxant drug. A small dose of

a potent narcotic (e.g., fentanyl, 2 µg/kg) may be given at the start of the surgery. Little analgesia is required once the skull is open. Controlled ventilation with d-tubocurarine has been widely used, but atracurium or vecuronium given by infusion while monitoring neuromuscular blockade and are very satisfactory and can be readily reversed. Monitor the neuromuscular block with a nerve stimulator or EMG.

4. Give a diuretic as the skull is being opened (*see* page 145).
5. Give dexamethasone, 0.15 mg/kg IV (maximum dose 10 mg), to minimize focal cerebral edema.
6. Discontinue volatile anesthetic agents before the end of surgery so that the patient is wide awake and responding before leaving the OR.

Anterior and Middle Fossa Surgery
1. Use an armored orotracheal tube.
2. Position patient with a 15° head-up tilt.
3. Maintain anesthesia with N_2O-O_2 and isoflurane (0.5–0.75%) and a muscle relaxant.
4. Control ventilation to provide a $PaCO_2$ of 30–35 mmHg; confirm by end-tidal CO_2 and blood gas analysis.
5. Set up monitors: esophageal stethoscope, BP, ECG, pulse oximeter, body temperature, and urine output.
   (a) Use a nerve stimulator or EMG as a guide to administration of relaxant drugs.
   (b) If massive blood loss is likely (e.g., with vascular malformations), insert CVP line and an arterial pressure line.
6. Watch for arrhythmias and/or changes in BP, especially during dissections in the region of the pituitary gland and hypothalamus. If these occur, alert the surgeon to discontinue surgery until the situation resolves. Atropine IV may be required for bradycardia.

Posterior Fossa Surgery (Prone Position)
1. Use a nasotracheal tube.
2. The patient should lie prone on a frame, with a 15° head-up tilt and with thorax and abdomen hanging free.
3. Anesthetize as for anterior or middle fossa surgery (*see above*).

Postoperative
1. The patient must have recovered fully from the effects of anesthesia before leaving the OR.
2. Order routine postcraniotomy nursing care.
3. Do not give narcotic analgesics.
4. Body temperature may rise, and measures to restore normothermia may be required.

ANEURYSM OF THE VEIN OF GALEN

1. Infants may be in severe congestive cardiac failure preoperatively. This can sometimes be improved by embolizing some of the aberrant vessels.
2. The mortality rate is high, usually owing to uncontrollable bleeding or intraoperative cardiac arrest. The use of profound hypothermia with circulatory arrest has been attempted, but the results were poor. Careful intraoperative management of the cardiovascular parameters may improve the outlook.
3. It is important that hypovolemia or hypotension be avoided before the vessels are clipped. The AV shunt through the lesion places a great stress on the heart; failure is common and myocardial perfusion is threatened by the low diastolic pressure. If the diastolic pressure falls, myocardial perfusion will be inadequate and cardiac arrest will occur. Hypotensive techniques are contraindicated. Aggressive cardiovascular monitoring is recommended to acurately observe the intraoperative status and replace fluids as needed.
4. Nitrous oxide should be avoided as it may depress the myocardium and elevate pulmonary vascular resistence. High-dose fentanyl anesthesia is recommended.
5. When the aneurysm is clipped, left ventricular afterload will suddenly rise and decompensation may occur. Vasodilators and inotropic agents should be prepared to compensate for this if necessary.

ELECTROCORTICOGRAPHY AND OPERATIONS FOR EPILEPSY

Many older children (over 8 years) cooperate adequately during neuroleptanalgesia for electrocorticography and operations for epilepsy (e.g., temproal lobectomy).

Special Anesthetic Problems

1. Drugs that modify the EEG significantly must not be given (e.g., barbiturates).
2. The patient must be awake and cooperative (including being able to speak).
3. Anesthetic techniques must be designed to provide optimal intracranial conditions for surgery.
4. Blood losses (a) are difficult to measure and (b) may be considerable.
5. Postoperatively, the patient must be free of residual effects of anesthesia to permit accurate neurologic assessment and monitoring.

Anesthetic Management
Preoperative
1. At the preoperative visit, assess the child and judge the likelihood of cooperation.
2. Explain to the patient the anesthetic technique proposed and the reasons for it. Encourage enthusiastic cooperation in the procedure (i.e., tell the patient that he will be in a dreamy state and will feel no pain but he himself must help make the operation a success).
3. Do not give premedication.
4. Omit anticonvulsant drugs the morning of surgery.
5. Check that blood is available for transfusion.

Perioperative
1. Ensure that equipment is at hand for emergency intubation and ventilation.
2. Start a large-bore IV infusion (use a local analgesic).
3. Give atropine IV followed by Innovar, 0.04 ml/kg.
4. Allow surgeons to:
   (a) Shave the head.
   (b) Insert a urinary catheter (ensure that lidocaine jelly is used).
5. Perform a scalp block on the side of surgery with 1% lidocaine with 0.25% bupivacaine.
6. Monitor the BP and arterial blood gases via an indwelling cannula.
7. During craniotomy give increments of fentanyl (2 μg/kg) to provide additional analgesia and give O_2 via a nasal catheter.
8. Talk with the patient and encourage regular deep breathing (to avoid hypoventilation).
9. While the skull is being opened, give mannitol, 1–2 g/kg, or furosemide, 0.6 mg/kg, and dexamethasone, 0.2 mg/kg (see page 145).
10. If excessive respiratory depression occurs, reverse this with levallorphan, 0.05 mg/kg.
11. When electrocorticography and excision of the lesion are complete, give an additional dose of Innovar (0.02 ml/kg).

Postoperative
1. If the patient remains excessively drowsy, give a small dose of naloxone (0.005 mg/kg).
2. Order routine postcraniotomy nursing care.

Suggested Additional Reading
Alfery DD, HM Shapiro, and RL Gagnon: Cardiac arrest following rapid drainage of CSF fluid in a patient with hydrocephalus. Anesthesiology 52:443, 1980.

Creighton RE, JES Relton, and HW Meridy: Anaesthesia for occipital encephalocoele. Can Anaesth Soc J 21:403, 1974.

Fitch W, GG Ferguson, D Sengupta, and J Garibi: Autoregulation of cerebral blood flow during controlled hypotension [abstract]. Stroke 4:324, 1973.

Fitch W, J Barker, WB Jennett, and DG McDowall: The influence of neuroleptanalgesic drugs on cerebrospinal fluid pressure. Br J Anaesth 41:800, 1969.

Frost EAQ: Anesthesia for elective intracranial procedures. Anesth Rev 7:13, 1980.

Harris MM, TA Yemen, A Davidson, et al: Venous air embolism during craniectomy in supine infants. Anesthesiology 67:816–819, 1987.

Lam AM, and AW Gelb: Cardiovascular effects of isoflurane-induced hypotension for cerebral aneurysm surgery. Anesth Analg 62:742, 1983.

*Lassen NA, and MS Christensen: Physiology of cerebral blood flow. Br J Anaesth 48:719, 1976.

McComish PB, and PO Bodley: Anaesthesia for Neurological Surgery. London, Lloyd-Luke, 1971.

McLeod EM, RE Creighton, and RP Humphreys: Anesthesia for cerebral arteriovenous malformations in children. Can Anaesth Soc J 29:299, 1982.

McLeod EM, RE Creighton, and RP Humphreys: Anaesthetic management of arteriovenous malformations of the vein of Galen. Can Anaesth Soc J 29:307, 1982.

Meridy HW, RE Creighton, and RP Humphreys: Complications during neurosurgery in the prone position in children. Can Anaesth Soc J 21:445, 1974.

Peacock WJ, LJ Arens, and B Berman: Cerebral palsy spasticity. Selective posterior rhizotomy. Pediatr Neurosci 13:61–66, 1987.

Rasch DK, DE Webster, J Hutyra, et al: Anesthetic management of hemodynamic changes during vein of Galen clipping. Anesthesiology 69:993–995, 1988.

Robertson JT, RW Schick, F Morgan, and DD Matson: Accurate placement of ventriculo-atrial shunt for hydrocephalus under electrocardiographic control. J Neurosurg 18:255, 1961.

Rockoff MA: Anesthesia for children with hydrocephalus. Anesthesiol Rev 6:28–34, 1979.

Shapiro HM: Intracranial hypertension: therapeutic and anesthetic considerations. Anesthesiology 43:445, 1975.

Turner JM, and DG McDowall: The measurement of intracranial pressure. Br J Anaesth 48:735, 1976.

Wood CC, DD Spencer, T Allison, et al: Localisation of human sensorimotor cortex during surgery by cortical surface recording of somatosensory evoked potentials. J Neurosurg 68:99–111, 1988.

---

* Key article

NEURORADIOLOGY

COMPUTED TOMOGRAPHY

1. CT requires absolute immobility of the patient throughout. For this reason, it is often necessary to sedate infants (except the very small), young children, and mentally retarded patients. Very rarely, a general anesthetic may be required. Older children of normal intelligence can cooperate and do not require any form of sedation or anesthetic, and small infants can be bundled and restrained during the procedure.
2. If general anesthesia is required, use only plastic materials in the breathing circuit, as metal interferes with x-ray imaging.
3. Intravenous pentobarbital is useful for sedation. An IV infusion is started, and 3 mg/kg of pentobarbital is given. After 3 minutes, further doses of 1 mg/kg may be titrated to a maximum of 7 mg/kg. The patient should be monitored with a pulse oximeter, and all equipment to establish an airway and ventilate should be on hand.

OTHER NEURORADIOLOGIC PROCEDURES

General anesthesia is often necessary for pediatric patients, as the procedure may be long and uncomfortable and the patient must be immobile.

Special Anesthetic Problems

1. ICP may be increased.
2. The radiologic examination may require special positioning and tilting of the patient.
3. It may be difficult to maintain body temperature of infants.
4. Reactions to contrast media may occur.
5. Patients must recover rapidly so that their neurologic status can be checked.

Anesthetic Management
Preoperative

1. Assess the patient's neurologic status carefully.
2. Check for a history of allergy, asthma, or previous reactions to x-ray contrast media.
3. Do not give sedatives or narcotics.
4. If metrizamide or iopamidol contrast medium is to be used in the sub-

arachnoid space, ensure that phenothiazine drugs have not been given during the past 48 hours.

Perioperative

1. An IV induction is preferred. Give thiopental (3–5 mg/kg) with atropine followed by succinylcholine.
2. For patients with increased ICP, give lidocaine, 1.5 mg/kg IV, to attenuate the hypertensive response to laryngoscopy and intubation.
3. Insert an endotracheal tube. A nasal or armored tube should be used if the positioning or movement of the patient might result in kinking of an oral tube (e.g., for air studies, myelograms).

Arteriography

1. If a tumor or AV malformation is suspected, maintain anesthesia with N_2O and a relaxant, or 0.5% halothane, with ventilation controlled to produce a PCO_2 of 30 mmHg (confirm by sampling from the arterial catheter). This degree of hypocapnia improves radiographic definition, by constricting normal vessels.
Note. If an AV malformation is suspected, preoperative management and induction of anesthesia should be as outlined on page 155.
2. Chart the total volume of contrast medium and flush fluid carefully, especially in small infants. Beware of fluid overload, especially in small infants with AV malformations.
3. A transient bradycardia with hypotension may occur at the time of injection into the carotid artery owing to baroreceptor activity; atropine prevents this.

Myelography

1. Maintain anesthesia with N_2O and halothane, allowing spontaneous ventilation unless need for assistance is indicated (e.g., for patients with severe kyphoscoliosis).
2. Monitor BP carefully during tilting; if hypotension occurs, level the table.

Postoperative

1. The patient must be awake before being moved to the PAR.
2. Do not give narcotic drugs.
3. Check arterial puncture sites frequently, and if a limb artery was used, check the circulation to that extremity.
4. Do not given phenothiazines for postoperative nausea following myelogram; these drugs may precipitate seizures.

ADDITIONAL POSSIBLE COMPLICATIONS

In addition to the complications that may develop during administration of any anesthetic, some special problems may occur during neuroradiologic procedures:

1. Accidental extubation owing to change in position of patient.
2. Hypothermia owing to difficulty maintaining blankets and heating lamps in place during frequent changes in the patient's position.
3. Acute rise in ICP, leading to coning of the brain stem. In this event:
   (a) Hyperventilate the patient.
   (b) Request that ventricular tap be performed as soon as possible.
   (c) Give an osmotic diuretic (mannitol, 2 g/kg, or furosemide, 0.6 mg/kg) and full doses of atropine to counter bradycardia.
4. Allergic reaction to contrast media. Recently, nonionic contrast media containing iodine have been introduced (e.g., Isovue, iopamidol). Such agents have a much lesser tendency to trigger adverse reactions. However, such a possibility must always be anticipated, especially in the patient with a history of allergy or asthma.

REACTIONS TO CONTRAST MEDIA

1. Reactions to intra-arterial contrast media are very rare in pediatric patients. However, the anesthesiologist must be prepared for this possibility.
2. Reactions are more common in patients with a history of asthma or other allergic phenomena.
3. Minor allergic reactions (e.g., skin rashes) may be treated with diphenhydramine, 1 mg/kg IM.
4. Major anaphylactic shock (very rare) must be treated aggressively with cardiopulmonary resuscitation as required plus appropriate drug therapy (steroids, epinephrine, etc.) (*see* page 411).
5. Contrast media may cause sickling in patients with sickle cell disease.

METRIZAMIDE-RELATED COMPLICATIONS

Metrizamide is still used for myelography in some institutions.

1. Nausea and vomiting are very common.
2. Convulsions (rare) may occur up to 8 hours after subarachnoid injection of metrizamide.
3. Phenothiazine drugs and related compounds (including droperidol) may reduce the threshold for seizures.

Suggested Additional Reading

Fitch W, and DG McDowall: Anaesthesia for neuroradiological investigations. Proc R Soc Med 64:75, 1971.

Pyles ST, and AG Pashayan: Anesthesia and neuroradiology: considerations regarding metrizamide. Anesthesiology 58:590, 1983.

Strain JD: I.V. administered pentobarbital sodium for sedation in pediatric CT. Radiology 161:105–108, 1986.

6

Ophthalmology

GENERAL PRINCIPLES

1. Children cannot usually be expected to cooperate during eye surgery. Therefore, general anesthesia is required.
2. Intraocular surgery and surgery of the nasolacrimal duct and eyelids require a bloodless field. Although induced hypotension is seldom indicated for these operations, all measures should be taken to ensure that the anesthetic does not increase bleeding. Smooth general anesthesia—with optimal airway, good positioning of the patient, and quiet emergence without coughing or straining—is important.
3. The oculocardiac reflex is powerful in children but can be readily blocked by giving atropine intravenously (IV) in usual dosage (0.02 mg/kg) at the time of induction. Do not rely on atropine given intramuscularly (IM) or on local anesthetic (retrobulbar) blocks to avoid this reflex. *Monitor the heart rate carefully during manipulation of the eyes.* In the very rare event that atropine is contraindicated, remember that the oculocardia reflex is more likely to be triggered by a sudden pull than by a gradually applied progressive traction. Remember also that the reflex usually fatigues rapidly, that is, a second pull does not elicit the same powerful effect.
4. Some children may be under treatment with long-acting plasma cholinesterase inhibitors (e.g., Phospholine). These are given as eyedrops to children with glaucoma and some patients with strabismus (esotropia). Significant systemic absorption occurs and may result in toxic symptoms (nausea, vomiting, abdominal pain) and prolonged apnea following succinylcholine administration. Timolol maleate topical (a β-blocking agent) is also used as an antiglaucoma agent in children. It is absorbed from the conjunctiva and may cause bradycardia refractory to atropine and bronchospasm. Children with asthma are made worse by this drug.
5. Drugs applied to the conjunctivae during surgery may cause systemic effects. Epinephrine and phenylephrine may cause hypertension and arrhythmias, effects that are potentially dangerous especially during halothane anesthesia. Phenylephrine drops cause fewer problems, especially if the concentration is limited to 2.5%; but if instilled on a hyperemic conjunctiva, they may cause hypertension. Monitor the heart rate and blood pressure carefully with drug instillation and be prepared to discontinue the halothane.
6. The effects of anesthetic drugs and techniques on the intraocular pressure (IOP) must be remembered:
   (a) Atropine causes only a very slight increase in IOP when given IM, IV, or orally (PO). Its use as a premedicant is not contraindicated in patients with glaucoma.

(b) All potent inhalation anesthetic agents cause a dose-related fall in IOP.

(c) Barbiturates and narcotic analgesics lower the IOP by facilitating aqueous outflow.

(d) Nondepolarizing muscle relaxants lower the IOP.

(e) Succinylcholine IV causes an increase in IOP that is not reliably prevented by pretreatment with d-tubocurarine or gallamine triethiodide. The increased IOP occurs within 30 seconds, and the pressure usually returns to normal within 6 minutes. Succinylcholine is usually omitted in patients undergoing intraocular surgery. The rise in IOP may be less in patients with already increased IOP (glaucoma), but it seems prudent to omit succinylcholine in such patients, especially if measurement of IOP is a part of the operation. The use of succinylcholine for patients with penetrating eye trauma has been controversial. Originally thought contraindicated, it has been shown to be safe in at least one large series. It has recently been shown that, when given with thiopental in a rapid sequence induction, succinylcholine causes no increase in IOP. Hence, it is now recommended that, when there is real concern about the danger of a full stomach, succinylcholine should be used.

(f) Ketamine has little effect on IOP.

(g) Endotracheal intubation, coughing, and straining all increase IOP. This effect may be modified by the prior administration of 1 mg/kg lidocaine IV.

(h) Hypercapnia increases IOP, and hypocapnia decreases it.

(i) Diuretic drugs decrease IOP and may reduce the increase in IOP following succinylcholine administration.

7. Succinylcholine causes contracture of the extraocular muscles and interferes with forced duction testing if performed within 15 minutes.

8. Anesthesia for ophthalmology must be deep enough to ensure that the eyes are immobile and fixed centrally. Smooth extubation without coughing can be effected by administration of lidocaine, 1–2 mg IV, before removing the tube.

9. Postoperative pain may be troublesome after eye operations, requiring full doses of analgesics. Unfortunately, nausea and vomiting are also common postoperatively but may be reduced by the intraoperative administration of a small dose of droperidol (75 μg/kg IV) before manipulation of the eyes or by the use of metoclopramide, 0.15 mg/kg IV immediately postoperatively. Metoclopramide does not cause sedation and is appropriate if adjustable sutures are being used.

CORRECTION OF STRABISMUS

Correction of strabismus is the commonest eye operation in children.

Associated Conditions

Malignant hyperpyrexia is very rare, but strabismus may be an associated clinical condition. Be constantly aware of this possibility (*see* page 133).

Special Anesthetic Problems

1. Oculocardiac reflex: severe bradycardia and even cardiac arrest can occur as a result of traction on the extraocular muscles (*see above*).
2. Oculogastric reflex: vomiting after eye muscle surgery is very common and should be prevented as outlined above.
3. Postoperative pain may be considerable.
4. If adjustable sutures are used the surgeon requires that the patient can be assessed postoperatively; excessive sedation should not be ordered. If a second anesthetic may be required to adjust the suture, an IV line or a heparin lock should be left in situ to facilitate the second induction. Do not use droperidol in such patients as they will then be too drowsy to cooperate, metoclopramide is preferred (*see below*).

Anesthetic Management

Preoperative

1. *Do not give heavy sedation.*
   (a) The surgeon may wish to examine the patient immediately before the operation.
   (b) Narcotics can increase the tendency to vomit postoperatively.
2. Give atropine, preferably IV, at induction.

Perioperative

1. Induction preferably IV, with thiopental-atropine-succinylcholine.
2. If induction was by inhalation, give atropine IV before the start of surgery.
3. Before orotracheal intubation, spray the larynx with lidocaine.
4. Maintain anesthesia with N_2O-O_2-halothane; allow spontaneous ventilation.
5. From the start of surgery, listen to the patient's heart sounds continuously via a precordial stethoscope and monitor the electrocardiogram. If bradycardia occurs, ask the surgeon to discontinue manipulation until you have given a further dose of atropine IV.

6. Give droperidol, 75 µg/kg IV, after induction of anesthesia to reduce postoperative vomiting, or give metoclopramide, 0.15 mg/kg, immediately postoperatively. Aspirate the stomach before extubation.

Postoperative
1. Extubate before the patient coughs or strains on the tube to prevent subconjuctival hemorrhage. Therefore, extubate the patient deeply anesthetized or give lidocaine, 1.5 mg/kg, to prevent laryngospasm.
2. Order analgesics for pain (e.g., codeine IM or acetaminophen PO or PR).
3. If nausea and/or vomiting occur, order an antiemetic (e.g., dimenhydrinate).

INTRAOCULAR SURGERY AND EUA FOR GLAUCOMA OR TUMOR

Children may require general anesthesia for cataract surgery, treatment of detached retina, or examination under anesthesia (EUA) for glaucoma or tumor.

Special Anesthetic Problems
1. The oculocardiac reflex: *see above*.
2. Intraocular pressure may be affected by anesthetic drugs and techniques (*see above*).
3. *Coughing and straining may elevate the IOP*. (Induction of and emergence from anesthesia should be as quiet and smooth as possible.)

Anesthetic Management
Preoperative
1. Give adequate sedation (*see above:* Special Anesthetic Problem 3).
2. It is safe to give atropine to patients with congenital open-angle glaucoma.

Perioperative
1. Induce anesthesia as smoothly as possible, IV or by inhalation of N_2O and halothane.
2. *Do not give succinylcholine*.
3. Deepen anesthesia and spray the larynx with lidocaine before intubation.
4. Maintain anesthesia with N_2O-O_2-halothane. Allow spontaneous ventilation for short procedures; otherwise, control the ventilation.

5. At the end of surgery, suction the pharynx carefully and extubate the patient while he is still deeply anesthetized. Lidocaine, 1.5 mg/kg IV, prior to extubation decreases the risk of coughing or straining during emergence.
6. Reapply the mask and give O_2 only until the patient wakens (quietly).

Postoperative
1. Order adequate sedation and analgesics.
2. Order an antiemetic as required.

PROBING THE NASOLACRIMAL DUCT

In most cases, lacrimal duct probing is done on an outpatient basis and no special problems arise. Endotracheal intubation is usually unnecessary, and the probing usually can be performed with an anesthesia mask in place. If it appears that the procedure may be more difficult and prolonged, intubation is preferred.

PENETRATING EYE TRAUMA

Penetrating eye trauma is a relatively common injury in children.

Special Anesthetic Problems
1. Any increase in IOP may result in loss of vitreous humor. The patient should be prevented from crying, coughing, and straining as much as possible. Sedate as necessary. There is now good evidence that succinylcholine can safely be given to patients with eye trauma; if there is concern about a full stomach, a rapid-sequence induction should be performed. Lidocaine IV will prevent an increase in IOP caused by laryngoscopy.
2. It may be difficult to position a mask if the eye is covered with a dressing.
3. The patient may have a full stomach.

Anesthetic Management
Preoperative
1. Give analgesics as required.
2. As early as possible before induction, give metoclopramide (Maxeran), 0.1 mg/kg IV, to expedite gastric emptying.

3. Give atropine IV at induction. (**Note:** atropine blocks the effect of metoclopramide and so should not be given earlier.)

Perioperative

1. Give 100% O_2 by mask for 4 minutes. Then:
2. Inject IV: lidocaine, 1 mg/kg, thiopental with atropine, and succinylcholine.
3. Have an assistant apply cricoid pressure.
4. Intubate the patient without prior lung inflation. Aspirate the stomach.
5. Control ventilation and maintain anesthesia with N_2O-O_2-halothane.

Postoperative

1. Extubate the patient in the lateral position when the patient is fully awake.

Suggested Additional Reading

Abramowitz MD, PT Elder, DS Friendly, WL Broughton, and BS Epstein: Antiemetic effectiveness of intraoperatively administered droperidol in pediatric strabismic out-patient surgery. Anesthesiology 53S:323, 1980.

Apt L, S Isenberg, and WL Gaffney: The oculocardiac reflex in strabismus surgery. Am J Ophthalmol 76:533, 1973.

Arthur DS, and KMS Dewar: Anaesthesia for eye surgery in children. Br J Anaesth 52:681, 1980.

Ausinsch B, SA Graves, ES Munson, and NS Levy: Intraocular pressures in children during isoflurane and halothane anesthesia. Anesthesiology 42:167, 1975.

Ausinsch B, RL Rayburn, ES Munson, and NS Levy: Ketamine and intraocular pressure in children. Anesth Analg 55:773, 1976.

Benjamin KW: The toxicity of ocular medications. Int Ophthalmol Clin 19:199, 1978.

Broadman LM, W Cerruzi, PS Patane, et al: Metoclopramide reduces the incidence of vomiting following strabismus surgery in children. Anesthesiology 69A:747, 1988.

Brown EM, D Krishnaprasad, and BG Smiler: Pancuronium for rapid induction technique for tracheal intubation. Can Anaesth Soc J 26:489, 1979.

Carballo AS: Succinylcholine and acetazolamide (Diamox) in anaesthesia for ocular surgery. Can Anaesth Soc J 12:486, 1965.

Craythorne NWB, HS Rottenstein, and RD Dripps: The effect of succinylcholine on intraocular pressure in adults, infants and children during general anesthesia. Anesthesiology 21:59, 1960.

Edmondson L, SL Lindsay, LP Lanigan, M Woods, and HER Chew: Intraocular pressure changes during rapid sequence induction of anaesthesia. Anaesthesia 43:1005–1010, 1988.

Eustis S, J Lerman, and DR Smith: Effect of droperidol pretreatment on post-anesthetic vomiting in children undergoing strabismus surgery: the minimum effective dose. J Pediatr Opthalmol Strabismus 24:165–168, 1987.

France NK, TD France, JD Woodburn, and DP Burbank: Alteration of forced duction testing by succinylcholine. Anesthesiology 51S:326, 1979.

Fraunfelder FT, and AF Scafidi: Possible adverse effects from topical ocular 10% phenylephrine. Am J Ophthalmol 85:447, 1978.

Jedeikin RJ, and S Hoffman: The oculocardiac reflex in eye-surgery anesthesia. Anesthesiology 21:59, 1960.

Lansche RK: Systemic reactions to topical epinephrine and phenylephrine. Am J Ophthalmol 61:95, 1966.

Libonati MM, JJ Leahy, and N Ellison: The use of succinylcholine in open eye surgery. Anesthesiology 62:637–640, 1985.

Litwiller RW, CA Difazio, and EL Rushia: Pancuronium and intraocular pressure. Anesthesiology 42:750, 1975.

Meyers EF, T Krupin, M Johnson, and H Zink: Failure of nondepolarizing neuromuscular blockers to inhibit succinylcholine-induced increased intraocular pressure: a controlled study. Anesthesiology 48:149, 1978.

Meyers EF, and SA Tomeldan: Glycopyrrolate vs atropine in prevention of oculocardiac reflex during eye surgery. Anesthesiology 51:350, 1979.

Murphy DF: Anesthesia and intraocular pressure. Anesth Analg 64:520–530, 1985.

Samuel JR, and A Beaugie: Effect of carbon dioxide on the intraocular pressure in man during general anesthesia. Br J Ophthalmol 58:62, 1974.

Samuels SI, and M Maze: Beta receptor blockade following the use of eye drops. Anesthesiology 52:369, 1980.

Wellwood M, and GV Goresky: Systemic hypertension associated with topical administration of 2.5% phenylephrine HCl. Am J Ophthalmol 93:369, 1982.

Wynands JE, and DE Crowell: Intraocular tension in association with succinylcholine and endotracheal intubation: a preliminary report. Can Anaesth Soc J 7:39, 1960.

7

Anesthesia for Dental Surgery

GENERAL PRINCIPLES
Suggested additional reading

GENERAL PRINCIPLES

1. Children require general anesthesia more frequently than adults for dental procedures.
2. Many children who present for general anesthesia for dentistry have had previous failed attempts at dental treatment under local analgesia and consequently are very apprehensive.
3. Some children have behavior disorders or retardation syndromes and require special consideration (*see* page 130).
4. Some children have other medical conditions that require special consideration (congenital heart disease, etc.).
5. Endotracheal intubation (usually via the nose) should be performed for all children having dental surgery in the hospital. (Nasal intubation per se causes bacteremia and is an indication for prophylactic antibiotics if heart disease is present.)
6. The use of air turbine dental drills has been a cause of intraoperative subcutaneous and mediastinal emphysema, leading to airway obstruction and possible pneumothorax. The anesthesiologist must be alert for this danger; if facial swelling occurs, discontinue N_2O, check for pneumothorax, and be prepared to support ventilation.
7. Special care must be taken to ensure that no foreign bodies remain in the airway at the end of the procedure (especially throat packs). *All* children should have a gentle, direct laryngoscopy performed before extubation to ensure that the airway is clear.
8. Dental procedures may be prolonged when extensive disease is present. In such instances, recovery to a normal appetite is not as brisk as following short operations. Therefore, patients should receive fluids intravenously (IV) to restore their calculated deficit and to provide maintenance fluids. We prefer to limit the length of general anesthesia for the outpatient to a maximum of 4 hours and to book such patients to commence at 0800 hours. They should stay for a recovery period at least equal to the duration of anesthesia.

Anesthetic Management
Preoperative
1. A complete medical history should be obtained and a routine preoperative physical examination performed.
2. Special investigations and treatments, as appropriate, should be ordered for children with other diseases.
3. No sedative premedication is usually ordered, as these children are most frequently treated as outpatients. Very upset children may benefit from a suitable dose of oral diazepam 1.5 hours preoperatively. Every effort should be made to reassure and gain the confidence of the upset child.

4. Make sure that all special drugs have been ordered and are administered at the right time (e.g., antibiotics for patients with heart disease).
5. For very upset or uncooperative retarded children, it may be helpful to insert an IV line in the preoperative area with the parents present. The use of rectal methohexital for induction may be considered for the child under 4 years old.

Perioperative
1. Apply monitors (precordial stethoscope, blood pressure cuff, electro-cardiogram, pulse oximeter, and axillary thermistor probe).
2. Induce anesthesia with thiopental IV or, for very upset young children (<4 years), with rectal methohexital.
3. Give succinylcholine, oxygenate, and perform nasotracheal intubation. Children over 5 years of age should receive *d*-tubocurarine, 0.05 mg/kg IV, prior to the thiopental to prevent postsuccinylcholine muscle pains (*see* page 53). If such pretreatment is administered, the dose of succinylcholine should be increased to 2 mg/kg to ensure good relaxation for intubation.
4. Maintain anesthesia with N_2O and halothane in oxygen. Allow spontaneous ventilation. For very prolonged procedures, controlled ventilation may be appropriate; if so, reduce the inspired halothane level to 1% and monitor blood pressure carefully.
5. Establish an IV infusion and give maintenance fluids, including those calculated to replace deficits caused by fasting. After all but very minor dental surgery, a delay in resuming oral intake can be anticipated, and hence any deficit should be corrected.
6. At the end of the procedure, when all dental instrumentation is removed, perform a gentle laryngoscopy to ensure a clear airway prior to extubation.

Postoperative
1. Order analgesics as required. (Dental nerve blocks with bupivacaine reduce the requirement.) Codeine, 1–1.5 intramuscularly, mg/kg is usually adequate.
2. Continue IV fluids until ready for discharge.

Suggested Additional Reading
Berry FA, WL Blankenbaker, and CG Ball: A comparison of bacteremia occurring with nasotracheal or orotracheal intubation. Anesth Analg 52:873, 1973.
Milne B, H Katz, J Rosales, et al: Subcutaneous facial emphysema complicating dental anaesthesia. Can Anaesth Soc J 29:71, 1982.
Scott JD, and D Allan: Anaesthesia for dentistry in children: a review of 101 surgical procedures. Can Anaesth Soc J 17:391, 1970.

8

Otorhinolaryngology

Although much of it is simple and commonplace, otorhinolaryngologic surgery has a disproportionately large potential for anesthetic and surgical complications. It demands meticulous attention to all aspects of the patient's perioperative care.

GENERAL PRINCIPLES

1. Because many of these operations involve the airway, the anesthesiologist must be prepared to provide good surgical access to that area while maintaining a safe ventilatory pathway for the patient.
2. The advent of the surgical microscope has permitted development of delicate and precise surgery for the middle ear. Anesthesia for such procedures must provide quiet operating conditions with minimal bleeding, smooth emergence from anesthesia, and minimal disturbance postoperatively.
3. After surgery involving the airway, skilled nursing care in the postanesthesia room (PAR) is essential, so that signs of impending complications can be detected early and appropriate treatment instituted immediately.
4. The use of the laser to treat lesions of the larynx has added some additional potential problems of anesthesia management (*see* page 190). In these patients, as in all others, the simplest techniques are the safest.

TONSILLECTOMY AND ADENOIDECTOMY

Chronic inflammation and hypertrophy of lymphoid tissues in the pharynx may necessitate surgery to relieve obstruction or remove the focus of infection. Repeated middle ear infections may be improved by adenoidectomy. Rarely, acute infection of a tonsil may result in a peritonsillar abscess (quinsy).

In very rare instances, severe chronic airway obstruction by adenoidal tissue may lead to pulmonary hypertension and right heart failure (cardiorespiratory syndrome [CRS]). This condition usually occurs in males and is more common in black children. There is usually a history of symptoms for a year or more. The child is usually febrile with tachycardia and tachypnea. Chest radiographs show cardiomegaly, and the electrocardiogram (ECG) indicates (right) ventricular enlargement. Children with CRS may be critically ill and require emergency intubation to relieve the obstruction. Once this is done and the failure is controlled with digitalis and diuretics, tonsillectomy and adenoidectomy should be performed.

Less rarely, chronic obstruction resulting from lymphoid hyperplasia may result in obstructive sleep apnea. Affected children are often obese, show daytime somnolence and behavior problems, snore at night, and sweat profusely. If such a history is obtained preoperatively, special care must be taken, as post-tonsillectomy complications (including apnea) are more common. The child should have sleep studies preoperatively to detect periods of apnea or hypopnea. The child should be closely monitored before and after operation, avoiding heavy narcotic sedation. Postoperative sleep studies show that 90% or more are improved. Those that do not improve should be investigated for residual soft tissue obstruction and may need uvulopalatopharyngoplasty.

Salicylate ingestion during the days prior to operation has been demonstrated to increase blood loss at tonsillectomy. If such a history is obtained, a bleeding time should be performed, and if it is prolonged (>10 min), the operation should be deferred.

Postoperatively, the presence of small amounts of blood in the pharynx may lead to laryngospasm, especially if halothane has been used. For this reason, isoflurane may be preferred for tonsillectomy, since emergence with this drug may be slightly more rapid with less potential for severe laryngospasm. Always ensure that the pharynx is suctioned clear prior to extubation.

Tonsillectomy is still one of the most common procedures in children and should be very safe. Unfortunately, deaths from tonsillectomy do still occur: the usual causes are excessive sedation of children with airway compromise and mismanagement of postoperative bleeding.

Surgical Procedures

1. Tonsillectomy.
2. Adenoidectomy.
3. Incision of peritonsillar abscess (quinsy).

Special Anesthetic Problems

1. Sharing the airway with the surgeon.
2. When acute infection or extreme lymphoid hypertrophy is present, intubation may be difficult.
3. Danger of bleeding postoperatively (*see* page 181).
4. A history of bleeding or recent salicylate therapy.
5. A history suggestive of sleep apnea.

Anesthetic Management

Preoperative

1. Patients with acute infection (e.g., quinsy) should be closely observed for impending airway obstruction.
2. Do not give sedation, particularly to patients with any degree of airway obstruction.
3. Check for history of recent (<10 days) salicylate ingestion. If so, check the bleeding time; if prolonged (>10 min), defer surgery.
4. Arrange sleep studies if indicated.

Perioperative

Tonsillectomy and/or Adenoidectomy

1. Induce anesthesia intravenously (IV) with thiopental and atropine, followed by succinylcholine.
2. Perform endotracheal intubation with a tube one size smaller than usual for the patient's size and age.
3. Maintain anesthesia with N_2O and isoflurane. Meperidine, 1.5 mg/kg, administered *intramuscularly* (IM) during anesthesia will provide for immediate postoperative analgesia.
4. Allow spontaneous ventilation, but be alert that some assistance may be required for a few minutes after administration of the meperidine.
5. An IV infusion should be given to replace the calculated fasting deficit: replace half this deficit in the first hour, and replace the other half over the next 2 hours. In addition, give 3 ml of IV fluid for every milliliter of blood lost. Discontinue the IV after 3 hours provided the patient is not bleeding or vomiting. It is particularly important to ensure that children having tonsillectomy and adenoidectomy performed as day care patients are well hydrated prior to discharge.
6. Measure and chart blood losses carefully.
7. Extubate the patient when the patient is fully awake.

Tonsillar Abscess or Other Airway Problem

1. Give atropine, 0.02 mg/kg IV.
2. Induce anesthesia by inhalation of N_2O and halothane. Maintain spontaneous ventilation.
3. Do not give muscle relaxants. (Airway obstruction may occur.)
4. When the patient is deeply anesthetized, give 1 mg/kg lidocaine IV and then perform endotracheal intubation. Be careful not to rupture the abscess during instrumentation.
5. Maintenance is as for tonsillectomy (*see above*).
6. Extubate the patient in a lateral position when the patient is fully awake. **N.B.** Sometimes inflamatory swelling may involve the suprag-

lottic structures and postextubation obstruction may occur. Close observation is essential.

Postoperative
1. Order an analgesic—not salicylate, which may precipitate bleeding. Tylenol, 10 mg/kg orally, is usually adequate if meperidine has been given intraoperatively.
2. Order fluids by mouth (e.g., cola and popsicles) when the patient is awake.
3. Closely monitor children who have a possible history of sleep apnea. Constant nursing attention should be provided (i.e., retain in PAR overnight or admit to special unit).
4. Beware of ordering extra narcotic analgesics for the restless child, especially if adenoid packing has been inserted. Restlessness may be a symptom of hypoxia secondary to obstruction, and narcotics may produce apnea.

REOPERATION FOR POST-TONSILLECTOMY BLEEDING

Special Anesthetic Problems
1. The stomach may contain blood, which may be regurgitated during induction of anesthesia.
2. Hypovolemia may be present and is easily underestimated.
3. Has the child a bleeding disorder that has been missed?

Anesthetic Management
Preoperative
1. Ensure that sufficient cross-matched blood has been transfused to restore blood volume and that additional blood is available in case of need.
2. Check coagulation indices.
3. Restrain the child gently if examination, insertion of packing, or ligation of bleeding vessels is attempted without anesthesia. (In the rare event that this is not possible, general anesthesia will be required.)

Perioperative
1. Prepare all equipment for a rapid-sequence induction.
2. Check again that the child has been adequately transfused. Surgery is

virtually never so urgent and bleeding never so brisk that complete restoration of intravascular volume is impossible.
3. Give 100% O_2 by mask.
4. Rapidly inject thiopental, 4 mg/kg, with atropine, followed immediately by succinylcholine.
5. Have an assistant apply cricoid pressure.
6. Intubate the trachea as quickly as possible.
7. Maintain anesthesia as for tonsillectomy (*see above*).
8. Extubate the patient when the patient is fully awake.

Postoperative
1. Check the patient's hemoglobin level to confirm adequacy of blood replacement.
2. Be alert to the possibility of further bleeding.
3. Order suitable doses of analgesic (not acetylsalicylic acid), but bear in mind that if the surgeon has inserted a pack:
   (a) Oversedation could result in complete obstruction of the airway.
   (b) Restlessness may indicate hypoxia rather than a need for sedation.

Suggested Additional Reading
Davies DD: Re-anesthetizing cases of tonsillectomy and adenoidectomy because of persistent postoperative hemorrhage. Br J Anaesth 36:244, 1964.
Eliaschar I, P Lavie, E Halperin, et al: sleep apneic episodes as indications for adenotonsillectomy. Arch Otolaryngol 106:492–496, 1980.
Goertz KE, and L Mattioli: Cardiorespiratory syndrome manifestations in children with chronic upper airway obstruction. J Kans Med Soc 80:126–129, 1979.
Mandel EM, and CF Reynolds: Sleep disorders associated with upper airway obstruction in children. Pediatr Clin North Am 28:897–903, 1981.
Spaur RE: The cardiorespiratory syndrome: cor pulmonale secondary to chronic upper airway obstruction from hypertrophied tonsils and adenoids. Ear Nose Throat J 62:562–570, 1982.
Tate N: Deaths from tonsillectomy. Lancet 2:1090, 1963.

CHOANAL ATRESIA

If complete (as in 90% of cases), choanal atresia (membranous or bony occlusion of the posterior nares) causes respiratory distress immediately after birth. As neonates are obligate nose breathers, nasal obstruction by choanal atresia must be relieved immediately by establishing an oral route with an oropharyngeal airway. The diagnosis can be confirmed by the inability to pass even a fine nasal catheter. Once the diagnosis is established, the passage of an orogastric tube will not only maintain an oral airway but will enable the infant to be fed.

Associated Conditions

The CHARGE syndrome consists of coloboma, congenital heart disease, choanal atresia, growth and mental retardation, ear anomalies, the genitourinary abnormalities with genital hypoplasia.

Surgical Procedures

1. Transpalatal repair—usually performed at age 1–2 days in the healthy term infant. Stents are left in for 3–6 months.
2. Transnasal puncture may be performed in the preterm infant or those with associated significant disease, for example, the CHARGE association.

Special Anesthetic Problems

1. Maintenance of the airway until completion of surgery.

Anesthetic Management

Preoperative

1. Adequate ventilation requires continued use of oropharyngeal airway.
2. Do not order sedatives.
3. Give atropine IM before induction or IV at induction.

Perioperative

1. Neonates: observe all special precautions (*see* page 94).
2. Leave the oropharyngeal airway in place: give 100% O_2 by mask.
3. Perform awake intubation, using an oral RAE* or similar tube.
4. Induce anesthesia with N_2O and halothane; allow spontaneous ventilation.
5. Suction the pharynx very carefully at the end of the operation.
6. Do not extubate the patient until the patient is fully awake and the stents are clear and secure.

Postoperative

1. Order humidified oxygen. The stents must be regularly suctioned with a fine catheter to keep them clear.

---

* Performed tube: Mallinckrodt Canada Inc., Pointe Claire, Quebec, Canada.

2. Constant observation is essential, as aspiration of food is likely after repair of choanal atresia.

Subsequent repairs may be necessary during later childhood for restenosis but present no other special anesthetic problems.

OTOLOGIC CONDITIONS

Special Anesthetic Problems
1. The child may have had repeated procedures and thus be very apprehensive.
2. The child's hearing may be impaired, making communication difficult.
3. During middle ear procedures even a small amount of bleeding may interfere with surgery. Position the child carefully and avoid anesthetic causes of bleeding. However, induced hypotension is not warranted for this type of surgery in children.
4. The surgeon may wish to use vasoconstrictor drugs (e.g., epinephrine, cocaine). In such cases, halothane should be avoided and isoflurane substituted.
5. Some otologic procedures are lengthy, and if so, the patient's ventilation should be controlled.
6. In rare cases, the patient's cooperation is required during surgery (*see* Neuroleptanalgesia, page 186).
7. Postoperative nausea secondary to labyrinthine disturbance is common.

MAJOR OTOLOGIC PROCEDURES

Anesthetic Management
Preoperative
1. Order adequate sedation, especially for children who have had surgery previously.

Perioperative
1. Induce anesthesia IV with thiopental and atropine, followed by succinylcholine.
2. Spray the larynx with lidocaine; then insert an orotracheal tube.
3. Maintain anesthesia with N_2O-O_2-halothane and allow spontaneous ventilation. Anesthesia must be deep enough to prevent any possibility of bucking on the tube, which increases bleeding.

4. Position the patient with a 15° head-up tilt to minimize bleeding.
5. If epinephrine is to be infiltrated, use isoflurane for maintenance.
6. The patient may be nauseated postoperatively; therefore, start an IV drip during surgery and give maintenance fluids.
7. For tympanoplasty: while the graft is being positioned, delete N_2O from the inspired mixture (N_2O bubbles might float the graft off the desired position).
8. Smooth extubation, without coughing, is essential. Therefore, remove the tube while the patient is still anesthetized.

Postoperative
1. Order analgesics and antiemetics as required.

MINOR OTOLOGIC PROCEDURES

Minor otologic procedures are usually performed in the outpatient department. Nitrous oxide has been shown to pass into the middle ear cavity if air is present and may modify findings at the time of surgery, but in general, its use is not contraindicated. N_2O does not increase the incidence of postoperative vomiting.

Special Anesthetic Problems
1. Some patients who require repeated minor otologic procedures have associated congenital deformities of the upper airway that predispose to their ear disease (e.g., cleft palate, Pierre Robin syndrome). Check carefully for potential airway problems during anesthesia.
2. Many of these children present for anesthesia with signs of an upper respiratory infection (URI). In such instances, the decision to proceed must be based on the urgency of surgery (e.g., acute middle ear infection) versus the severity of the URI. If the child's temperature is normal and no abnormal signs are present in the chest, the decision is usually to proceed.

Anesthetic Management
Preoperative
1. Sedation is usually unnecessary and is contraindicated for outpatients (*see* page 106).

Perioperative
1. Induce anesthesia IV with thiopental, mixing atropine in the same syringe.

2. Maintain anesthesia with N_2O and halothane by mask.
3. Intubation is not required, but a laryngoscope and tubes should be at hand in case of unexpected difficulties.

Postoperative
1. Analgesics are not usually required.

NEUROLEPTANALGESIA FOR EAR SURGERY

For certain operations (e.g., ossicular reconstruction), the surgeon may wish to assess hearing during the surgical procedure. Most older children cooperate well if such operations are performed under a combination of neuroleptanalgesia and local analgesia.

Anesthetic Management
Preoperative
1. Explain to the patient in detail what will happen during the operation and reassure the patient that no pain will be felt.
2. Order diazepam, to be given orally, to ensure a degree of sedation preoperatively.

Perioperative
1. Establish an IV line with a local analgesic.
2. Give atropine in the usual dosage, followed by Innovar, 0.04 ml/kg.
3. Ensure that the patient is positioned comfortably and warn the patient not to cough or move the head.
4. Supplement analgesia as required with increments of fentanyl, 2 μg/kg. Talk with the patient periodically to assess the effects of the drugs.
5. Monitor ventilation and periodically remind the patient to breathe deeply.

Postoperative
1. Smaller than usual doses of analgesics are effective in most cases.
2. The continuing antiemetic effect of the neuroleptanesthetic agent usually minimizes postoperative nausea.

SURGERY OF THE NOSE

The commonest procedures for nasal surgery are reduction of nasal fractures, septoplasty, rhinoplasty, and excision of nasal polyps.

Special Anesthetic Problems
1. The nasal airway may be blocked.
2. Children with nasal polyps usually have them as a complication of cystic fibrosis (*see* page 140).

Anesthetic Management
Preoperative
1. Assess the nasal airway.
2. If the patient has cystic fibrosis, order appropriate preoperative care (*see* page 140).

Perioperative
1. Induce anesthesia IV with thiopental and atropine, followed by succinylcholine.
2. If the nose is blocked, insert an oropharyngeal airway before attempting mask ventilation.
3. Perform orotracheal intubation, preferably with a cuffed tube.
4. Insert a throat pack to prevent blood from pooling in the pharynx and esophagus.
5. Position the patient with a slight head-up tilt.
6. Extubate the patient when the patient is fully awake.

Postoperative
1. Order analgesics as required.
2. Administer humidified oxygen by mask.

ENDOSCOPY

Endoscopy is often indicated in infants and children for diagnosis (e.g., stridor) or therapy (e.g., removal of a foreign body).

Procedures
1. Laryngoscopy.
2. Bronchoscopy: alone and for bronchography.
3. Esophagoscopy.

Special Anesthetic Problems
1. Existing airway problem or tracheotomy.
2. Difficulty maintaining optimal ventilation during endoscopy, particularly in a patient with a very small airway.

3. Possibility of complete airway obstruction during some procedures (e.g., removal of foreign body).
4. Postoperative reduction in airway lumen by subglottic edema.

Note. Many conditions for which endoscopy is performed can progress to complete obstruction under anesthesia. Always have a selection of laryngoscopes and endotracheal tubes prepared; from the start of anesthesia, ensure that the endoscopist is at hand in case tracheotomy becomes urgently necessary.

General Anesthetic Management
1. *Spontaneous ventilation* is usually preferred during endoscopy in children (but *see below*). This is safer than controlled ventilation and allows the endoscopist to examine structures as they appear during almost normal breathing.
2. *Controlled ventilation* is necessary for patients who are in respiratory failure and already on a ventilator.

LARYNGOSCOPY

In neonates, laryngoscopy can usually be performed without anesthesia, but observe all special precautions (*see* page 94). Most older infants and children require general anesthesia.

Anesthetic Management
Preoperative
1. Do not give heavy sedation to patients with airway problems. Diazepam given orally is useful for older children having repeated endoscopy.
2. Give atropine IV to all of these patients.

Perioperative
1. Apply monitors, including pulse oximeter, and induce anesthesia by inhalation of N_2O and O_2 with halothane.
2. When the patient is asleep, discontinue the N_2O and continue with halothane in O_2. When the patient is deeply anesthetized, perform laryngoscopy and spray the larynx and supraglottic structures with lidocaine (maximum dose 5 mg/kg).
3. Replace the mask until the lidocaine becomes effective (2–3 minutes). During the surgical procedure, insufflate O_2 with halothane into the pharynx. Place an open suction tube at the mouth to scavenge gases.
4. Monitor ventilation carefully with a stethoscope.

Postoperative
1. Observe the patient closely until he wakens.
2. Order humidified oxygen postoperatively.
3. Order "nothing by mouth" (NPO) until 2 hours after application of the lidocaine spray.

N.B. The above method of anesthesia, employing insufflation and topical analgesia with spontaneous ventilation, is considered overall the safest and most satisfactory method. Endotracheal tubes get into the surgeon's field of vision, "jet injector" methods may be dangerous in children, and all other methods are cumbersome and complicated and hence may fail.

The only problem of the above method is that it may cause some operating room (OR) pollution with anesthetic cases. However, we can minimize the escape of gases and scavange most of these with a well-placed suction tube at the mouth.

Special Considerations
1. *Laryngomalacia* is a common cause of inspiratory stridor in the new-born. This can be diagnosed during laryngoscopy while the infant is awake or is awakening from anesthesia. The stidor usually disappears during deeper levels of anesthesia. In this condition, there is incomplete maturation of the cartilages of the larynx and a tendency for the epi-glottis or one of the arytenoid cartilages to prolapse into the glottis on inspiration, causing marked inspiratory stridor. The condition is self-limiting, and no special treatment is required. However, laryngoscopy is indicated to rule out other causes of stridor (cysts, etc).
2. *Congenital cysts* may occur in the region of the epiglottis and arytenoepiglottic folds. There may be inspiratory and expiratory stridor and a poor cry. The diagnosis is usually confirmed by radiography. Treatment is by excision or marsupialization.
3. *Subglottic hemagioma* may show with crouplike symptoms and a barking cough. The child frequently has other visible hemangiomata. The symptoms will persist or recur, and diagnosis is confirmed at endoscopy. Current treatment is by laser destruction of the tumor.
4. *Laryngeal papillomas*, this (fortunately rare) condition is caused by a virus, and the cauliflowerlike papillomas may cause very serious obstruction to ventilation. Various treatments have been tried, including cryoprobing, ultrasound, and immune sera. The presently preferred therapy is resection by laser. Children with this condition usually present at 2–4 years of age and return for repeated laryngoscopy and resection. Recurrences are almost certain until adolescence, when the lesions usually spontaneously regress. Increasing hoarseness and dys-

pnea are the usual indications for reoperation, and on each occasion the extent of regrowth is impossible to determine prior to laryngoscopy. Sometimes very extensive papillomas completely obscure the glottis. A very cautious approach to all these patients is indicated. Provide humidified gases postoperatively.

Special Anesthetic Problems

1. Acute airway obstruction may occur during induction of anesthesia.
2. The glottic opening may be difficult to visualize. Therefore, barbiturates and relaxants are contraindicated.
3. The surgical treatment by laser demands an unobstructed view of the larynx and immobile vocal cords.
4. Instrumentation of the trachea below the glottis should be avoided, as this may "seed" papillomas into the lower airways. Hence, endotracheal tubes should be avoided if possible, and tracheostomy is contraindicated.

Anesthetic Management for Laser Surgery

The safest plan is as outlined above: no premedication, careful inhalation induction followed by laryngoscopy, and lidocaine spray to the larynx. If obstruction develops during induction (rare but not unknown), an endotracheal tube must be inserted to establish the airway. This can be removed when the patient is deeply anesthetized and the bulk of the papillomas have been resected. Usually intubation is not necessary, and laser resection can proceed once topical analgesia has been applied. Maintain anesthesia by insufflation of halothane via a side arm on the laryngoscope.

N.B. Jet ventilation may be very dangerous in obstructing lesions of the airway. Laryngeal obstruction during jet ventilation may lead to pneumomediastinum and pneumothorax. If jet ventilation is used, extreme care must be taken to avoid barotrauma: the jet must not be advanced beyond the lumen of the laryngoscope, and distal airway pressure should be monitored whenever possible.

Special Precautions For Use of the Laser

1. Cover the patient's eyes.
2. Use reduced concentrations of O_2 (<30% if this provides satisfactory oxygenation) to limit the conflagration at the lesion. Nitrous oxide also supports combustion and should be avoided. If the use of an endotracheal tube is essential, use a nonflammable tube (e.g., flexometallic or

the laser shielding tube*). Alternatively, if these are not available a plastic tube may be wrapped in aluminum foil or packed away from the line of the laser by using damp gauze. If a tube should ignite, it must be immediately disconnected from the anesthetic circuit and withdrawn from the patient. Injury results both from the burn and from the products of tube combustion.

3. All personnel in the OR should wear eyeglasses for protection in case the laser beam is accidentally reflected in their direction. Post a warning sign on the door that the laser is in use.

BRONCHOSCOPY

Bronchoscopy may be performed for various indications, for example, removal of foreign body, diagnosis of respiratory disease, removal of secretions, or treatment of atelectasis. (For bronchoscopy in patients with cystic fibrosis, *see also* page 140.) General anesthesia is usually required.

Special Anesthetic Problems

1. Difficulty maintaining adequate ventilation during the procedure, when the airway must be shared with the endoscopist.
2. Existing impairment of ventilation in some cases.

Anesthetic Management

Preoperative

1. Assess respiratory status carefully.
2. Do not give heavy narcotic premedication.
3. Give atropine to all patients: IM preoperatively or (preferably) IV at induction.

Perioperative

Spontaneous ventilation is preferred for all patients except those who have respiratory insufficiency.

1. Induce anesthesia by inhalation of N_2O and halothane in O_2.
2. Discontinue the N_2O and maintain anesthesia with halothane in O_2.
3. When the patient is adequately anesthetized, remove the mask and perform laryngoscopy. Spray the larynx, trachea, and bronchi with lidocaine (maximum 5 mg/kg).
4. Replace the mask; continue anesthesia with O_2 and halothane until the

---

* Phycon laser shielding tube, Fuji Systems Corp, Tokyo, Japan.

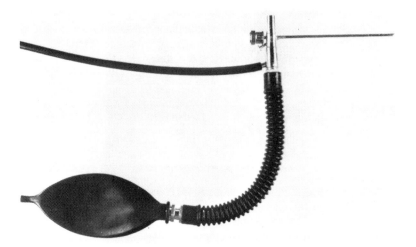

Fig. 8-1. Pediatric bronchoscope with attachments for Jackson Rees T-piece, for use during controlled ventilation.

lidocaine takes effect (2–3 minutes), at which time the bronchoscope can be inserted.

5. Supply O_2 and halothane to the side arm and allow spontaneous ventilation, but remember that when a telescope is in use through a small Storz bronchoscope the resistance to ventilation is high. Hence, at such times, ventilation should be assisted.

6. Monitor the ventilation and heartbeat through two stethoscopes: one is taped to the precordium; the other is moved over the lung fields. Monitor oxygenation continuously with a pulse oximeter.

7. Be alert to the possibility of pneumothorax, a rare complication of bronchoscopy.

8. When controlled ventilation is essential, as for patients in respiratory failure, use a Venturi device (e.g., Sanders injector), but remember that patients in whom severe chronic respiratory disease has reduced their lung compliance may not ventilate well with this method (*see* page 190). For such patients, use a bronchoscope with special attachments for controlled ventilation (Fig. 8-1).

Postoperative

1. Order NPO for at least 2 hours (after lidocaine spray).
2. Order humidified O_2.
3. Watch for signs of stridor.

BRONCHOSCOPY FOR BRONCHOGRAPHY

When bronchoscopy is done for bronchography, the child is anesthetized and a bronchoscope is inserted. Under direct vision, a small amount of contrast medium (e.g., a thin solution of barium) is introduced through a catheter into the lobe(s) to be examined. Radiographs will be of best quality if the contrast medium is introduced during quiet, shallow, spontaneous ventilation. Coughing results in poor-quality films.

Anesthetic Technique

1. Proceed as outlined under Bronchoscopy (*see above*).
2. Before the contrast medium is introduced, give fentanyl, 2 μg/kg IV or meperidine, 0.2 mg/kg IV. This produces quiet, shallow ventilation.
3. At the end of the procedure, reverse the narcotic-induced ventilatory depression with naloxone if necessary.

ESOPHAGOSCOPY

In children, esophagoscopy is usually performed to dilate a stricture or for removal of a foreign body.

Special Anesthetic Problems

1. The child may have undergone esophagoscopy repeatedly and thus be very apprehensive.
2. In small infants, passage of an esophagoscope may compress the trachea and obstruct ventilation, even when an endotracheal tube is in place.
3. Coughing or other movements can result in esophageal perforation during the procedure. Patients must be anesthetized adequately to maintain complete immobility.
4. Lower esophageal strictures or achalasia may have resulted in esophageal dilation higher up. Food and secretions accumulated in the dilated segment may be aspirated during anesthesia.

Anesthetic Management
Preoperative

1. Order adequate sedation, especially for children who have had esophagoscopy previously (in which case, delay bringing the child to the OR until all preparations are made).
2. Check whether the radiographs show esophageal dilation and/or retained material.

Perioperative

1. Give 100% O_2 by mask.
2. Induce anesthesia IV and secure the airway rapidly. (Use cricoid pressure whenever there is a risk of regurgitation and aspiration.)
3. Deepen the anesthesia before permitting the endoscopist to proceed.
4. Monitor the ventilation carefully through a precordial stethoscope.

Postoperative

1. Observe the patient until the patient is fully awake.
2. Be alert for signs of esophageal perforation, especially if difficulty was encountered. Signs include:
   (a) Tachycardia.
   (b) Fever.
   (c) Signs of pneumothorax.
   (d) Radiographic evidence of pneumothorax or mediastinal air.
3. Order NPO until 2 hours after application of the lidocaine spray.

CROUP

Croup is usually due to inflammation in the region of the larynx, but other causes must be kept in mind (e.g., a foreign body). The inflammation may be:

1. Supraglottic—epiglottitis.
2. Subglottic—laryngotracheobronchitis.

EPIGLOTTITIS

Epiglottitis is commonest in children 3–7 years old but may also occur in infants or adults. It is accompanied by severe systemic illness with pyrexia and leukocytosis. In addition to the epiglottis, all the supraglottic structures are swollen and inflamed, contributing to the obstruction. Blood cultures are almost always positive for the infective agent, which is usually *Haemophilus influenzae*. The common symptoms are sore throat, dysphagia, and drooling; severe airway obstruction may develop rapidly. Typically, the patient appears toxic and anxious and sits in a tripod position with chin extended and mouth open. In infants the presentation is less typical, and patients have presented with sudden apnea during investigation of a high fever. Thus, epiglottitis should be considered in the differential diagnosis of the infant with pyrexia and any respiratory difficulty.

Extraepiglottic infection may occur: pneumonia, cervical adenitis, otitis media, septic arthritis, and meningitis are described in association with epiglottitis.

Anesthetic Management

Preoperative

1. The child should be disturbed as little as possible. No venipunctures or painful injections should be done: the child may cry and become acutely obstructed. Do not try to visualize the pharynx, as acute obstruction may result. Gently apply a mask and give O_2.
2. The child must be attended constantly by a physician capable of establishing an emergency airway and equipped to do so.
3. Assemble the team and transfer the patient rapidly to the OR and give the patient O_2, allowing the patient to remain in the chosen posture.
4. Soft-tissue radiographs of the neck may be misleading and are unnecessary in the typical case. If radiographs are required to make the diagnosis, the patient must be accompanied to the radiology department by a physician as the patient's airway may become obstructed during the examination. The patient should not be made to lie down for the radiographs.
5. The OR should be prepared for emergency bronchoscopy and possible tracheotomy.

If apnea occurs (at any time):

1. Try to ventilate the patient with O_2 by bag and mask. This is usually successful.
2. If unsuccessful, proceed to an immediate attempt at laryngoscopy and intubation, and prepare for emergency tracheotomy if intubation proves impossible.

Perioperative

1. Apply a precordial stethoscope, pulse oximeter, and ECG electrodes.
2. Do not lay the patient down. Induce anesthesia with O_2 and halothane by placing the mask gently over the child's face while the child is sitting up, either on the OR table or on the anesthetist's knee.
3. When anesthesia is induced, gently lay the patient down. Assisted ventilation may be necessary at this time.
4. Apply other monitors and establish an IV infusion; administer IV atropine and obtain a blood culture.

5. Administer lidocaine, 1 mg/kg IV, to minimize the risk of coughing and laryngospasm; then perform laryngoscopy and orotracheal intubation. In the rare event that the glottis is obscured by the swelling and distortion of the supraglottic structures, apply external pressure to the chest. This usually expels a bubble through the larynx, providing a guide to intubation.
6. When the patient is anesthetized and well oxygenated:
    (a) Remove the oral tube.
    (b) Insert a nasotracheal tube (one size smaller than predicted for age) and tape it securely in position. (The initial passage of a tube will have defined the airway, making replacement by another tube much easier.)
7. Very rarely, pulmonary edema may occur following intubation for epiglottis. This is thought to be due to hypoxia, elevated catecholamines, and disturbed alveolar-capillary pressure gradient. Treatment is with controlled ventilation, positive end-expiratory pressure, diuretics.

Postoperative

1. Constant (24 hr/day) nursing care in an intensive care unit is essential. Accidental extubation is a serious early complication and must be prevented by suitable restraints and adequate sedation.
2. Ensure adequate humidification of inspired gases and regular suctioning of the nasotracheal tube. Blockage of the tube may result from tracheal secretions.
3. Commence antibiotic therapy. Ampicillin was the drug of choice, but resistant strains of *H. influenzae* necessitated the addition of chloramphenicol to the initial therapy pending culture results. More recently, cefuroxime, a cephalosporin with a high margin of safety and good cerebrospinal fluid penetration, has been used. The total daily IV dose of antibiotics for epiglottitis consists of ampicillin (250 mg/kg/day) plus chloramphenicol (100 mg/kg/day), or cefuroxime (200 mg/kg/day).
4. Extubate the patient when the pyrexia has resolved (usually within 12–36 hours). Some physicians perform repeat laryngoscopy prior to extubation.
5. Observe the patient after extubation for several hours—very rarely a patient will require reintubation for recurrent obstruction.

Suggested Additional Reading

Battaglia JD, and CH Lockhart: Management of acute epiglottitis by nasotracheal intubation. Am J Dis Child 129:334, 1975.
Blackstock D, RJ Adderley , and DJ Steward: Epiglottitis in young infants. Anesthesiology 67:97–101, 1987.

Diaz J: Croup and epiglottitis in children: the anesthesiologist as diagnostician. Anesthesiology 64:621–633, 1985.

Edelson PJ: Radiograpic examination in epiglottitis. J Pediatr 81:1036, 1972.

Epiglottitis in adults [editorial]. Br Med J 3:204, 1971.

Hawkins DB, AH Miller, GB Sachs, et al: Acute epiglottitis in adults. Laryngoscope 83:1211–1220, 1973.

Sendi K, and WS Crysdale: Acute epiglottitis: a decade of change—a 10 year experience with 242 children. J Otolaryngol 16:196–202, 1987.

Schloss MD, JA Gold, JK Rosales, and JD Baxter: Acute epiglottitis: current management. Laryngoscope 93:489–493, 1983.

Travis KW, ID Todres, and DC Shannon: Pulmonary edema associated with croup and epiglottitis. Pediatrics 59:695–698, 1977.

LARYNGOTRACHEOBRONCHITIS

"Acute infectious croup," or laryngotracheobronchitis, is caused by a virus, most commonly in children 2–5 years old. Inspiratory stridor is the principal symptom. Treatment varies according to the severity of the disease.

1. In mild cases, conservative measures (e.g., humidification of inspired gases) may be effective.
2. In most other cases, epinephrine inhalations delivered by intermittent positive-pressure breathing (IPPB) results in improvement.
3. Rarely, nasotracheal intubation or tracheotomy is required.

IPPB WITH EPINEPHRINE

IPPB with epinephrine is widely reported to be efficacious. It seems that both the positive-pressure ventilation and the inhaled epinephrine contribute to the success.

Method

1. Prepare the nebulizer solution of epinephrine: add 0.5 ml of 2.25% racemic epinephrine to 3.0 ml of distilled water.
2. Attach a suitable pediatric-size anesthesia mask to a patient-triggered ventilator. Add the solution to the nebulizer attachment and deliver it at 15–20 cm H_2O pressure and high inspiratory flow rate.
3. These patients are hypoxic. During IPPB, add at least 40% O_2 to the inspired gases; patients usually then settle well and accept the mask quietly.
4. Monitor ventilation and heart rate via a precordial stethoscope. Some increase in heart rate may occur, but other arrhythmias are very rare.

5. Give the treatment for 20 minutes, by which time considerable improvement is usually apparent. (If not, the diagnosis of croup should be reconsidered.)
6. After IPPB, observe the patient carefully. Rarely, the stridor increases rapidly, necessitating immediate establishment of an artificial airway.
7. Some patients require more than one treatment. Total failure to respond with any improvement is an indication to review and question the diagnosis. The use of racemic epinephrine is contraindicated in infants with tetralogy of Fallot as a severe blue spell may be precipitated.

NASOTRACHEAL INTUBATION

If conservative measures and epinephrine inhalations with IPPB fail to relieve symptoms, an artificial airway may be required. Nasotracheal intubation has been used very successfully in many centers, with only a small incidence of complications reported. The critical factor seems to be the diameter of the endotracheal tube, which should be very small (e.g., 3.5 mm). The tube is left in place for 7–10 days. Constant (24 hr/day) expert respiratory care is essential.

The presence of a small tube and thick secretions renders accidental blockage very likely.

A few patients may not respond as favorably to nasotracheal intubation and cannot be successfully extubated after the standard time. This occurs most commonly in patients under 1 year of age, in those with branchial arch deformities or a history of congenital subglottic stenosis, and in those with a history of repeated croup. Tracheotomy may be necessary for these patients.

TRACHEOTOMY

Tracheotomy may become necessary in the treatment of upper airway obstruction or to facilitate respiratory care in other conditions.

Anesthetic Management
Preoperative
1. Give 100% O_2 by mask and assist ventilation manually.
2. Do not give sedatives or narcotics.
3. Give atropine IV.

Perioperative
1. Continue 100% O_2 by mask.
2. (a) If the airway obstruction is severe, insert an endotracheal tube or

pass a bronchoscope before inducing anesthesia; (b) otherwise, induce anesthesia with halothane and O_2 and assist ventilation as required.
3. Tracheotomy is usually performed with a bronchoscope in place. (This facilitates surgery and enables the anesthesiologist to see that the tracheotomy tube has been passed into the lumen of the trachea.)

Postoperative

All Patients
1. As soon as possible, obtain a chest radiograph: check that the tube is positioned correctly and that pneumothorax has not developed (this is a rare complication of tracheotomy).
2. Be alert to the possibility of accidental extubation before the track into the trachea becomes established. If this happens, it may be very difficult to reinsert the tube.

Patients with Croup
3. Add appropriate concentration of O_2 to the inspired gases (to overcome the continuing danger of hypoxemia).
4. Insist upon close, constant observation of the child until the tracheotomy tube can be removed (usually 7–10 days).
   (a) Establishment of the airway does not result in immediate return to normal pulmonary function.
   (b) Respiratory arrest may occur during the postoperative period.

Suggested Additional Reading

Adair JC, WH Ring, WS Jordan, and RA Elwyn: Ten-year experience with IPPB in the treatment of acute laryngotracheobronchitis. Anesth Analg 50:649, 1971.
Allen TH, and IM Steven: Prolonged nasotracheal intubation in infants and children. Br J Anaesth 44:835, 1972.
Mitchell DP, and RL Thomas: Secondary airway support in the management of croup. J Otolaryngol 9:419, 1980.
Newth CJL, H Levison, AC Bryan: The respiratory status of children with croup. J Pediatr 81:1068, 1972.

Subglottic Stenosis

Subglottic stenosis is one of the most common causes of chronic airway obstruction in infants and children. The stenosis may be congenital or acquired—usually a complication of prolonged endotracheal intubation. Severe subglottic stenosis requires tracheotomy followed by surgery to reconstruct the subglottic space.

The surgical procedure generally involves division of the cricoid cartilage and insertion of a cartilage graft to increase the diameter. A stent may then be left in place to maintain the lumen.

Associated Conditions (Congenital Type)
1. Congenital heart disease.
2. Down syndrome.
3. Tracheoesophageal fistula.

Anesthetic Management
Preoperative
1. A tracheostomy is in place, and all care and monitoring of this should be continued until the child arrives at the OR.

Perioperative
1. Administer atropine IV.
2. Anesthetize via the tracheotomy tube with halothane in N_2O-O_2.
3. Remove the tracheotomy tube and insert an armored tube via the stoma; suture this firmly in place. (**N.B.** The lumen of the trachea will take a larger tube than is expected.)
4. Check ventilation to both lungs frequently (with two stethoscopes).
5. Maintain anesthesia with N_2O and halothane.
6. Blood loss is minimal.

Postoperative
1. Replace tracheotomy tube.
2. Administer humidified O_2.
3. Some IV fluids may be required for 1–2 days postoperatively until a fluid diet can be taken.
4. A full diet can be resumed in a week.
5. The stent is removed and laryngoscopy is performed under general anesthesia 3 months later.
6. The tracheotomy is left in place until the patient is able to tolerate plugging of the inner cannula.

Suggested Additional Reading
Crysdale WS: Subglottic stenosis in children: a management protocol plus surgical experience in 13 cases. Int J Pediatr Otorhinol 6:23, 1983.
Friedberg J, and MD Morrison: Paediatric tracheotomy. Can J Otolaryngol 3:147, 1974.

Kim IG, WM Brummit, A Humphry, SW Siomra, and WB Wallace: Foreign body in the airway: a review of 202 cases. Laryngoscope 83:347, 1973.

*Maze A, and E Bloch: Stridor in pediatric patients. Anesthesiology 50:132, 1979.

---

* Key article

9

Plastic and Reconstructive Surgery

Many children require plastic surgery to correct congenital deformities, and in most pediatric hospitals this type of surgery constitutes at least 10% of the operations. The head and neck are commonly affected, which may introduce special problems for the anesthesiologist. In addition, some children undergo plastic surgery for acquired lesions (e.g., burn scars and contractures, dog bites).

GENERAL PRINCIPLES

1. Many of these children have psychological upsets stemming from both the deformity and multiple surgical procedures. Thus, a very careful, considerate approach by the anesthesiologist is essential.
2. Smooth general anesthesia with quiet emergence lessens the risk of damage to grafted areas and delicately sutured repairs.
3. Many patients requiring plastic surgery have potentially serious airway problems that require careful assessment and special management.
4. Congenital structural anomalies commonly affect more than one body system. If congenital heart disease (CHD) is present, ensure that the child is given prophylactic antibiotic therapy preoperatively.

CLEFT LIP AND PALATE

Cleft lip and palate are present in various combinations in as many as 1 in 1,000 liveborn infants. Thus, their repair constitutes a large part of pediatric plastic surgery. Infants with these lesions may be both anemic and malnourished because of feeding difficulties and may have had repeated respiratory infections.

Associated Conditions
1. Congenital heart disease.
2. Pierre Robin syndrome.
3. Treacher Collins syndrome. } *see* Syndromes, Appendix I
4. Subglottic stenosis.

Surgical Procedures
1. Cleft lip repair—usually performed at 10–12 weeks.
2. Cleft palate repair—usually performed at 12–18 months.
3. Palatoplasty and pharyngoplasty—usually performed at 5–15 years.

Special Anesthetic Problems

1. Airway problems, including difficulty with intubation.
2. Blood loss (during cleft palate repair).
3. Problems related to associated conditions (e.g., CHD).

Anesthetic Management

Preoperative

1. Carry out very careful assessment.
   (a) Direct special attention to the airway, lungs, and other systems that may be affected in congenital syndromes.
   (b) Check especially carefully for upper respiratory tract infection; if this is present, surgery must be postponed.
   (c) Check for anemia.
2. Check for a history of recent medication with salicylates. If positive, determine the bleeding time to detect continuing drug effects on coagulation.
3. For cleft palate surgery, check that at least 1 unit of blood is available.
   4. If induction by inhalation is planned, order atropine to be given intramuscularly (IM) 30 minutes before surgery.

Perioperative

1. If there is any doubt about the ease of endotracheal intubation, perform an inhalation induction.
2. Give N_2O and O_2 with halothane until the patient is anesthetized adequately for laryngoscopy. Give lidocaine, 1.5 mg/kg intravenously (IV), prior to insertion of the laryngoscope to minimize the risk of coughing or laryngospasm.
3. If the cleft is large or bilateral, pack it with moist sterile gauze to prevent trauma during laryngoscopy and intubation.
4. For orotracheal intubation, use a RAE preformed tracheal tube. Check carefully that bilateral ventilation of the lungs is present after the mouth gag is positioned. Insertion of the gag tends to advance the tube toward the bronchi.
5. Monitor air entry continuously during surgery, paying special attention each time the gag is repositioned or the patient is moved.
6. Maintain anesthesia with N_2O plus relaxant and controlled ventilation, with a low concentration of halothane (0.75%) or isoflurane (1%) added. This volatile agent should be discontinued before the end of the operation so that the patient awakens promptly upon reversal of the relaxant drug.
7. Monitor blood loss carefully and replace if indicated.

8. Inspect the mouth and pharynx carefully at the end of surgery; use a laryngoscope and remove all blood and clots.
9. Extubate the patient when the patient is fully awake.

Postoperative

1. Order constant observation in the postanesthesia room (PAR) for 24 hours, as airway problems or bleeding may occur.
2. Order nursing in a croup tent.
3. Order analgesics—codeine is preferred; definitely do not use acetylsalicylic acid.
4. Acute swelling of the tongue causing obstruction has been reported following cleft palate repair. Examine the mouth, and if any signs of swelling exist, the patient should be left intubated.

PHARYNGOPLASTY

Pharyngoplasty is performed to reduce velopharyngeal incompetence and improve speech. The procedure inevitably increases resistance to ventilation.

Special Anesthetic Problems

1. Postoperative airway obstruction may occur in the PAR.
2. Chronic airway obstruction may persist after the operation and lead to pulmonary hypertension and/or obstructive sleep apnea.

Anesthetic Management
Preoperative

As for cleft palate (*see above*).

Perioperative

As for cleft palate (*see above*).

Postoperative

1. Observe closely in the PAR for airway obstruction and/or bleeding for at least 12 hours.
2. Do not order heavy narcotic sedation—IM codeine is adequate for analgesia.
3. Continuing supervision for signs of obstruction during sleep is suggested, and postoperative sleep studies should be performed.

Suggested Additional Reading

Bell C, TH Oh, and JR Loeffler: Massive macroglossia and airway obstruction after cleft palate repair. Anesth Analg 67:71–74, 1988.

Kravath RE, CP Pollak, B Borowiecki, and ED Weitzman: Obstructive sleep apnea and death associated with surgical correction of velopharyngeal incompetence. J Pediatr 96:645, 1980.

Lee JTR, and HGG Kingston: Airway obstruction due to massive lingual oedema following cleft palate surgery. Can Anaesth Soc J 32:265–267, 1985.

Levin RM: Anesthesia for cleft lip and cleft palate. Anaesthesiol Rev 6:25–30, 1979.

Wallbank WA: Cardiac effects of halothane and adrenaline in hare-lip and cleft palate surgery. Br J Anaesth 42:548, 1970.

Whalen JS, and AW Conn: Anaesthetic management for repair of cleft lips and cleft palates. Can Anaesth Soc J 10:584, 1963.

Whalen JS, and AW Conn: Improved technics in anesthetic management for repair of cleft lips and palates. Anesth Analg 46:355, 1967.

CYSTIC HYGROMA

Cystic hygroma is in fact a cystic lymphangioma that usually occurs in the neck and less commonly in the axilla. Intraoral extension of this benign tumor may cause airway obstruction. Three percent of cervical tumors extend into the mediastinum.

Special Anesthetic Problems

1. Existing airway obstruction.
2. Difficulty with intubation owing to distortion of the airway.
3. Complete removal of tumor may involve extensive dissection and be accompanied by major blood loss.

Anesthetic Management

Preoperative

1. Assess the patient carefully, looking especially for evidence of intrathoracic extension of the tumor.
2. Do not give heavy sedation. Order atropine to be given IM.
3. Ensure availability of blood and blood products for transfusion.
4. Prepare a selection of tubes and laryngoscope blades.

Perioperative

1. Induce anesthesia cautiously by inhalation of N_2O and halothane. Maintain spontaneous ventilation.
2. When the patient is anesthetized, establish a reliable large-bore IV route.
3. Before attempting intubation, discontinue N_2O and give O_2 and halothane for 2 minutes. Coughing and breath-holding and/or laryngospasm during attempts at intubation may be minimized by giving lidocaine, 1.5 mg/kg IV.
4. Intubate, preferably using an armored tube, and secure this firmly. For some patients, if intraoral dissection is planned, a nasal tube may be preferable. For a difficult intubation, insert an oral tube first and then change to a nasal tube.
5. Maintain anesthesia with N_2O plus relaxant and low concentrations of halothane (0.75%) or isoflurane (1%) with controlled ventilation.
6. For large tumors requiring extensive dissection, an arterial line should be inserted.
7. Beware of vagal reflexes during dissection in the neck. Give atropine IV if these occur.
9. Replace blood losses carefully, with appropriate fluids, guided by the blood pressure (BP) and the measured blood losses.
10. After the operation, extubate the patient smoothly; prevent excessive coughing and bucking, which might cause bleeding at the surgical site.
11. If extensive surgery has been performed adjacent to the airway, extubation should be delayed until the extent of postoperative swelling is determined. If this is significant, intubation will be required until it resolves. A few cases may require tracheotomy.

Postoperative

1. If extubated;
   (a) Order close observation in the PAR overnight (because of the danger of bleeding into the surgical site or compression of the airway).
   (b) Avoid large doses of narcotic analgesics.
2. If intubated:
   (a) Confirm the position of the endotracheal tube by radiography.
   (b) Order appropriate humidified oxygen in air and continuing care.

Suggested Additional Reading

MacDonald DJF: Cystic hygroma: an anaesthetic and surgical problem. Anaesthesia 21:66, 1966.
Brooks JC: Cystic hygroma of the neck. Laryngoscope 83:117–128, 1973.

FRACTURED MANDIBLE

Surgical Procedures
1. Interdental wiring.
2. Open reduction and wiring.

Special Anesthetic Problems
1. The patient may have a full stomach.
2. Intubation may be difficult because of tissue damage and distortion.
3. Foreign bodies may be present in the airway (e.g., teeth).
4. The mouth is wired closed after the procedure; therefore, postoperative vomiting is virtually lethal.

Anesthetic Management
Preoperative
1. Assess the patient carefully.
2. Determine the more-patent nostril for intubation.
3. For patients with a full stomach, delay surgery if possible and give metoclopramine IV (to hasten gastric emptying).
4. Do not give heavy sedation.

Perioperative
1. Use a rapid-sequence induction with cricoid pressure.
2. Examine the pharynx quickly but carefully during laryngoscopy to search for foreign debris.
3. Use an orotracheal tube initially and then change this to a nasotracheal tube. (If you attempt to place the nasotracheal tube initially, you may start a nosebleed—then the patient will have a full stomach plus a nosebleed.) Once the oral tube is in, pass a nasal tube through the nose, repeat the laryngoscopy, and change tubes.
4. Insert a nasogastric tube and aspirate. Pack throat with sterile gauze.
5. Maintain anesthesia with N_2O and relaxant, using controlled ventilation. (This permits rapid reawakening and minimal postoperative nausea.)
6. Before final fixation of jaws, remove the pack and inspect the pharynx with a laryngoscope; remove blood clots and other debris.
7. Keep the nasotracheal tube in place during transportation to the PAR.
8. Leave the nasogastric tube in situ for use during the postoperative period.

Postoperative
1. Order close observation of patient.
2. Do not remove the nasotracheal tube until the patient is fully awake.
3. Ensure that wire cutters are at hand at all times.

Removal of Interdental Wiring

General anesthesia is usually required for removal of the wiring and arch bars when the fracture is healed. The wires holding the jaws together can be removed before induction of anesthesia. However, jaw movement remains extremely restricted because of the prolonged immobilization rendering laryngoscopy and intubation extremely difficult.

Ensure that the patient has been fasted preoperatively. After removal of the securing wires, induce anesthesia by inhalation of N_2O and halothane until a nasopharyngeal tube can be inserted for maintenance.

Exercise great care to maintain the airway and have equipment for emergency intubation and/or tracheotomy immediately at hand.

RECONSTRUCTIVE SURGERY FOR BURNS

After the acute phase of their injury, children who have extensive burns require repeated anesthesia for plastic and reconstructive surgery.

Special Anesthetic Problems
1. Contractures resulting from burns of the face and neck may make intubation and maintenance of the airway during anesthesia very difficult.
2. Succinylcholine is contraindicated for 2–3 months after severe burns. (It may cause cardiac arrest secondary to hyperkalemia.)
3. Severe emotional problems may have resulted from the accident, disfigurement, and the repeated surgical procedures.
4. Blood losses may be large during grafting of extensive burns.
5. Temperature homeostasis is impaired, and special measures must be taken to avoid excessive heat loss.
6. Infection of burns is a serious hazard at this stage. Observe great care in handling the patient to prevent cross infection; use reverse-isolation techniques in the operating room (OR) and postoperatively.
7. Hepatic dysfunction may follow burns; recovery takes several weeks.
8. Emergence from anesthesia should be quiet to avoid damage to recently grafted areas.

Anesthetic Management

Ketamine is a very valuable agent for use during reconstructive surgery in burned patients (*see* page 51) and in some centers has been used as the sole anesthetic. Provided emergence reactions are avoided (by appropriate premedication), ketamine is highly suitable for repeated use in these children; in fact, many request "the same anesthetic as last time" (i.e., ketamine). In addition, this agent causes less disturbance of appetite and feeding than do conventional anesthetics, an important feature for these patients.

Be aware that, although unlikely, airway obstruction may occur during ketamine anesthesia; be prepared to reestablish ventilation.

Other advantages of ketamine in patients with burns are

1. Profound analgesia is provided without respiratory or cardiovascular system depression. (Cardiac output is increased and is maintained during changes in position.)
2. Analgesics are not usually required postoperatively. Emergence is quiet, with minimal risk to grafted areas.
3. Unlike halothane, ketamine has no immunosuppressive action.

General endotracheal anesthesia is the other alternative. If this is used there are some special considerations:

1. A 40% higher dose of thiopental is required in children with fresh burns and during convalescence. This dose may cause cardiovascular effects if the patient is at all hypovolemic. Ketamine may be preferred for induction of such patients.
2. Succinylcholine is contraindicated in all burn patients.
3. The dose requirements for nondepolarizing muscle relaxants are increased in proportion to the magnitude of the burn. Relaxants should be titrated to achieve the desired effect, and if possible, a neuromuscular blockade monitor should be used.
4. If there has been airway involvement in the burn, progressive stenosis may develop, usually in the subglottic area. Carefully select an endotracheal tube and do not be surprised if a smaller tube is required at a subsequent operation. Severe stenosis may, of course, require tracheostomy.
5. Severely ill patients may not tolerate volatile agents; in such cases, narcotic analgesics (e.g., fentanyl) with relaxants and controlled ventilation are preferred.

Preoperative

1. Assess the patient's condition carefully and examine the anesthetic history.

2. Take time to talk with the patient: encourage questions, answer them honestly, and reassure the patient about the planned procedure.
3. Preoperative fasting must be rigidly observed, even if you plan to use ketamine.
4. Order adequate sedation (e.g., pentobarbital, 2 mg/kg, or diazepam, 0.2–0.4 mg/kg) to be given orally (PO) 2 hours preoperatively.
5. Atropine should be given to prevent bradycardia and copious secretions, which may complicate ketamine anesthesia.
6. Make sure that the OR is warmed to 25°C.

Perioperative

1. Ketamine: as for acute burns (*see* page 334).
2. Alternatively, use general endotracheal anesthesia:

If no airway problems

(a) Induce anesthesia IV with thiopental or by inhalation of N_2O-halothane.
(b) Perform intubation under deep halothane anesthesia after spraying with lidocaine.
(c) Maintain anesthesia with N_2O and halothane. Insert a reliable IV line.
(d) Monitoring must be adapted to the site and extent of the burn area, that is, BP cuff placed on any uninjured limb. An esophageal stethoscope is usually suitable and can incorporate electrocardiogram (ECG) leads.* Attempt to monitor all the usual parameters. Pulse oximetry can be obtained from the tongue if there is no other site.
(e) Measure blood losses and be prepared to replace these. If massive transfusion is required, be alert to the possibility of hypocalcemia, which is more common in burn patients.

If there are airway deformities (cervical contractures, etc.)

(a) If the chin cannot be extended or the mouth opened, direct visual intubation may be impossible. Select from the following alternatives.

(i) Blind nasal intubation: proficiency demands much experience, and this approach may be particularly difficult if scar tissue has distorted the airway.
(ii) After release of scar tissue under local analgesia, induce anesthesia and perform direct-vision intubation.

---

* For example, Esophagocardioscope: Portex, Inc., Wilmington, MA.

(b) Once the airway is established, anesthesia can be maintained as above.

Postoperative

1. Emergence from anesthesia should be quiet. Order adequate analgesic drugs if required.
2. If ketamine has been used, be aware of the possibility of psychotic emergence reactions (*see* page 51). Order constant observation until patient has fully recovered and is fit to return to the ward.

Suggested Additional Reading

Cote GJ, and AJ Petkau: Thiopental requirements may be increased in children reanesthetised at least one year after recovery from extensive thermal injury. Anesth Analg 64:1156, 1985.

Martyn JAJ, LMP Liu, SK Szyfelbein, et al: Pancuronium requirements in burned children. Anesthesiology 59:561–564, 1983.

Martyn JAJ, RS Matteo, and DJ Greenblatt: Comparative pharmacodynamics of *d*-tubocurarine in burned and non-burned man. Anesth Analg 61:241–246, 1982.

Szyfelbein SK, LG Drop, and JAJ Martyn: Persistent ionized hypocalcemia during resuscitation and recovery phases of body burns. Crit Care Med 9:454–458, 1981.

Tolmie, JD, TH Joyce, and GD Mitchell: Succinylcholine danger in the burned patient. Anesthesiology 28:467, 1967.

Wilson RD, RJ Nichols, and NR McCoy: Dissociative anesthesia with CI-581 in burned children. Anesth Analg 46:719, 1967.

Zook EG, RP Roesch, LW Thompson, and JE Bennett: Ketamine anesthesia in pediatric plastic surgery. Plast Reconstr Surg 48:241, 1971.

MAJOR CRANIOFACIAL RECONSTRUCTIVE SURGERY

Extensive reconstruction is now possible for children with severe facial deformities. The improvement in appearance frequently has a major beneficial effect on the child's future life. Much of this surgery is now being performed during infancy or early childhood. The objective is to allow the child to go to school looking as normal as possible.

GENERAL PRINCIPLES

1. A team approach is essential for successful performance of this type of surgery.
2. Operations involving the jaws are usually delayed until dentition is complete (i.e., 13 years or older).

3. Operations not involving dentition (e.g., for craniofacial dysostosis) are usually performed at an earlier age.

Special Anesthetic Problems

1. Intubation of the airway may be very difficult if the deformity is severe. Some patients require tracheotomy preoperatively (using local analgesia); in such cases beware of pneumothorax.
2. Blood loss may be very extensive from the surgical site and bone graft donor site (e.g., pelvic girdle or ribs).
3. Surgery is of long duration, and special precautions must be taken to protect the patient against complications of prolonged anesthesia (e.g., pressure sores).
4. Surgical manipulation involving the orbit and face may initiate the oculocardiac reflex.
5. Surgical manipulations may damage the endotracheal tube intraoperatively (rare).
6. Patient must awaken rapidly postoperatively so that the surgeon can check cranial nerve function.
7. Extensive postoperative swelling may dictate the need for prolonged intubation after the operation.

Anesthetic Management

Preoperative

1. Examine the patient very thoroughly, particularly for airway abnormalities and cardiopulmonary disease.
2. Consider the possibility of associated congenital defects or other features of a syndrome that may have implications for anesthesia (*see* Appendix I). Some children (e.g., Apert's syndrome or Crouzon's disease) may have sleep apnea and should be investigated in a sleep laboratory.
3. Check all laboratory results, especially for indications of coagulopathy.
4. Order any further tests necessary to assess the patient fully before surgery.
5. Ensure that adequate supplies of blood and blood products will be available and that serum has been saved for further cross-matching should this be necessary.
6. Reassure the patient and explain the planned procedures, including postoperative care.
7. Order preoperative sedation: diazepam, 0.5 mg/kg PO (maximum 10 mg).

Perioperative

1. Induce anesthesia:
   - (a) If there are no intubation problems, induce with thiopental IV; then proceed to intubation with a relaxant.
   - (b) If difficulty is anticipated, use an inhalation induction (*see* page 68).
   - (c) If intubation is judged impossible, induce anesthesia after tracheotomy under local analgesia.
2. The endotracheal tube should be sutured in position, with due consideration being given to the movements of the facial bones that will accompany the surgery. The tube should either be sutured to a structure that will not be moved or it should be so positioned in the trachea to allow for the effects of movement as its point of fixation.

   An armored tube should be used when possible. The SWAY* tube, which is armored only in the proximal extratracheal segment, may be useful if prolonged intubation is anticipated.
3. Maintain anesthesia with N_2O and narcotic (e.g., fentanyl, 2–3 µg/kg/hr) and a suitable relaxant drug.
4. Control ventilation to a $PaCO_2$ of 25–30 mmHg.
5. Position the patient with 10–15° head-up tilt.
6. Pad all pressure areas well, including occiput and areas compressed by the endotracheal tube (e.g., nares or lip).
7. Place ointment in eyes (the surgeon will usually perform tarsorrhaphy).
8. Monitor:
   - (a) Ventilation and heart rate, via stethoscope.
   - (b) ECG, pulse oximeter, and end-tidal CO_2.
   - (c) Central venous and arterial BP by direct means.
   - (d) Serial determinations of acid-base, blood gas, and hematocrit (Hct).
   - (e) Temperatures.
   - (f) Coagulation indices (during transfusion if this is massive).
   - (g) If major blood loss expected or diuretics are to be administered, insert a urinary catheter.
9. Be prepared for massive blood replacement.
10. If reduction in brain mass is required, given furosemide, 1 mg/kg IV.
11. When indicated, induce hypotension with either isoflurane or sodium nitroprusside (*see* page 148).
12. The patient should be fully awake in the OR at the end of surgery, so that the surgeon can check the patient's vision and ascertain whether cranial nerve injury has occurred during surgery.

---

* Phycon SWAY tube, Fuji Systems Corp, Tokyo, Japan.

Postoperative

1. Order routine postcraniotomy nursing care when applicable.
2. Leave endotracheal tube in place until:
   (a) The patient is fully awake *and*
   (b) There is no further danger that postoperative tissue swelling might obstruct the airway. (Many patients require intubation for 24–48 hours postoperatively.)
3. Observe caution when using narcotic analgesics.
4. Check hemoglobin and Hct to ensure adequacy of blood replacement.

Suggested Additional Reading

Davies DW, and IR Munro: The anesthetic management and intraoperative care of patients undergoing major facial osteotomies. Plast Reconstr Surg 55:50, 1975.

Diaz JH, and CE Henling: Pneumoperitoneum and cardiac arrest during craniofacial reconstruction. Anesth Analg 61:146, 1982.

Handler SD: Craniofacial surgery: otolaryngological concerns. Int Anesthesiol Clin 26:61–63, 1988.

Handler SD, ME Beaugard, and LA Whitaker: Airway management in the repair of craniofacial defects. Cleft Palate J 16:16, 1978.

Munro IR: Craniofacial surgery: airway problems and management. Int Anesthesiol Clin 26:73–78, 1988.

Robideaux V: Oculocardiac reflex caused by midface disimpaction. Anesthesiology 49:433, 1978.

Schafer ME: Upper airway obstruction and sleep disorders in children with craniofacial anomalies. Clin Plastic Surg 9:555, 1982.

For implications for anesthesia in relation to congenital defects, see the relevant entry and references in Appendix I.

10

General and Thoracoabdominal Surgery

COMMON MINOR SURGICAL PROCEDURES
Division of "tongue-tie"
Inguinal herniotomy
Orchidopexy
Circumcision
 Suggested additional reading
Neonatal necrotizing enterocolitis
 Suggested additional reading
Organ transplantation
 Care of the donor
 Suggested additional reading

GENERAL PRINCIPLES

1. Many of the patients are neonates, some preterm, and thus demand special considerations (*see* page 94).
2. In many cases, the pathophysiology of the surgical disease dictates the optimal anesthestic management. The anesthesiologist should understand the effects of the lesion on normal physiology.
3. Surgery is very rarely required immediately. Usually, some time is available for preoperative resuscitation. The optimum time for surgery must be decided by consultation among anesthesiologist, neonatologist, and surgeon.
4. For emergency abdominal surgery, the problem of the full stomach must be considered. (Even if the patient has not eaten for some time, secretions accumulate in the stomach, and emptying may be delayed by obstruction or ileus.) Children admitted for emergency surgery have high volume and acidity of gastric contents. Children with a history of gastroesophageal reflux may be at special risk. Remember:
   (a) The effects of drugs on the barrier pressure (lower esophageal pressure [LES] minus gastric pressure); it is reduced by atropine, diazepam, nitrous oxide, and volatile agents. Barrier pressure is increased by metoclopramide, pancuronium, and vecuronium; it is little changed by succinylcholine.
   (b) Drugs can also be used to reduce the volume and acidity of gastric contents: cimetidine (oral or rectal), ranitidine, metoclopramide, sodium citrate.
   Possible plans of action:
      (i) Whenever possible pretreat with drugs to reduce volume and acidity of gastric contents. Pass a gastric tube when appropriate.
      (ii) Newborn and small infants at high risk: aspirate stomach contents through a gastric tube, preoxygenate, and perform awake intubation.
      (iii) Older children: aspirate stomach contents (if appropriate) and perform a rapid-sequence induction combined with cricoid pressure (Sellick maneuver). Cricoid pressure must be commenced as soon as any drugs are given that may reduce LES pressure. There is still no relaxant that can replace succinylcholine for speed of onset and intensity of neuromuscular block.
   (c) **Remember:** For crash induction in children (under 10 years), succinylcholine does not increase intra-abdominal pressure at this age, and pretreatment with curare is not indicated.

5. During thoracoabdominal surgery, blood loss may be considerable; be prepared to handle major blood transfusion.

6. For major abdominal surgery, always place intravenous (IV) lines in the upper limbs. The inferior vena cava (IVC) may become occluded during the operation, and thus transfusion via the lower limb veins would be useless.

7. During lung surgery bronchial secretions (often sanguineous) may accumulate and interfere with ventilation. Perform perioperative tracheobronchial toilet whenever this becomes necessary.

8. During thoracotomy, $\dot{V}/\dot{Q}$ ratios in the lungs are disturbed. Therefore, increase the inspired oxygen concentration to maintain a safe level of oxygen saturation.

9. In infants and small children, retraction of the lungs may obstruct major airways, impairing ventilation, or it may compress the heart and great veins, leading to a precipitous fall in cardiac output and hence blood pressure (BP). Constant breath-by-breath monitoring via stethoscope is essential, and a Doppler flowmeter should be used to monitor the pulse and measure BP. In the event of bradycardia, hypotension, or impaired ventilation:
    (a) Ask the surgeon to remove all retractors immediately.
    (b) Ventilate the patient with 100% O_2.

10. Patients requiring minor surgery (e.g., herniotomy) may be preterm and/or have other conditions (e.g., anemia) that may complicate anesthesia and require special precautions. Remember the special problems of the ex-preterm infant (*see* page 96).

Suggested Additional Reading

Cotton BR, and G Smith: The lower oesophageal sphinctor and anaesthesia. Br J Anaesth 56:37–46, 1984.

Hunt PCW, BR Cotton, and G Smith: Barrier pressure and muscle relaxants. Anaesthesia 39:412–415, 1984.

Manchikanti L, JA Colliver, TC Marrero, and JR Roush: Assessment of age-related acid aspiration risk factors in pediatric, adult, and geriatric patients. Anesth Analg 64:11–17, 1985.

Schurizek BA, L Rybro, NB Boggild-Madsen, and B Juhl: Gastric volume and pH in children for emergency surgery. Acta Anaesthesiol Scand 30:404–408, 1986.

Sehhati GH, R Frey, and EG Star: The action of inhalation anesthetics upon the lower oesophageal sphincter. Acta Anaesth Belg 2:91–98, 1980.

Tryba M, F Yildiz, K Kuhn, M Dziuba, and M Zenz: Rectal and oral cimetidine for prophylaxis of aspiration pneumonitis in paediatric anaesthesia. Acta Anaesthesiol Scand 27:328–330, 1983.

Young ET, NG Goudsouzian, and A Shah: Effect of ranitidine on intra-gastric pH in children. Anesth Analg 65S:170, 1986.

CONGENITAL DEFECTS THAT MAY NEED SURGERY DURING THE NEONATAL PERIOD

CONGENITAL LOBAR EMPHYSEMA

Abnormal distention of a lobe (usually upper or middle) compresses the remaining normal lung tissue and displaces the mediastinum: respiratory distress and cyanosis result. When severe, this presents as an extreme emergency during the early neonatal period.

Obstruction of the bronchus supplying the distended lobe may be extrinsic (e.g., abnormal blood vessels) or intraluminal, or it may be due to a defect of the bronchial wall (bronchomalacia). The chest radiograph demonstrates a hyperlucent area with sparse lung markings (differentiation from pneumothorax) and mediastinal shift. Less severe forms of this condition may pass unnoticed for months or even years (*see* page 222).

Associated Condition

1. Congenital heart disease—an incidence of up to 37% in reported series.

Surgical Procedure

1. Lobectomy (if no intraluminal or extrinsic cause can be found).

Special Anesthetic Problems

1. Respiratory failure owing to compression of normal lung tissue.
2. The possibility of a "ball valve" effect, further increasing the size of the affected lobe during positive-pressure ventilation.
3. Nitrous oxide may cause further distention of the lobe and is contraindicated.

Anesthetic Management

1. Observe special precautions for neonates.

Preoperative

1. The patient is nursed semiupright.

2. Give O_2 by hood. Do not apply intermittent positive-pressure ventilation (IPPV) (ball valve effect).
3. Insert a gastric tube and apply continuous suction. This prevents gastric distention from further compromising ventilation.
4. Order blood for transfusion.
5. Sudden serious deterioration of the patient's condition may demand immediate emergency thoracotomy to exteriorize the affected lobe and allow normal lung tissue to ventilate.

Perioperative

1. Bronchoscopy to exclude intraluminal obstruction is usually done before thoracotomy.
2. Give atropine IV.
3. Give 100% O_2 by mask for at least 4 minutes and then perform awake intubation (or allow the surgeon to pass the bronchoscope).
4. Induce and maintain anesthesia with isoflurane or halothane in oxygen.
5. After bronchoscopy and before thoracotomy, change to an endotracheal tube.
6. Allow spontaneous ventilation until the thorax is open. At this time, the affected lobe usually balloons out of the chest, and ventilation must be controlled.
7. Once the thorax is open, a nondepolarizing neuromuscular blocking drug can be given to facilitate controlled ventilation and minimize the need for inhaled anesthetic vapors. N_2O can be added to the inspired gases at this time, but a high FiO_2 ($>50\%$) should be maintained.
8. After the affected lobe has been excised, the remaining lung tissue will gradually expand to fill the thorax.

Postoperative

1. Discontinue all anesthetic drugs and administer 100% O_2. Reverse relaxant drugs.
2. When the infant is wide awake, suction the endotracheal tube and remove it.
3. Place the infant in a heated incubator and supply O_2 as required to maintain arterial oxygenation.
4. A chest drain (connected to underwater drainage and suction) is required for 48 hours.

OLDER CHILDREN

In approximately 10% of cases, a congenital emphysematous lobe is discovered at an older age. These children should be anesthetized before intubation but otherwise managed as outlined above. Do not start controlled ventilation until the chest is open.

Suggested Additional Reading

Cote CJ: Anesthetic management of congenital lobar emphysema. Anesthesiology 49:296, 1978.

Mart JT: Case history number 93: congenital lobar emphysema. Anesth Analg 55:869, 1976.

Murray GF: Congenital lobar emphysema. Surg Gynecol Obstet 124:611, 1967.

Raynor AC, MP Capp, and WC Sealy: Lobar emphysema of infancy: diagnosis, treatment, and etiological aspects. Ann Thorac Surg 4:374, 1967.

CONGENITAL DIAPHRAGMATIC HERNIA

The incidence of congenital diaphragmatic hernis is 1 in 4,000 live births. There are several types. The commonest is posterolateral, through the foramen of Bochdalek, usually on the left side. Herniation of abdominal contents into the thorax leads to respiratory distress, mediastinal displacement ("dextrocardia"), and a scaphoid abdomen. Breath sounds are absent over the affected side. Bowel sounds are very rarely heard over the thorax. The radiographic appearance is usually diagnostic but may be indistinguishable from that of congenital lobar emphysema.

In many patients with congenital diaphragmatic hernia the lungs are severely hypoplastic. It was thought that compression of the developing lung caused this hypoplasia. It is now also suggested that there may be a primary failure of lung development associated with secondary failure of the diaphragm to develop normally. The infant is often in severe respiratory distress at, or soon after, birth.

In recent years, the diagnosis has usually been made in utero by fetal ultrasound.

Associated Conditions

1. Malrotation of the gut (40% of cases).
2. Congenital heart disease (15%).
3. Renal abnormalities (less common).
4. Neurologic abnormalities (less common).

Surgical Procedures

1. Reduction of hernia and repair of the diaphragmatic defect: usually a transabdominal procedure.

Special Anesthetic Problems

1. Optimal preoperative preparation of the patient

The trend in recent years is not to rush to surgery. Relief of compression of the lungs by herniated abdominal contents will not usually solve the problem. Indeed, there is evidence that respiratory mechanics are worse postoperatively. It is now preferred to treat the respiratory insufficiency by muscle paralysis, controlled ventilation, and therapy to control pulmonary vasoconstriction. The operation can then be performed as an elective procedure when the infant is improving.

Preoperative Management

This requires the facilities and trained staff of a specialist unit. The infant is nursed in a semiupright, semilateral position, facing toward the involved side. A gastric tube is passed and maintained on low suction to prevent further distention of intrathoracic abdominal viscera. All but the exceptionally fit older infant will require intubation and ventilation preoperatively. Muscle paralysis following intubation will facilitate controlled ventilation and minimize struggling, thereby decreasing the O_2 demand. It will also reduce airway pressure and further lung damage, and diminish the danger of pneumothorax. The infant should be hyperventilated if possible, but avoiding the use of unnecessary high pressure. The possible role for high-frequency ventilation in patients with diaphragmatic hernia is as yet undefined. Pneumothorax is an ever-present danger and must be watched for and immediately treated. The pulmonary vascular resistance may be reduced by hyperventilation, fentanyl infusion, and minimal handling of the child. Drugs such as tolazoline have been given as pulmonary vasodilators but may also result in systemic hypotension and myocardial failure.

Aggressive invasive monitoring with arterial and pulmonary artery line is required to ensure optimal treatment of the pulmonary status.

The best ventilatory predictor of the degree of pulmonary hypoplasia, and hence the likely outcome, is suggested to be the $PaCO_2$ related to the ease of ventilation. Those patients who are easy to hyperventilate survive, and those who are hypercarbic and hypoxic despite hyperventilation do not; it is possible that extracorporeal membrane oxygenation may increase survival of the latter group.

Anesthetic Management

1. Observe special precautions for neonates (*see* page 94).

Perioperative

1. Induce and maintain anesthesia with appropriate doses of fentanyl. Ventilate with oxygen plus air to maintain oxygen saturation. Do not give N_2O (it could further distend gas-containing herniated viscera).
2. Monitor airway pressure. This should not exceed 25–30 cm H_2O (higher pressures may cause further lung damage).

3. Do not try to expand the lungs following reduction of the hernia (lung damage).
4. Monitor blood gas and acid-base status frequently, and correct as indicated.

Postoperative

1. Return the patient to the intensive care unit (ICU) for continued ventilation and therapy to maintain pulmonary perfusion.
2. Most patients should be expected to have a stormy course and require aggressive intensive therapy as outlined in the preoperative management.
3. Unfortunately, some infants who have been salvaged by heroic intensive care measures may remain O_2 dependent for years.

Suggested Additional Reading

Bray RJ: Congenital diaphragmatic hernia. Anaesthesia 34:567, 1979.

Bonn D, M Tamura, D Perrin, G Barker, and M Rabinovitch: Ventilatory predictors of pulmonary hypoplasia in congenital diaphragmatic hernia, confirmed by morphological assessment. J Pediatr 111:423–431, 1987.

Collins DL, JJ Pomerance, KW Travis, SW Turner, and SJ Pappelbaum: A new approach to congenital posterolateral diaphragmatic hernia. J Pediatr Surg 12:149, 1977.

Dibbins AW: Neonatal diaphragmatic hernia: a physiologic challenge. Am J Surg 131:408, 1976.

Ein SH, G Barker, P Olley, B Shandling, JS Simpson, CA Stephens, and RM Filler: The pharmacologic treatment of newborn diaphragmatic hernia—a 2-year evaluation. J Pediatr Surg 15:384, 1980.

German JC, AB Gazzaniga, R Amlie, et al: Management of pulmonary insufficiency in diaphragmatic hernia using extracorporeal circulation with a membrane oxygenator (E.C.M.O.). J Pediatr Surg 12:905, 1977.

Kitagawa M, A Hislop, EA Boyden, and L Reid: Lung hypoplasia in congenital diaphragmatic hernia: a quantitative study of airway, artery, and alveolar development. Br J Surg 58:342, 1971.

Levin DL: Congenital diaphragmatic hernia: a persistent problem. J Pediatr 111:390–392, 1987.

Redmond C, J Heaton, J Calix, E Graves, et al: A correlation of pulmonary hypoplasia, mean airway pressure, and survival in congenital diaphragmatic hernia treated with extracorporeal membrane oxygenation. J Pediatr Surg 22:1143–1149, 1987.

Sakai H, M Tamura, Y Hosokawa, AC Bryan, GA Barker, and DJ Bohn. Effect of surgical repair on respiratory mechanics in congenital diaphragmatic hernia. J Pediatr 111:432–438, 1987.

Shocat SJ, RL Naeye, WDA Fort, et al: Congenital diaphragmatic hernia—new concept in management. Ann Surg 190:332, 1979.

Wooley MM: Congenital posterolateral diaphragmatic hernia. Surg Clin North Am 56:317, 1976.

TRACHEOESOPHAGEAL FISTULA AND ESOPHAGEAL ATRESIA

Tracheoesophageal fistula and esophageal atresia, interrelated conditions, may present in several combinations. The overall incidence is 1 in 3,000 live births.

The commonest form is esophageal atresia with a fistula between the trachea and the distal segment of the esophagus. This condition is often detected when the neonate chokes at the first feeding but ideally should be diagnosed at birth by the inability to pass a soft rubber catheter into the stomach. Plain radiography confirms the diagnosis, showing the catheter curled in the upper esophageal pouch and an air bubble in the stomach indicating a fistula. Contrast medium should not be used since it may be aspirated and further damage the lungs.

The second and commonest form is the H-type fistula without atresia, the diagnosis of which may be more difficult and hence delayed. In many cases, there is a history of repeated respiratory infections.

Associated Conditions

1. Prematurity (30–40%).
2. Congenital heart disease (22%).
3. Additional gastrointestinal (GI) abnormalities (e.g., pyloric stenosis).
4. Renal and genitourinary (GU) abnormalities.
5. The VATER association: vertebral defects, anal atresia, transesophageal fistula (TEF), esophageal atresia, radial and renal dysplasia.

Surgical Procedures

The infant's general condition and the anatomy of the defect govern the choice of surgical management.

1. Primary repair (ligation of fistula and esophageal anastomosis), which is preferred.
2. Staged repair (gastrostomy followed by division of the fistula and later esophageal repair).

Special Anesthetic Problems

1. Pulmonary complications secondary to aspiration.
2. Possibility of intubating the fistula.
3. Anesthetic gases may inflate the stomach via the fistula.

4. Surgical retraction during repair may obstruct ventilation.
5. Subglottic stenosis or tracheal stenosis may be present.

Anesthetic Management
1. Observe special precautions for neonates (*see* page 94).

Primary repair

Preoperative
1. The baby is nursed in a semiupright position.
2. The proximal esophageal pouch is suctioned continuously to prevent aspiration of secretions.
3. Institute intensive respiratory care to reduce pulmonary complications. (Even so, the lung condition seldom improves until after ligation of the fistula; therefore, surgery should not be delayed in the hope that pulmonary status will improve.)
4. Order blood for transfusion (250 ml).
5. Give maintenance fluids IV (but bear in mind that dehydration is unlikely to be a major problem, as neonatal fluid requirements are low during the first 24 hours and electrolyte depletion does not occur with esophageal obstruction).
6. In the preterm infant with respiratory distress syndrome and poor lung compliance, there is a real danger of massive distension of the stomach (or massive leak from the gastrostomy) and failure to ventilate. Rupture of the stomach and pneumoperitoneum may occur. It has been suggested that the leak through the fistula in such cases may be controlled by a Fogarty catheter passed via a gastrostomy into the lower esophagus.

Perioperative
1. Suction the upper pouch.
2. Perform awake intubation, inserting the tube with the bevel facing posteriorly (to avoid intubating the fistula). Beware of the possibility of subglottic stenosis—have small tube sizes available. In extreme narrowing, a large venous cannula may have to be used as an endotracheal tube.
3. Immediately after intubation, check ventilation throughout the lung fields. *If ventilation is unsatisfactory*, remove the tube, give O_2, and reinsert the tube. It is advantageous to place the tube with its tip just above the carina; this can be done by advancing the tube into a bronchus and withdrawing until bilateral ventilation is heard. This should place the tip of the tube below the fistula in most cases. More com-

plicated methods to position the tube have been described but are not necessary in our experience.

4. When satisfactory intubation has been achieved, oxygenate and perform tracheobronchial suction.

5. Maintain anesthesia with N_2O, O_2, and halothane or isoflurane with spontaneous ventilation. *If spontaneous ventilation is inadequate*: initiate controlled ventilation cautiously, watching for inflation of the stomach.

    (a) If inflation occurs, discontinue N_2O and allow the patient to breathe spontaneously (with careful manual assistance) until the chest is open. Then the fistula must be ligated as soon as possible.

6. When the chest is open, give a muscle relaxant and control the ventilation manually in the usual manner.

7. Monitor the ventilation carefully during surgical manipulation: large airways may be kinked by retraction, especially as the fistula is being approached.

Postoperative

1. If the chest is clear and the patient is awake and moving vigorously, extubate the patient.

2. If there are pulmonary complications or any doubts about the adequacy of ventilation, continue controlled ventilation.

3. The pharynx is suctioned with a soft catheter that has a suitable length clearly marked: it must not reach (and damage) the anastomotic site.

4. Prolonged intensive respiratory care may be required. (Swallowing is not normal postoperatively, and aspiration may be frequent.)

5. Prognosis after the repair depends on the maturity of the infant and on whether other congenital anomalies are present and/or pulmonary complications develop. In the absence of these conditions, the mortality rate should be nil.

Staged repair

If staged repair is planned, preliminary gastrostomy is performed under local or general anesthesia. Management of the second stage (ligation of the fistula) should follow the sequence outlined above. Further surgery (to repair the atresia) may be done later when the patient's condition is optimal.

Late Complications

1. Diverticulum of the trachea, at the site of the old fistula, is common in patients who had a TEF repaired during infancy. Be aware of this possibility and the danger of intubating the diverticulum during anesthesia in later life.

2. The tracheal cartilage structure is abnormal, and tracheomalacia may cause symptoms during infancy following TEF repair. Episodes of stridor, dyspnea, and cyanosis ("dying spells") characteristically occur during feeding. This is due to compression of the soft trachea between the dilated esophagus and the arch of the aorta. Severe symptoms require surgical treatment by aortopexy or tracheoplasty with an external splint (*see* page 277).
3. Stricture may develop at the site of the esophageal anastomosis and require repeated dilatations and/or resection.

Suggested Additional Reading

Baraka A, and M Slim: Cardiac arrest during IPPV in a newborn with tracheoesophageal fistula. Anesthesiology 32:564, 1970.

Bray RJ, and WH Lamb: Tracheal stenosis or agenesis in association with tracheo-oesophageal fistula and oesophageal atresia. Anaesthesia 43:654–658, 1988.

Calverley RK, and AE Johnston: The anaesthetic management of tracheo-esophageal fistula: a review of ten years' experience. Can Anaesth Soc J 19:270, 1972.

Davies MRQ, and S Cywes: The flaccid trachea and tracheo-esophageal congenital anomalies. J Pediatr Surg 13:363, 1978.

Filler RM, PJ Rossello, and RL Lebowitz: Life threatening anoxic spells caused by tracheal compression after repair of esophageal atresia: correction after surgery. J Pediatr Surg 11:739, 1976.

Karl HW: Control of life threatening leak after gastrostomy in an infant with respiratory distress syndrome and tracheoesophgeal fistula. Anesthesiology 62:670–672, 1985.

Salem MR, AY Wong, YH Lin, HV Firor, and EJ Bennett: Prevention of gastric distention during anesthesia for newborns with tracheoesophageal fistulas. Anesthesiology 38:82, 1973.

Templeton JM, JJ Templeton, L Schnaufer, HC Bishop, et al: Management of esophageal atresia and tracheoesophageal fistula in the neonate with severe respiratory distress syndrome. J Pediatr Surg 20:394–397, 1985.

CONGENITAL HYPERTROPHIC PYLORIC STENOSIS

Congenital hypertrophic pyloric stenosis, a common surgical problem of infancy, may occur in up to 1 in 300 live births in some populations, the incidence having considerable geographic variation. First-born male infants are more commonly affected. Hypertrophy of the muscle of the pyloric sphincter causes obstruction, leading to persistent vomiting. Dehydration, hypochloremia, and alkalosis develop. If the diagnosis is promptly made, severe derangements are avoided.

Associated Condition

1. Jaundice (2%): no special treatment is required, and the jaundice clears after pyloromyotomy.

Surgical Procedure

1. Pyloromyotomy.

Special Anesthetic Problems

1. Ensuring that dehydration and electrolyte imbalance are fully corrected prior to surgery (pyloromyotomy is not an emergency procedure).
2. Danger of vomiting and aspiration during anesthesia.

Anesthetic Management

1. Observe special precautions for neonates (*see* page 94).

Preoperative

1. Insert a gastric tube and apply continuous suction.
2. Rehydrate the patient, correcting the electrolyte imbalance: this may require 24–48 hours.
   (a) Give 2:1 dextrose:saline solution and/or normal saline as indicated by serum electrolyte values. Add KCl supplements (3 mEq/kg/day) when urine flow is established.
   (b) Delay surgery until the infant appears clinically well hydrated and has normal electrolyte levels, acid-base balance, and good urine output.
3. Immediately preoperatively reassess the patient to ensure that the fluid status is now satisfactory:
   (a) Check for clinical signs of hydration (skin turgor, fontanelle, vital signs, activity, moist tongue).
   (b) Check urine output.
   (c) Check biochemistry—values should be: pH 7.3–7.5, Na >132, Cl >90, K >3.2, bicarbonate <30 mmol/L).

Perioperative

1. Give atropine IV.
2. Place the patient in the left lateral position and aspirate the stomach with a soft catheter, even if the patient has been on continous gastric suction.

3. Give 100% O_2 by mask.
4. Perform awake intubation or rapid-sequence induction with cricoid pressure.
5. Induce and maintain anesthesia with N_2O and halothane (0.5%) or isoflurane (0.75%).
6. Give a muscle relaxant and control the ventilation. (This permits the use of minimal amounts of anesthetic agents.) The choice of relaxant is dictated by the probable duration of surgery (i.e., the speed of the surgeon). Atracurium, 0.3 mg/kg IV, is useful for short procedures.
7. Ensure that the infant is well relaxed and immobile while the pyloric muscle is being split. (Coughing or movement could result in surgical perforation of the mucosa.)
8. At the end of the operation, the patient must be wide awake and in a lateral position for extubation.

Postoperative

1. Maintain IV infusion of fluids until oral intake is adequate (usually 25 hours). Oral feeding is started with clear fluids 6–12 hours postoperatively.
2. Hypoglycemia has been reported if IV fluids containing glucose are discontinued before oral intake is adequate.

Suggested Additional Reading

Bennett EJ, HL Augee, and MT Jenkins: Pyloric stenosis. Clin Anesth 3:276, 1968.
Conn AW: Anaesthesia for pyloromyotomy in infancy. Can Anaesth Soc J 10:18, 1963.
Daly AM, and AW Conn: Anaesthesia for pyloromyotomy: a review (The Hospital for Sick Children, Toronto). Can Anaesth Soc J 16:316, 1969.
Shumake LB: Postoperative hypoglycemia in congenital hypertrophic pyloric stenosis. South Med J 68:223, 1975.

OMPHALOCELE AND GASTROSCHISIS

In omphalocele and gastroschisis, there is herniation of abdominal contents through the anterior abdominal wall. In gastroschisis, the defect is lateral to the umbilicus (usually on the right), the umbilical cord is situated normally, and other congenital defects are rare. In omphalocele, the umbilical cord is continuous with the apex of the sac, and associated congenital defects are common (± 75%). The incidence of these conditions is

Gastroschisis 1 in 30,000 live births

Omphalocele 1 in 5,000 to 1 in 10,000 live births

Gastroschisis is often an isolated defect; omphalocele is usually accompanied by other congenital malformations.

Associated Conditions (WITH OMPHALOCELE)
1. Prematurity (30%).
2. Other GI malformations (malrotation, diaphragmatic hernia, etc.) (25%).
3. GU anomalies (25%).
4. Congenital heart disease (10%).
5. Beckwith-Wiedemann syndrome (omphalocele, macroglossia, and severe hypoglycemia). These infants are usually large and have visceromegaly of the liver, kidney, and pancreas.

Surgical Procedures
The size of the abdomen in relation to the lesion determines the surgical procedure.

1. Primary closure—preferred if possible since there is less risk of infection and other complications. Primary closure does, however, increase intra-abdominal pressure, and this may lead to hypotension, reduced cardiac output, postoperative ventilatory failure, bowel ischemia, and anuria. It has been recommended that intragastric pressure may be a guide to the safety of primary closure: pressures over 20 mmHg are associated with increased complications.
2. Skin closure only.
3. Staged procedure—initial closure with a prosthetic pouch, followed by progressive daily reduction of this to the level of the abdominal wall and subsequent full-thickness closure.

Special Anesthetic Problems
1. Heat loss from exposed viscera.
2. Severe fluid and electrolyte disturbance and hypovolemic shock from transudation of fluid into bowel. Hypoproteinemia may occur.
3. Possibility of hypoglycemia.
4. Postoperative compromise of ventilation and circulation with primary closure owing to high intra-abdominal pressure.

Anesthetic Management
1. Observe special precautions for neonates (*see* page 94).

Preoperative
1. The patient is nursed in a semiupright position with exposed viscera

wrapped in sterile plastic film, covered by towels to minimize heat and fluid losses.
2. Insert a gastric tube to decompress the bowel.
3. Monitor the blood glucose; if hypoglycemic (<40 mg/dl), infuse glucose continuously (6–8 mg/kg/min). **N.B.** Severe rebound may occur after bolus doses of glucose.
4. Rehydrate the patient and correct the hypovolemia and electrolyte and oncotic status. Initial fluid requirements are high (up to 140 ml/kg/24 hr), and normal saline plus colloid (plasma or albumin) is required to correct the hypovolemia.
5. Order blood for transfusion (250 ml).

Perioperative
1. Ensure that the operating room (OR) is warmed to ≥24°C and that heating lamps and blankets are in place.
2. Local analgesia may be used for some patients (*see* page 103). If so:
   (a) Maintain check on total dose given.
   (b) Alert the surgeon if toxic dose is approached.

   For general anesthesia:

1. Give atropine IV.
2. Aspirate the gastric tube.
3. Give 100% oxygen by mask.
4. Perform awake intubation or rapid-sequence induction with cricoid pressure.
5. Induce and maintain anesthesia with halothane (0.5–1.0%) or isoflurane (0.75–1.5%) in O_2 and air.
   (a) Do not give N_2O, as it will cause further bowel distention.
6. Give small doses of muscle relaxants and control ventilation.
7. It may be planned to measure intragastric pressure during abdominal closure. Pressures of over 20 mmHg are usually poorly tolerated.

Postoperative
1. Assess spontaneous ventilation; if in any doubt, change to a nasotracheal tube and continue controlled ventilation for 24–48 hours.
2. Continue nasogastric suction.
3. Continue IV fluids. Some infants require a prolonged period of IV hyperalimentation, as bowel function may be impaired for a long time (weeks or months).

Suggested Additional Reading
Dierdorf SF, and G Krishna: Anesthetic management of neonatal surgical emergencies. Anesth Analg 60:204, 1981.
Goudsouzian NG: Omphalocele. *In*: Common Problems in Pediatric Anes-

thesia (LC Stehling, ed.) Chicago, Year Book Medical Publishers, 1982, p. 14–18.

King DR, R Savrin, and ET Boles: Gastroschisis update. J Pediatr Surg 15:553, 1980.

Mollitt DL, TVN Ballantine, JL Grosfeld, and P Quinter: A critical assessment of fluid requirements in gastroschisis. J Pediatr Surg 13:217, 1978.

Seashore JH: Congenital abdominal wall defects. Clin Perinatol 5:61, 1978.

Yaster M, JR Buck, DL Dudgeon, et al: Hemodynamic effects of primary closure of omphalocele gastroschisis in human newborns. Anesthesiology 69:84–88, 1988.

BILIARY ATRESIA

Biliary obstruction in the newborn most commonly results from neonatal hepatitis or biliary atresia. Atresia of the extrahepatic bile ducts may be congenital or due to postnatal inflammation. The incidence of biliary atresia is 1 in 25,00 live births. The problem in the persistently jaundiced newborn with direct (mixed hyperbilirubinemia is to rule out other causes and confirm the diagnosis of atresia of the bile ducts. This is usually achieved by radioisotope scanning and percutaneous liver biopsy.

Associated Anomalies

1. Malrotation.
2. Situs inversus viscerum.

Surgical Procedure

1. Hepatic portoenterostomy (Kasai procedure). The major preoperative survival determinant seems to be the age at which surgery is performed. If the infant is over 12 weeks, success is less likely.

Anesthetic Problems

1. Hepatic function is impaired.
2. Hypoprothrombinemia develops and leads to impaired coagulation, especially in older infants.
3. Blood loss may be extensive.
4. Intraoperative radiographs may be needed, and hence a heating blanket cannot be used.

Anesthetic Management

Preoperative

1. Observe all considerations for the neonate (*see* page 94) preoperatively.
2. Check the coagulogram and that the patient has received a vitamin K_1 injection.

3. Check the adequate blood and fresh frozen plasma are available for transfusion.

Perioperative

1. Give atropine IV.
2. Administer 100% O_2 by mask.
3. Intubate awake or following a very small dose of thiopental (3 mg/kg) and succinylcholine (1 mg/kg).
4. Induce and maintain anesthesia with N_2O and halothane (0.5%) or isoflurane (0.75%).
5. Administer a relaxant (atracurium is preferred) and control the ventilation.
6. Insert generous IV lines into upper limbs or neck.
7. Monitor the BP carefully; be alert to the possibility of sudden hypotension resulting from IVC obstruction during surgical manipulation. Placing the infant in a slight head-down position may minimize falls in BP during manipulations of the liver.
8. Monitor the temperature; if necessary, use an overhead heater, in addition to all other measures, to maintain normothermia.

Postoperative

1. Prolonged IV hyperalimentation may be required.
2. Ascending cholangitis is common, and portal hypertension may develop.
3. Many children develop esophageal varices and suffer repeated bleeds.
4. The use of salicylates is very dangerous and is contraindicated in these children.

Suggested Additional Reading

Kasai M, S Kimura, Y Asakura, H Suzaki, Y Taira, and E Ohashi: Surgical treatment of biliary atresia. J Pediatr Surg 3:665, 1968.

Barkin RM, and JR Lilly: Biliary atresia and the Kasai operation; continuing care. J Pediatr 96:1015, 1980.

INTESTINAL OBSTRUCTION IN THE NEWBORN

Intestinal obstruction in the newborn may result from various lesions (e.g., duodenal atresia, duplication, midgut volvulus or malrotation) or accumulation of viscid meconium ("meconium ilus").

Associated Conditions

1. Prematurity.
2. Down syndrome—and hence congenital heart disease (18%).
3. Cystic fibrosis (invariably accompanies meconium ileus).
4. Subglottic stenosis with duodenal atresia.

Special Anesthetic Problems

1. Hypovolemia; acid-base and electrolyte imbalance.
2. Gross abdominal distention in some cases.
3. Risk of regurgitation and aspiration.

Anesthetic Management

1. Observe special precautions for neonates (*see* page 94).

Preoperative

1. Check that the patient has had adequate fluid volume replacement.
2. Check acid-base and electrolyte status and correct any imbalance as far as possible.
3. Ensure that the GI tract has been decompressed as much as possible (via an indwelling gastric tube).

Perioperative

Local Anesthesia

In some very sick neonates, laparotomy is performed under local analgesia. If anesthesia stand-by is requested:

1. Be alert to the possibility of regurgitation and aspiration during surgery—even under local analgesia. (It is preferable to intubate the patient and assist ventilation during surgery.)
2. Monitor the total dose of local analgesic administered and warn the surgeon if toxic levels are approached.

General Anesthesia

1. Give atropine IV.
2. Aspirate the stomach contents via the gastric tube.
3. Give 100% O_2 by mask.
4. Perform awake intubation. Beware of the possibility of subglottic stenosis.
5. Induce and maintain anesthesia with halothane (0.5%) or isoflurane (0.75%) in an air-O_2 mixture. Do not give N_2O, as this may cause further distention.

6. Give small doses of relaxant drugs (atracurium is preferred) and control the ventilation.
7. Despite apparently adequate preoperative fluid resuscitation, some patients become hypotensive once the abdomen is open, especially those with small bowel atresia or midgut volvulus. They may need surprisingly large volumes of IV fluid (even blood or plasma) to restore the BP. Be prepared.

Postoperative
1. Do not extubate the infant until the child is fully awake and vigorous. Then extubate in the lateral position.
2. Prolonged IV or gastrostomy feeding may be required.
3. Following meconium ileus, prolonged bowel dysfunction, sepsis, and pneumonia must be anticipated.

Suggested Additional Reading

Lynn HB: Duodenal obstruction: atresia, stenosis, and annula pancreas. *In*: Pediatric Surgery, 3rd ed. (MM Ravitch, KJ Welch, CD Benson, E Aberdeen, and JG Randolph, eds.) Chicago, Year Book Medical Publisher, 1979.
Sears BE, J Carlin, and WP Tunnell: Severe congenital subglottic stenosis in association with congenital duodenal obstruction. Anesthesiology 49:214, 1978.
Stevenson RJ: Neonatal intestinal obstruction in children. Surg Clin North Am 65:1217–1234, 1985.

OTHER MAJOR THORACOABDOMINAL LESIONS AND PROCEDURES

NEUROBLASTOMA AND GANGLIONEUROMA

Neuroblastoma is one of the commonest malignant tumors of children. More than 50% are in the retroperitoneal space, but they may occur anywhere along the sympathetic chain.

Ganglioneuromas are benign tumors arising from sympathetic ganglia.

Special Anesthetic Problems
1. Massive blood loss may occur during surgery (especially with neuroblastoma).
2. Catecholamine levels may be increased, and the BP may rise (but cardiac arrhythmias are very rare).

3. Thoracic tumors may compress the lungs and produce respiratory failure.

Anesthetic Management

1. **Important.** Adequate supplies of blood for transfusion must be available, together with facilities to measure (and replace) blood losses.
2. Details of anesthetic management depend on the patient's age and the tumor's location.
3. Although some of these tumors secrete catecholamines, it is not necessary to give adrenergic blocking agents preoperatively (as would be necessary with pheochromocytoma).

Suggested Additional Reading

Evans AE, GJ D'Angio, and CE Koop: Diagnosis and treatment of neuroblastoma. Pediatr Clin North Am 23:161, 1976.
Farman JV: Death from neuroblastoma: a case report. Br J Anaesth 37:883, 1965.
Farman JV: Neuroblastomas and anaesthesia. Br J Anaesth 37:866, 1965.

LUNG SURGERY

Lung surgery may be indicated for:

Lung abscess
Bronchiectasis
Lung cysts
Bronchogenic cysts
Diagnostic biopsy (in children usually to confirm or exclude infection by virus, etc.)
Pulmonary arteriovenous (AV) malformation
Sequestrated pulmonary lobe
Pulmonary neoplasms
Chronic pulmonary infection

Special Anesthetic Problems

1. Once the thorax is open, major inequalities of ventilation and perfusion should be anticipated; increase the FIO_2 and monitor saturation closely.
2. Major hemorrhage may occur suddenly if large vessels are inadvertently cut or torn. Therefore, reliable large-bore infusion routes must be established and blood for transfusion must be immediately available in the OR.

3. Postoperative pain limits coughing and deep breathing, especially in older children, predisposing to atelectasis.
4. Pulmonary function may be seriously impaired, resulting in respiratory failure in some patients (e.g., those for lung biopsy). In such patients, even minor fluid overload may precipitate serious deterioration in lung function postoperatively.
5. Pus from purulent lesions (e.g., lung abscess, bronchiectasis) may become dispersed during surgery. Double-lumen tubes and bronchial blockers to isolate an infected segment of lung are not available for infants and small children. Selective intubation of the right or left main bronchus may be appropriate in a small percentage of patients; preoperative bronchoscopy to remove accumulated secretions is useful for many. If it is necessary to isolate a lung segment in a small child, a Fogarty catheter (positioned during bronchoscopy) can be used as a blocker.
6. Pulmonary AV malformation results in a very large right to left shunt, with a consequent low arterial O_2 tension that cannot be corrected by increasing the F_1O_2.

Anesthetic Management
Preoperative
1. Assess the patient very carefully, considering the history, physical examination, and laboratory and other studies.
   (a) Evaluate pulmonary function as fully as possible (only limited data may be obtainable for children too young or otherwise unable to cooperate in the full range of tests).
   (b) Check the results of blood gas studies.
In summary, ascertain whether the patient is in the best possible condition for the planned surgery.
2. Ensure that adequate supplies for transfusion have been ordered and serum saved for further cross-matching.
3. (a) Ensure that appropriate respiratory care is ordered.
   (b) For older patients, explain the value of preoperative breathing exercises and the need for postoperative respiratory care.
4. Order appropriate preoperative sedation, taking care to avoid causing respiratory depression in patients with impaired pulmonary function.

Perioperative
1. Apply monitors.
2. Give 100% O_2 by mask.
3. Induce anesthesia, usually with thiopental IV followed by succinylcholine.

4. Ventilate with 100% O_2 until patient is fully relaxed and then perform intubation.
5. Insert an esophageal stethoscope and thermistor probe.
6. Establish a reliable wide-bore (18 gauge or larger) IV route.
7. Insert an arterial line (except for "minor" procedures in healthy children).
8. Maintain anesthesia with N_2O and halothane, or N_2O with narcotic, adding sufficient O_2 to maintain the SaO_2 at >95%.
9. Give nondepolarizing muscle relaxant and control the ventilation (aim to maintain the $PaCO_2$ at 35–40 mmHg).
10. After the patient has been positioned for thoracotomy, recheck the ventilation of all areas of the lungs.
11. Suction the endotracheal tube as necessary to remove secretions during surgery.
12. If one-lung anesthesia is used:
    (a) Increase the concentration of O_2 in inspired gases.
    (b) Monitor arterial saturation continuously.
13. Inflate the lungs fully periodically during thoracotomy and as the chest is being closed.
14. When the chest is closed, ensure that chest drains are connected to a Heimlich valve or underwater drain.
15. At the end of surgery, before extubation, ensure that the patient is awake and responding and has adequate spontaneous ventilation. If in doubt, leave the endotracheal tube in place and continue artificial ventilation until it is safe to withdraw this support.

Postoperative
1. Provide analgesia: perform intercostal nerve blocks or cryopexy and/or order a narcotic infusion.
2. Ensure that chest drains are patent and are connected to an underwater seal and suction.
3. Order arterial blood gas determinations as necessary to assess the adequacy of ventilation.
4. Ensure that chest radiography is performed, and check this for pneumothorax or atelectasis.
5. Order hemoglobin (Hb) and hematocrit (Hct) determinations to assess the adequacy of blood replacement.

MEDIASTINAL TUMORS

Relatively common tumors of the mediastinum in children include the following:

1. Lymphoma, Hodgkin's disease, etc.

2. Dermoid cysts.
3. Neuroblastoma and ganglioneuroma (*see* page 237).
4. Thymoma (less common).

These children may need general anesthesia for excision of the mediastinal tumor or for cervical node or other biopsies to establish a diagnosis.

Special Anesthetic Problems

1. Acute airway obstruction may occur during anesthesia, even in patients with no history of dyspnea. Endotracheal intubation may fail to relieve the obstruction, and endobronchial intubation may be required to maintain ventilation. This is especially likely in patients with massive enlargement of hilar glands secondary to lymphoma, etc. Even during the simple procedure of cervical node biopsy, general anesthesia may be very dangerous.
2. The hilar mass may compress the heart and cause acute hypotension.
3. Major blood loss may occur during mediastinal surgery.
4. Myasthenic patients require special consideration (*see* page 242).

Anesthetic Management

Preoperative

1. Assess the patient carefully, looking particularly for potential airway problems. Enquire about any postural dyspnea—orthopnea is a sign of potential impending disaster.
2. Complete radiologic studies and computed tomography (CT) scans to define the extent of airway compromise and potential heart and great vessel compression by the tumor mass.
3. In cases of lymphoma, steroid hormones and cytotoxic drugs should be given preoperatively. These agents usually induce rapid regression of hilar node enlargement and lessen the danger of airway obstruction or cardiac compression.
4. For mediastinal surgery, ensure that blood is available for transfusion and that serum is saved for cross-matching any necessary additional units.
5. If there is a danger of airway obstruction, do not order premedication (except atropine).
6. If airway problems are anticipated, prepare a full range of endotracheal tubes and laryngoscope blades and have a bronchoscopist available.

Perioperative

N.B. Lymph node biopsy in the child with a symptomatic large mass at the hilum may be most safely performed with a local anesthetic with the patient in the sitting position.

For general anesthesia:

1. If problems with intubation are anticipated, induce anesthesia by inhalation. Otherwise, use IV induction.
2. Establish reliable IV routes for infusion.
3. Monitor ventilation continuously and check carefully after any changes in the patient's position.
4. Maintain anesthesia with N_2O and halothane. Spontaneous ventilation may be safer for cervical node biopsy. Otherwise, controlled ventilation will be required.
5. Monitor the cardiac rhythm closely during surgical dissection.
6. At the completion of surgery, check adequacy of ventilation before extubation.

Postoperative
1. Order analgesics as required.
2. Order maintenance fluids.
3. Check Hct for adequacy of blood replacement.
4. Obtain chest radiograph in the postanesthesia room (PAR): check for pneumothorax.

Suggested Additional Reading

Azizkhan RG, DL Dudgeon, JR Buck, et al: Life threatening airway obstruction as a complication to the management of mediastinal masses in children. J Pediatr Surg 20:816–822, 1985.

Bittar D: Respiratory obstruction associated with induction of general anesthesia in patient with mediastinal Hodgkin's disease. Anesth Analg 54:399–403, 1975.

Keon TP: Death on induction of anesthesia for cervical node biopsy. Anesthesiology 55:471–472, 1981.

MYASTHENIA GRAVIS

Myasthenia gravis presents in three forms in infants and children:

1. *Transient neonatal myasthenia.* This occurs in babies of myasthenic mothers. It presents within a few hours of birth, usually with hypotonia and difficulty in feeding. Improvemement occurs within a few weeks, but therapy with anticholinesterases is needed meanwhile.
2. *Neonatal persistent myasthenia.* This appears during the first few months of life and is progressive.

3. *Juvenile myasthenia gravis.* This may be generalized or limited to the ocular muscles.

The diagnosis can usually be confirmed by testing with edrophonium.

Associated Condition
Hyperthyroidism may be present.

Surgical Procedure
Thymectomy is performed in cases of generalized myasthenia gravis, even if there is no thymoma. The best remission of symptoms is seen in young patients who have thymic hyperplasia.

Special Anesthetic Problems
1. Muscle weakness may lead to ventilatory failure.
2. Therapy with anticholinesterases increases the respiratory tract secretions, which may accumulate.
3. Potential sudden deterioration in muscle power may be due to
   (a) A myasthenic crisis or
   (b) A cholinergic crisis induced by excessive dosage with anticholinesterase.
4. Postoperative pain may limit ventilation and coughing, compounding the problem.
5. Chest physiotherapy postoperatively rapidly fatigues the patient if it is too vigorous.
6. There may be abnormal responses to neuromuscular blocking drugs.

Anesthetic Management
Preoperative
1. The patient should be admitted to hospital for a period of rest and anticholinesterase drugs should be reduced or withdrawn.
2. Ensure that blood is available for transfusion.
3. Do not give heavy premedication—*no narcotic analgesics.*

Perioperative
1. Induce anesthesia by inhalation or with a small dose of thiopental IV (3–4 mg/kg).
2. Deepen anesthesia with N_2O and halothane.
3. Do not give any muscle relaxants; intubate when the patient is adequately anesthetized with halothane and after applying topical analgesic to the larynx.

4. Control ventilation.
5. Ensure reliable IV infusion routes.
6. At the completion of surgery, allow the patient to waken and resume spontaneous ventilation with the endotracheal tube in place. Check the vital capacity; if this is adequate (>20 ml/kg), proceed with extubation.

Postoperative

1. Expert observation and respiratory care in the ICU is essential.
2. Reduce or discontinue anticholinesterase therapy (to lessen the likelihood of a cholinergic crisis).
3. Edrophonium testing should be performed periodically as a guide to anticholinesterase therapy.
4. Give narcotic analgesics only very sparingly—regional nerve block or a field block is preferable.
5. Plan physiotherapy very carefully to avoid excessive fatigue of the patient. (Time it to take advantage of the increased muscle power after each edrophonium test.)
6. If fatigue and/or serious retention of secretions occurs, perform nasotracheal intubation and institute IPPV.

Suggested Additional Reading

Davies DW, and DJ Steward: Myasthenia gravis in children and anaesthetic management of thymectomy. Can Anaesth Soc J 29:253, 1973.
Millichap JG: Myasthenia gravis. *In*: Current Pediatric Therapy, Vol. 8 (SS Gellis and BM Kagan, eds). Philadelphia, WB Saunders, 1978, p. 459.
Millichap JG, and PR Dodge: Diagnosis and treatment of myasthenia gravis in infancy, childhood, and adolescence: a study of 51 patients. Neurology 10:1007, 1960.

SPLENECTOMY

See Idiopathic Thrombocytopenic Purpura (page 120) and Trauma (page 328).

PHEOCHROMOCYTOMA

Pheochromocytomas are rare in children (<5% of all cases); when it appears, it is usually in the adrenal medulla and is bilateral in 20%. The principal symptoms are headache, nausea, and vomiting, with sustained, or, less commonly, episodic hypertension. Abdominal pain may occur, and if undiagnosed, this might prompt an unnecessary and dangerous exploratory operation in an unprepared patient. The diagnosis is confirmed by the finding of increased catecholamines (or their metabolites) in the urine. Sustained hypertension with vasoconstriction contracts the intravascular volume and elevates the Hct.

Associated Conditions

1. Neurofibromatosis.
2. Thyroid tumor.
3. Multiple endocrine adenomatoses (e.g., Sipple's syndrome).

Special Anesthetic Problems

N.B. Anaesthesia is dangerous in the unprepared patient—violent swings in BP may occur.

1. Difficulty managing the BP—keeping it down before excision of the tumor and keeping it up afterward.
2. Potential for dangerous cardiac arrhythmias (extremely rare in children).
3. Major blood loss from extensive surgery performed to locate and remove multiple tumors.
4. Necessary avoidance of anesthetic drugs that might increase the release of catecholamines (e.g., succinylcholine) or sensitize the heart to them (e.g., halothane). Pancuronium or droperidol may cause a hypertensive crisis. Drugs that release histamine should be avoided, for example, *d*-tubocurarine, atracurium.

Anesthetic Management

General anesthesia may be required for special investigations to locate the tumor as well as for its extirpation.

Preoperative

1. The patient should be treated with α-blocking drugs for several days (e.g., phenoxygenzamine HCl, 0.25–1.0 mg/kg/day), until:
   (a) BP is consistently normal.
   (b) Hct has fallen (indicating expansion of intravascular volume).
       It is not necessary to β block children, and this is contraindicated in the inevitable presence of incomplete α blockade.
2. Ensure that adequate supplies of blood for transfusion are available.
3. Check that drugs are at hand to treat any disturbance of BP or cardiac rhythm. These drugs should include the following:
   (a) Phentolamine—to lower BP: usually necessary.

(b) Propranolol—to treat arrhythmias
(c) Isoproterenol—to increase heart rate $\left.\begin{matrix} \\ \\ \end{matrix}\right\}$ seldom necessary
(d) Norepinephrine—to increase BP

4. Give premedication on the ward, for example, pentobarbital, 2–4 mg/kg orally.

Perioperative

1. If the patient appears apprehensive on arrival in the OR anteroom, give diazepam IV and wait 5 minutes before taking the patient into the OR.
2. Attach monitors.
3. Induce anesthesia IV with thiopental, 5 mg/kg, adding atropine, 0.02 mg/kg.
4. Give vecuronium, 0.1 mg/kg IV.
5. Ventilate with N_2O, O_2, and 1% isoflurane.
6. Give lidocaine, 1.5 mg/kg IV, and when the patient is fully relaxed, intubate the trachea.
7. Maintain anesthesia with N_2O, O_2, and 0.75% isoflurane, with controlled ventilation.
8. Insert arterial and central venous pressure (CVP) lines.
9. Infuse fentanyl, 5 μg/kg, when surgery commences; and continue with an infusion of 2 μg/kg/hr of fentanyl.
10. Monitor arterial and venous pressures closely throughout.
11. When the tumor has been excised:
    (a) Transfuse fluids rapidly to maintain arterial pressure. Large volumes may be required.
    (b) Maintain CVP at 9–11 cm H_2O.
    (c) If hypertension persists, suspect additional tumors.
12. When tumor(s) are out:
    (a) Discontinue isoflurane.
    (b) Continue anesthesia with N_2O, O_2, fentanyl, and vecuronium until the end of surgery.

Postoperative

1. Check blood glucose levels frequently. (Hypoglycemia may occur owing to the fall in catecholamine level and a secondary rebound hyperinsulinism.)
2. Anticipate a rise in Hct as the effect of phenoxybenzamine wears off.
3. Order analgesics as required.
4. Order maintenance IV fluids; these should contain added dextrose.

Suggested Additional Reading

Bittar DA: Innovar induced hypertensive crises in patients with phaeo-chromocytoma. Anesthesiology 50:366, 1979.

Channa AB, AB Mofti, GM Taylor, MO Mekki, and MH Sheikh: Hypoglycaemic encephalopathy following surgery on phaeochromocytoma. Anaesthesia 42:1298–1301, 1987.

Jones RB, and AB Hill: Severe hypertension associated with pancuronium in a patient with pheochromocytoma. Can Anaesth Soc J 28:394, 1981.

Perry LB, and AB Gould, Jr: The anesthetic management of pheochromocytoma: effect of preoperative adrenergic blocking drugs. Anesth Analg 51:36, 1972.

Pullerits J, and JW Balfe: Anaesthesia for phaeochromocytoma. Can J Anaesth 35:526–533, 1988.

Stringel G, SH Ein, RE Creighton, D Daneman, N Howard, and RM Filler: Pheochromocytoma in children—an update. J Pediatr Surg 15:496, 1980.

WILMS' TUMOR

Wilms' tumors constitute 50% of the retroperitoneal masses in children and cause 6–8% of deaths from cancer in children under 12 years of age. They vary histologically but may grow large and usually present as an abdominal mass. Five percent are bilateral. Abdominal pain and fever are common symptoms. Hypertension may develop, possibly owing to ischemia of renal tissue adjacent to the tumor, but the BP may remain elevated after removal of the entire affected kidney.

Associated Conditions

1. Hemihypertrophy.
2. The Beckwith-Wiedemann syndrome.
3. Neurofibromatosis.

Special Anesthetic Problems

1. Massive blood loss may occur during surgery.
2. Surgical manipulations may kink the IVC and cause abrupt falls in cardiac output.
3. A thoracoabdominal approach may be required for large tumors. Whole body radiation may impair pulmonary function.
4. The child may have severe hypertension (rare).
5. Rarely, tumor may invade IVC and embolize during operation.
6. A coagulopathy, acquired von Willebrand's disease, may occur in association with Wilms' tumor. This improves after resection of the

tumor. Factor VIII concentrates may be required to reduce the bleeding time.

Anesthetic Management

Preoperative

1. Check that blood is available for transfusion (at least 2,000 ml) and that serum is saved for further cross-matching.
2. Be prepared for probable massive transfusion; check coagulation.
3. Do not palpate the patient's abdomen.

Perioperative

1. Induce anesthesia and apply monitors.
2. Start an IV infusion into an upper limb vein with a large-bore cannula (at least 18 gauge).
3. Maintain anesthesia with N_2O and isoflurane and a relaxant (atracurium preferred.)
4. Watch for an abrupt fall in BP (owing to surgical manipulation around the IVC causing kinking). Notify the surgeon immediately if this occurs.
5. If hypertension is a problem (unusual), control it by increasing the inspired isoflurane concentration.

Note. Significant blood losses may occur during wound closure: continue transfusion to match losses. (Do not relax as soon as the tumor is out.)

Postoperative

1. Hypertension may continue and require therapy (e.g., hydralazine).
2. Blood loss into the wound may continue, requiring continued tranfusion.

Suggested Additional Reading

Cobb ML, and RW Vaughan: Severe hypertension in a child with Wilms' tumor: a case report. Anesth Analg 55:519, 1976.

Jenking RDT: The treatment of Wilms' tumor. Pediatr Clin North Am 23:147, 1976.

Noronha PA, MA Hruby, and HS Maurer: Aquired von Willebrand disease in a patient with Wilms' tumor. J Pediatr 95:997–999, 1979.

"ACUTE ABDOMEN"

In children, an "acute abdomen" most commonly represents acute appendicitis, intussusception, or perforated Meckel's diverticulum.

SPECIAL ANESTHETIC PROBLEMS

1. Full stomach: even if the child has not eaten or drunk for several hours (and even if the child has vomited), do not assume that the stomach is empty. Gastric secretions accumulate rapidly when intestinal ileus is present.
2. Fluid and electrolyte disturbances may occur secondary to vomiting.
3. The patient may have a high temperature.

Anesthetic Management
Preoperative
1. Assess the patient's general condition carefully. Check the fluid intake, serum electrolytes, and urine output. Ensure that fluid replacement is sufficient to correct deficits and produce good urine output.
2. If the patient's temperature is elevated, the patient must not be given atropine intramuscularly (IM).
3. Prepare and check all equipment for a "crash induction" and have suitable assistance available.

Perioperative
1. Check that a reliable IV route is available.
2. Attach monitors.
3. Give 100% O_2 for 4 minutes.
4. Inject induction drugs directly into a free-running IV line: thiopental with atropine, followed immediately by succinylcholine.
5. Have an assistant apply cricoid pressure.
6. Do not ventilate via mask.
7. Insert an endotracheal tube as soon as the patient has fasciculated.
8. Maintain anesthesia with N_2O and halothane with a nondepolarizing muscle relaxant.
9. At the end of surgery, withdraw all anesthetic agents, reverse the relaxants, and ensure that the patient is fully awake.
10. Place the patient in a lateral position for extubation.

Postoperative
1. Order analgesics as required.
2. Order maintenance fluids to be given IV.

TORSION OF TESTIS

Testicular torsion requires immediate surgery. Therefore, in most cases it is not possible to prepare the patient. It is important to note that the volume and concents of the stomach in these patients are similar to those of the child with an acute abdomen; therefore, beware at induction.

Anesthetic Management

Preoperative

1. Prepare and check all equipment for a "crash" induction and have suitable assistance available.

Perioperative and Postoperative

1. As for "Acute Abdomen" (*see* page 248).

COMMON MINOR SURGICAL PROCEDURES

Note. Some children who require elective surgery have conditions that may complicate anesthesia:

1. Anemia detected at preoperative examination. (Remember, however, that the Hb level is normally at its lowest at 3 months of age.)
   (a) If the Hb level is below 10.0 g/dl, surgery should be deferred until the anemia has been investigated and treated. Transfusion should not be necessary preoperatively.
   (b) If surgery cannot be deferred (e.g., irreducible incarcerated hernia), use an anesthetic technique suitable to the patient's anemic state (*see* page 114). If the Hb level is very low, order a transfusion of packed cells to be given preoperatively.
2. History of prematurity and respiratory distress syndrome. These infants must not be considered absolutely normal, even if they are now apparently healthy. Pulmonary function is impaired during at least the first year of life. Apnea may occur postoperatively, especially in infants who are still under 45 weeks of postconceptual age.

DIVISION OF "TONGUE-TIE"

If the frenulum is so short that the patient has difficulty passing the tongue around the buccal sulcus, surgical division of the "tongue-tie" probably is advised. This is usually done as an outpatient procedure.

Special Anesthetic Problem

1. This is a very minor procedure, but the surgeon must have good access to the oral cavity.

Anesthetic Management
Preoperative
1. Premedication: order tropine only; preferably, give it IV at induction.

Perioperative
1. Induce anesthesia with thiopental with atropine followed by succinyl-choline.
2. Intubate and maintain anesthesia with halothane in 50% N_2O with O_2.
3. Suction the pharynx to remove blood. Apply lidocaine gel to the wound.
4. The patient should be fully awake before extubation and transfer to the PAR.

Postoperative
1. Further analgesics are not usually required.

INGUINAL HERNIOTOMY

Inguinal hernia is common during childhood, usually a result of patent processus vaginalis; its repair is the commonest elective general surgical procedure in children. Because these hernias readily become incarcerated during the first year of life, their repair should not be unduly delayed in this age group. Once incarceration has occurred, conservative treatment is usually instituted. Virtually all of these hernias can be reduced, and then, after 24–48 hours, herniotomy can be performed.

If emergency surgery is to be performed as an outpatient procedure, select suitable anesthetic techniques (*see* page 106).

Anesthetic Management
Preoperative
1. Assess the patient's general condition carefully.
2. Infants with a history of prematurity should be admitted for monitoring postoperatively.
3. All patients: give atropine IV at induction.

Perioperative
N.B. The small preterm infant may benefit from spinal analgesia for her-niotomy, especially if there is a history of residual pulmonary disease (*see* page 104).

Otherwise, for general anesthesia:

1. Induce anesthesia: by inhalation, rectal methohexital, or thiopental IV followed by succinylcholine.

2. Intubate and maintain anesthesia with N_2O and halothane.
3. Perform an ilioinguinal and iliohypogastric nerve block on the operative side(s).
4. Ensure that analgesia is adequate before allowing surgery to commence and during traction on the peritoneum.

Postoperative
1. Order additional analgesics as required; usually, acetaminophen, 10 mg/kg, is adequate.

Suggested Additional Reading

Langer JC, B Shandling, and M Rosenberg: Intraoperative bupivacaine during outpatient hernia repair in children: a randomised double blind trial. J Pediatr Surg 22:267–270, 1987.

ORCHIDOPEXY

Anesthetic management for orchidopexy is as for inguinal herniotomy (*see* page 251).

CIRCUMCISION

Indications for circumcision vary in different communities and from time to time. It remains a common (often outpatient) procedure in pediatric surgery.

Special Anesthetic Problem
1. Management of postoperative pain.

Anesthetic Management
Preoperative
1. Assess the patient's general condition carefully.

Perioperative
1. Induce and maintain anesthesia as for herniotomy (*see* page 251).
2. Provide for analgesia postoperatively. Perform:
    (a) Block of dorsal nerve of penis with 0.25% bupivacaine (Marcaine) without epinephrine: maximal dose 2 mg/kg. Or:
    (b) Apply lidocaine jelly to the wound.

Postoperative
1. If regional anesthesia is unsatisfactory: order narcotic analgesic (e.g., codeine, 1.5 mg/kg IM, which can be repeated in 4 hours if necessary).

Suggested Additional Reading

Bacon AK: An alternative block for post-circumcision analgesia. Anaesth Intensive Care 5:63, 1977.

Tree-Trakarn T, and S Pirayavaraporn: Postoperative pain relief after circumcision: comparison among morphine, nerve block, and topical analgeisa. Anesthesiology 62:519–522, 1985.

NEONATAL NECROTIZING ENTEROCOLITIS

Neonatal necrotizing enterocolitis, a disease of low-birth-weight infants (usually <34 weeks' gestation), is characterized by intestinal mucosal injury secondary to ischemia of the bowel. It may lead to perforation and peritonitis. Severe fluid and electrolyte disturbance, endotoxic shock, and coagulopathy resulting from thrombocytopenia may develop. The etiology is uncertain, but the disease usually affects infants with a history of birth asphyxia, respiratory distress syndrome, and shock. Umbilical artery catheterization and enteral feeding may be etiologic factors. The clinical picture is of abdominal distention, bloody diarrhea, temperature instability, and lethargy; apnea may occur. Abdominal radiographs may show intramural bowel or portal venous gas.

Special Anesthetic Problems

1. Prematurity and respiratory distress.
2. Shock, hypovolemia, and electrolyte disturbance.
3. Sepsis, acidosis, and coagulopathy.
4. Interstitial gas in the bowel wall.
5. Antibiotics may interact with relaxant drugs.

Anesthetic Management

Preoperative

1. Restore blood and fluid volumes: blood, plasma, and crystalloid solutions may be required.
2. Check coagulation: thrombocytopenia must be corrected by blood and platelet infusions.
3. Exchange transfusion may be required. Correct the acid-base status.
4. Monitor carefully for apnea.

Perioperative

1. Observe all special precautions for the premature infant (*see* page 96).
2. Perform awake intubation if not yet intubated.

3. Fentanyl in an appropriate concentration of oxygen is preferred. (Do not use N_2O, as this may expand intramural bowel gas.)
4. Administer small doses of vecuronium as required for relaxation.
5. Continue fluid resuscitation throughout surgery as dictated by clinical status and laboratory studies.

Postoperative
1. Return the patient to the neonatal ICU for continued respiratory care.

Suggested Additional Reading
Brown EG, and AY Sweet: Neonatal necrotizing enterocolitis. Pediatr Clin North Am 29:1149, 1982.
Haselby KA, SF Dierdorf, G Krishna, CC Rao, TM Wolfe, and WL McNiece: Anaesthetic implications of neonatal necrotizing enterocolitis. Can Anaesth Soc J 29:255, 1982.

ORGAN TRANSPLANTATION

Transplantation of solid organs is now becoming commonplace in pediatric practice. Though transplantation (apart from renal) is limited to a few specialist centers, organ procurement may be performed in many hospitals. The anesthesiologist has a major role to play in the care of the donor, to ensure that donated organs remain in optimal condition until harvesting.

CARE OF THE DONOR

When cerebral death occurs, a sequence of physiologic changes follows throughout the body that may compromise the survival of organs destined for transplantation. Hence, intensive measures to support these organs are indicated—this will involve the anesthesiologist caring for the donor during organ retrieval.

Following cerebral death, widespread vasodilation occurs and the patient tends to become pink and hypotensive. This hypotension may be compounded by hypovolemia secondary to the use of diuretics for previous attempts at cerebral resuscitation.

1. Restoration of the circulating volume should be rapidly performed. Large volumes of fluid may be required (20–40 ml/kg).
   (a) Lactated Ringer solution and 5% dextrose in normal saline. Use 5% dextrose in water if Na >150 mEq/L.

(b) Five percent albumin for refractory hypotension.

(c) Packed red blood cells for Hct <30.

Adequate volume expansion is indicated by a CVP >8 cm H_2O and a continuing satisfactory urine output.

2. If hypotension persists despite adequate volume expansion, then vasopressor therapy should be commenced.

(a) Dopamine is the drug of choice, in a dose of 5–15 μg/kg/min.

3. Renal function should be maintained by fluid loading.

(a) If urine output drops below 2 ml/kg/hr, give furosemide, 1 mg/kg, as necessary.

(b) Diabetes insipidus frequently occurs in brain-dead donors. High urine output may lead to hypovolemia, hypernatremia, and hypokalemia.

(i) DDAVP (desmopressin) 1–4 μg, may be given IV, or

(ii) a Pitressin (vasopressin) infusion, 0.01–0.02 units/kg/hr, titrated to maintain the desired output.

4. Hepatic function should be preserved by maintaining oxygenation and perfusion.

Additional measures to maintain the donor include

1. Measure esophageal and rectal temperature and maintain normal body temperature.

2. Frequent determination and correction of acid-base and electrolyte status.

3. Continued optimal ventilation; beware of pulmonary changes.

4. Careful aseptic technique. Prophylactic antibiotics may be used. Blood cultures are taken immediately prior to harvesting.

All of the above measures should be continued throughout the surgical procedure of organ procurement.

Suggested Additional Reading

Jordan CA, and JV Snyder: Intensive care and intraoperative management of the brain dead organ donor. Transplant Proc 19(suppl 3):21–25, 1987.

11

Cardiac Surgery and Cardiologic Procedures

Heart surgery in children is performed almost exclusively for congenital heart disease (CHD). The incidence of CHD is approximately 6 in 1,000 live births. The lesions listed in Table 11-1 account for almost 90% of all congenital heart defects.

THE CHILD WITH CONGENITAL HEART DISEASE (CHD)

Children with CHD usually present with dyspnea, cyanosis, or failure to thrive. Severe malformations may cause gross cardiac failure during the neonatal period. Cardiac failure results from the high pressures needed to compensate for obstruction (valve stenosis or coarctation) or high-volume flow through intracardiac (ventricular septal defect [VSD]) or extracradiac shunts (patent ductus arteriosus [PDA]). Dyspnea may result from cardiac failure or changes in pulmonary blood flow. Older infants and children with CHD are very prone to repeated respiratory infections.

Conditions that cause increased blood flow to the lungs, if uncorrected, eventually result in irreversible pulmonary hypertension. This may be prevented by pulmonary artery banding or radical repair during early life. Cyanotic conditions induce a series of compensatory changes in blood (principally polycythemia) that may also lead to complications (*see* page 262).

GENERAL PRINCIPLES

When appropriate, *see also* Special Considerations for Anesthesia of Neonates, pages 94 and 96.

1. The techniques used must minimize demands on the cardiovascular system (CVS).
   (a) Give adequate premedication to reduce anxiety, activity, and O_2 requirements.
   (b) Ensure rapid, smooth induction of anesthesia, with no crying or struggling.
   (c) Give adequate doses of analgesics or general anesthetic agents perioperatively. Prevent tachycardia and/or hypertension. High-dose narcotic anesthesia may also favorably influence the neuroendocrine and metabolic responses to surgery.

TABLE 11-1.   TYPES OF CONGENITAL HEART DEFECTS

Type	Lesion	Incidence (%)
Left-to-right shunt (acyanotic)	Ventricular septal defect	25
	Patent ductus arteriosus	17
	Atrial septal defect	7
Cyanotic	Tetralogy of Fallot	11
	Transposition of the great vessels	8
	Tricuspid atresia	3
Obstructive	Pulmonary stenosis	7
	Coarctation of the aorta	6
	Aortic stenosis	4

    (d) Apply controlled ventilation but maintain normocarbia.

    (e) Give adequate doses of muscle relaxants to prevent any risk of movement or ventilation.

    (f) When appropriate consider left ventricular (LV) afterload reduction and/or measures to reduce pulmonary vascular resistance (see below).

2. Optimal myocardial function and cardiac output must be maintained during surgery.

    (a) Do not give agents that cause excessive myocardial depression.

    (b) Adjust the fluid balance to provide optimal cardiac filling pressures.

    (c) Avoid producing hypocarbia, which:

        (i) Reduces cardiac output.

        (ii) Causes vasoconstriction and increases systemic resistance.

        (iii) Shifts the hemoglobin-oxygen (Hb-O_2) dissociation curve to the left.

        (iv) Decreases myocardial blood flow.

        (v) Decreases the serum K level.

        (vi) Favors development of arrhythmias.

        (vii) Decreases cerebral blood flow.

    (d) Serial measurements of all relevant indices, including blood gas analyses, should be made throughout surgery to achieve these objectives.

3. Detrimental changes in cardiac shunts must be prevented.

    (a) Use drugs that have minimal effects on peripheral vascular resistance.

(b) Be aware of the possible effects of intermittent positive-pressure ventilation (IPPV) on shunts; avoid high intrathoracic pressures, but maintain the lung volume as necessary by the use of positive end-expiratory pressure (PEEP). Pulmonary vascular resistance is least at an optimal lung volume and will increase at volumes above or below this optimal level.

(c) Drugs that produce a controllable degree of myocardial depression (e.g., halothane) may be useful when there is ventricular muscle obstructing blood flow (e.g., tetralogy of Fallot).

(d) Patients who are dependent on systemic-to-pulmonary shunts will desaturate if the systemic arterial pressure is allowed to fall.

4. Conditions that favor optimal myocardial perfusion must be maintained throughout surgery to avoid ischemic damage to the heart and subsequent impairment of cardiac function postoperatively. The duration of diastole and the diastolic pressure are important factors in maintaining perfusion of the myocardium, which is especially vulnerable if ventricular hypertrophy is present. Avoid producing tachycardia, which shortens diastole and thus may impair myocardial perfusion. Replace blood and give adequate fluids to maintain the diastolic pressure.

   During cardiopulmonary bypass (CPB) it is preferable to maintain a regular rhythm until aortic cross-clamping and cardioplegia administration. If ventricular fibrillation occurs, higher perfusion pressures are needed to ensure myocardial perfusion.

5. The cardiac work load must be minimized.
   (a) Prevent hypertension and tachycardia during anesthesia by ensuring adequate levels of analgesia and by use of vasodilators and/or β-adrenergic blockers when appropriate.
   (b) Do not give drugs that may produce hypertension (e.g., pancuronium).
   (c) Pulmonary hypertension must be controlled.

6. Heparin has a larger volume of distribution and a more rapid plasma clearance in infants compared with adults. Therefore, larger doses may be required initially and the level of heparinization should be checked frequently (every 30 minutes).

7. During CPB the myocardium may be protected by:
   (a) Cardioplegic solutions that are infused at a pressure of 100–150 mmHg into the coronary circulation following aortic clamping. Controversy exists about the most advantageous type of solution, but most contain high levels of potassium with added dextrose and buffers. The addition of free radical scavenger agents and calcium

ion channel blockers has been suggested. Repeated doses of cardioplegia are normally used at 15–20 minute intervals.

(b) Hypothermia—but remember that the heart has a great tendency to rewarm because of manipulation and heat from operating room (OR) lights. Therefore, during prolonged surgery, cold cardioplegic solutions should be repeated and a pericardial cooling bath used.

(c) Pre-bypass systemic corticosteroids may help preserve myocardial tissue during ischemic arrest periods, but this is controversial.

(d) An optimal reperfusate solution may be used following a period of ischemic arrest. This solution should be cold and alkaline and should contain a low concentration of ionized calcium and a slightly elevated potassium level. In practice, a repeat dose of cardioplegia is often given just before reperfusion.

SPECIAL PROBLEMS

1. *Large shunts* may be present.
   Right-to-left (R→L) shunts result in:
   (a) Low arterial O_2 tension—only minimally improved by increasing the FIO_2.
   (b) Delayed uptake of inhaled anesthetic agents.
   (c) Extreme danger of systemic emboli from venous air embolism.
   (d) Short arm-brain circulation time.
   (e) Danger of overdose with intravenous (IV) drugs.
   (f) Less efficient ventilation and gas exchange (large $PaCO_2$ − $PeCO_2$)

   Left-to-right (L→R) shunts result in:
   (a) Pulmonary vascular overperfusion, but good ventilatory efficiency and gas exchange initially.
   (b) Later pulmonary hypertension and congestive heart failure (eventually).

2. *Obstructive lesions* may result in:
   (a) Fixed cardiac output—and therefore the inability to compensate for changes in metabolic demand or peripheral vascular resistance.
   (b) Myocardial hypertrophy, with possible inadequacy of myocardial perfusion, especially to the subendocardium.
   (c) Congestive heart failure.
   (d) Sudden serious arrhythmias.

3. *Heart failure* is common in infants with CHD and is worsened by drugs that depress the myocardium (e.g., halothane).

4. *Electrolyte disturbance.*
   (a) Serum electrolyte (especially K^+) levels may be low, particularly in patients who have had prolonged diuretic therapy. (Hypokalemia predisposes to cardiac arrhythmias, particularly during hypothermia.)
   (b) Neonates with CHD may have low Ca^{2+} and glucose levels.
5. *Drugs* essential for CHD therapy may cause problems.
   (a) Digitalis: the therapeutic index is low—toxicity is an everpresent hazard, especially in young children. Hypothermia increases the risk of digitalis toxicity since the K^+ level will fall.
   (b) Diuretics: may deplete K^+, further increasing the risk of digitalis toxicity.
   (c) β-adrenergic blocking agents: may impair cardiac contractility. This is not usually a problem.
6. *Polycythemia.* A high hematocrit (Hct) level (over 55) (in cyanotic lesions) results in:
   (a) Increased viscosity of the blood, and therefore increased cardiac work.
   (b) Increased tendency to thrombosis.
   (c) Increased risk of thrombosis if dehydration or venous stasis develops.
   (d) Possible coagulopathy—primarily thrombocytopenia.
   (e) Predisposition to cerebral abscess.
   Despite the dangers of polycythemia, these children are very dependent on a high Hct to ensure adequate O_2 transport. Hemodilution to normal Hct levels may be followed by severe cardiovascular collapse. Lowering the Hct may also lead to increased R→L shunt. Hemodilution, if considered to be indicated, must be very carefully controlled and not taken to a Hct below 50.
7. Some patients with large L→R shunts are at risk of pulmonary hypertensive crises during and after surgery (e.g., VSD, truncus, arterioventricular canal). It is important to prevent these because they are difficult to reverse. The standard measures that are taken may include
   (a) Minimal handling of the child.
   (b) Controlled hyperventilation ($PaCO_2$ = 25–30).
   (c) Fentanyl infusion (e.g., 25 μg/kg loading dose plus 2 μg/kg/hr).
   (d) Sodium nitroprusside (SNP) infusion.
   (e) Phenoxybenzamine: 1 mg/kg loading dose followed by 1 mg/kg/day in divided doses.
   (f) Prostaglandin E_1 (PGE_1) infusion, 0.03–0.1 μg/kg/min.
   (g) Avoidance of nitrous oxide.

8. Some infants may be dependent on the patency of the ductus arteriosus as a route for shunting of blood until surgery can be performed (e.g., transposition of great arteries with intact septum, interrupted aortic arch). PGE_1 is used to keep the ductus open in such infants. An infusion of 0.03–0.1 μg/kg/min should be continued until the appropriate surgical procedure is completed.

9. *Associated malformations.* Many children with CHD have additional defects (e.g., cleft palate, Down syndrome, subglottic stenosis).

10. *Method of induction:* different methods do not seem to have markedly different effects on the oxygen saturation—even in cyanotic patients. Hence, the anesthesiologist should practice whatever he does best and seems most appropriate for a given patient.

11. *Muscle relaxants.* Nondepolarizing agents may take longer to have their full effect in patients with CHD; hence, a longer period of mask ventilation should be applied before attempting intubation.

12. *Temperature control* may be especially poor in neonates with cyanotic CHD as they cannot respond to heat losses as well as normal infants. Body temperature will fall rapidly if they are exposed to a cool environment.

13. *Sepsis* is a major threat to the success of cardiac surgery. Great care must be taken to observe strict asepsis when inserting invasive monitoring or infusion lines.

14. *Repeated surgery.* Some children need repeated surgery, which imposes a severe psychological stress on them and their parents. A very considerate, careful approach by the anesthesiologist is essential.

ROUTINE PRE-, PERI-, AND POSTOPERATIVE CARE

When appropriate, *see also* Special Considerations for Anesthesia of Neonates and Preterm Infants, pages 94 and 96.

PREOPERATIVE ASSESSMENT AND PREPARATION

Perform an independent physical examination, especially of the CVS and respiratory system, ear, nose, throat, teeth, and veins. Review the cardiology notes, echocardiogram, cardiac catheterization, and angiogram data. Note salient abnormalities and findings on the anesthesia chart. If the child has had a recent respiratory infection, elective surgery should be postponed for 2–3 weeks.

For children over 2–3 years of age, ensure that they have had explained to them the use of oxygen tent, IV lines, chest drains, sedation, and (when indicated) controlled ventilation.

Many patients with CHD take several medications regularly. Propranolol and other β-blockers should be discontinued the night before surgery. With rare exceptions, digitalis and diuretics should be withheld on the day of surgery.

If the patient requires O_2 therapy and/or maintenance of the sitting position during transit to the OR, order these specifically.

BLOOD SUPPLIES

During any type of cardiac surgery, blood must be immediately available (hanging or in the OR refrigerator). In many centers, ordering blood is the responsibility of the surgical service. However, the day before surgery the anesthesiologist should ensure that adequate supplies of blood and blood products will be available by operation time.

Some patients have special requirements, for example:

1. For cyanotic patients with a Hb >16 g/dl, plasma should be available.
2. For all infants, check that the blood to be supplied is less than 5 days old and tested for cytomegalovirus.
3. For infants undergoing CPB, ensure that packed cells, fresh-frozen plasma, and platelets (1 unit/5 kg) have been ordered.
4. For all children likely to require prolonged CPB (>1.5 hours), ensure that fresh-frozen plasma and platelets have been ordered.
5. For older children and those with initial high Hct, the "cell saver" may be used to conserve blood, and in many of these children having relatively "minor" surgery, blood transfusion may be avoided.

PREMEDICATION

Children with CHD require adequate preoperative sedation to reduce excitement, anxiety, and crying (and thus reduce O_2 consumption). Therefore, order a barbiturate for the evening before surgery for children over 8 years of age or who display anxiety and preoperative sedation for all children over 1 year or weighing more than 9 kg.

1. Children under 1 year of age or weighing <9 kg:
   (a) Atropine alone, to be given intramuscularly (IM) 30 minutes preoperatively.

2. Older children:
   (a) Pentobarbital: 2 mg/kg to be given 1.5 hours preoperatively—per rectum to children under 4 years and orally (PO) with a sip of water to older children.
   (b) Morphine: 0.2 mg/kg IM 1 hour preoperatively, *mixed with* (c).
   (c) Atropine in usual dosage to be given IM. (The tachycardia following IV administration is undesirable in patients with CHD.) This regimen of premedication does not cause significant falls in oxygen saturation levels preoperatively, even in the cyanotic patient.
3. For cyanotic children with a high Hct (>16), order maintenance IV fluids while ordering nothing by mouth prior to surgery.

Routine Anesthetic Management

Preoperative

1. Check all anesthesia and monitoring equipment before having the patient brought into the OR.
2. Prepare for use, in case of emergency, syringes containing the following drugs:
   (a) Sodium bicarbonate 7.5% solution: 20 ml.
   (b) Atropine solution diluted to 0.1 mg/ml: 4 ml.
   (c) Calcium gluconate 10% solution: 10 ml.
   (d) Epinephrine 1:10,000: 10 ml.
3. Check that preoperative medication has been given as ordered.
4. Apply monitors: precordial stethoscope, blood pressure (BP) cuff, electrocardiogram (ECG; use adhesive electrodes), and pulse oximeter. Record heart rate and rhythm and BP.

Perioperative

1. Administer oxygen by mask. Often the child will be happier if this is held slightly away from the face: use a high flow.
2. Induce anesthesia preferably IV (particularly in patients with a R→L shunt, which slows inhalation induction). For most patients, thiopental given slowly IV (2 to 4 mg/kg) produces a smooth induction with minimal cardiovascular effects. Otherwise, for the very unstable patient, fentanyl up to 30 μg/kg IV and diazepam up to 0.2 mg IV may be administered for induction.
3. Drugs given IV should be administered in small doses, *slowly*. (If a R→L shunt is present, they act very rapidly, but if the circulation time is slow, their effect may be less rapid.)
4. For intubation:

(a) Give succinylcholine, 1 mg/kg IV. If the circulation time is slow (so that the drug is partly metabolized before reaching the muscles), double the dose (2 mg/kg IV).

OR:

(b) Give an initial dose of nondepolarizing relaxant and ventilate the patient until relaxation is adequate; vecuronium, 0.1 mg/kg, produces good conditions for intubation within 2 minutes (see also item 10, below).

5. Use a cuffed endotracheal tube if size 6 mm or larger is required.
6. Insert an esophageal stethoscope and esophageal and rectal thermometers.
7. Maintain anesthesia with a suitable mixture of N_2O and O_2. (It is rarely necessary to use more than 50% O_2. If a large R→L shunt is present, increasing the F_IO_2 will have very little effect on the PaO_2.) Avoid N_2O in the patient with pulmonary hypertension.
8. If myocardial function is good, use isoflurane (0.5–0.75%). Otherwise, add narcotics (e.g., fentanyl or sufentanil).
9. Control ventilation but avoid respiratory alkalosis, which reduces cardiac output, impairs myocardial blood flow, and may cause arrhythmia. $PaCO_2$ should be in the physiologic range (35–40 mmHg). Note that end-tidal CO_2 is a satisfactory means to means to monitor $PaCO_2$ in acyanotic patients but may underestimate the $PaCO_2$ in children with cyanotic CHD.
10. The choice of muscle relaxant for use during maintenance of anesthesia should be influenced by the following:
    (a) Vecuronium has very little effect on cardiovascular parameters and is probably the agent of choice for most infants and some children.
    (b) If some decrease in afterload might be advantageous, d-tubocurarine is still a very useful drug.

Therefore:

    (i) If a mild degree of hypotension and afterload reduction may be advantageous, use d-tubocurarine.
    (ii) For least change in CVS indices, use vecuronium.

11. Give maintenance fluids as outlined on page 268. Many of these children are polycythemic preoperatively, in which case plasma is preferable to blood as replacement fluid. A Hct of 35–40% by the end of surgery is usually desirable.
12. Use a blood warmer for all infusions.

At End of Operation. The following is only a brief outline of the extreme care necessary in the postoperative management of all patients who have undergone cardiac surgery. For detailed information, the anesthesiologist should consult a standard text on postoperative cardiac care [*see also* Postoperative (in the Intensive Care Unit), page 268].

1. Plan to continue artificial ventilation for patients who have:
   (a) Hypoxemia despite a high FiO_2.
   (b) Low cardiac output (*see also* Postoperative, page 269).
   (c) Pulmonary hypertension.
   (d) Diminished lung compliance.
   (e) Persistent arrhythmias.
   (f) Hypothermia (below 34°C).
   (g) Continuing hemorrhage.
Also:
   (h) If you have any doubt about the patient's ability to maintain adequate ventilation.
Note. Many other patients also may benefit from a period of mechanical ventilation during the immediate postoperative period. This permits the more liberal use of narcotic analgesics and hence a more comfortable early recovery phase.

2. If IPPV is to be continued:
   (a) Change to a nasotracheal tube if the patient's condition is judged stable enough to tolerate it. (During some types of surgery, blood-stained secretions may accumulate in the tube. Hence, the change is advisable to provide the child with a clean tube at the start of IPPV in the intensive care unit [ICU].)
   (b) Otherwise, continue ventilation via the orotracheal tube.
Note. It is preferable to change tubes at the end of the procedure, rather than pass a nasotracheal tube initially (which could cause nosebleed perioperatively, especially if the patient is heparinized).

3. During transportation:
   (a) Give oxygen by mask, or if the patient is still intubated, continue controlled ventilation with O_2. Make sure that an adequate supply of O_2 is available for the journey to the ICU. Monitor with a portable pulse oximeter if available.
   (b) Use a portable monitor for the ECG and arterial pressure.
   (c) Leave the Doppler flowmeter in place over the radial artery to continuously monitor the pulse.
   (d) Continue the infusions of inotropic drugs and/or vasodilators with a battery-powered syringe pump. Beware of interruptions to the flow of these drugs during and following transport to the ICU.

Postoperative (in the Intensive Care Unit)

1. Ensure that the patient's ventilation is adequate on the ventilator by auscultating the chest. Order a suitable inspired O_2 concentration and confirm ventilation and oxygenation by blood gas determination as soon as the patient is settled.

2. Order a narcotic analgesic and sedative drugs:
   (a) Morphine may be given IV q2h or, preferably, as a continuous infusion (rate 10–30 μg/kg/min).
   (b) Diazepam, 0.1 mg/kg IV q2h as needed, or midazolam infusion (*see* page 49)

3. Order maintenance fluids: 5% dextrose with 0.3 N saline initially (with added KCl, 2 mEq/kg/24 hr—provided urine output is 1 ml/kg/hr or more; otherwise, withhold the KCl).

4. Check blood loss via drainage tubes; instruct the nurses to replace this and further losses with "whole blood."

5. If bleeding persists, order coagulation studies. Based on the results of these, administer fresh frozen plasma or platelet concentrates as indicated.

PRINCIPLES OF POSTOPERATIVE CARDIAC CARE

RESPIRATORY SYSTEM

The status of the respiratory system following cardiac surgery in infants and children may be determined by the following factors:

1. Pre-existing status.
   (a) Immaturity of respiratory system in young patients (especially infants).
   (b) Effects of the cardiac disease on the lungs (e.g., hyperperfusion).
2. Effects of anesthesia, operation, and CPB.
   (a) Decreased lung volume.
   (b) Increased lung water.

Therefore, most children benefit from a period of controlled ventilation and/or PEEP or constant positive airway pressure (CPAP). This assists in restoring the lung volume to normal and improves gas exchange. Levels of added oxygen and PEEP or CPAP can be reduced as the pulmonary status improves. Diuretic therapy may be indicated to reduce lung water. Special measures to control pulmonary vascular resistance (PVR) may be required in patients with pulmonary hypertension (*See* page 262).

CARDIOVASCULAR SYSTEM

After cardiac surgery, the cardiovascular status is determined by:

1. Pre-existing status.
   (a) Immaturity of the heart and circulatory system in infants (*see* page 22).
   (b) Effects of the cardiac disease on the CVS.
2. Effects of anesthesia, surgery, and CPB. These are dictated by:
   (a) The duration of anesthesia and surgery.
   (b) The duration of CPB.
   (c) The duration of induced cardiac arrest.
   (d) The success of myocardial protection techniques (*see* page 260).

After all but the most minor cardiac operations, a deterioration in cardiac function is to be expected. This deterioration progresses for the first few hours after surgery, probably associated with edema of the myocardium and other changes. The result is a decrease in compliance of the ventricles and a decrease in contractility. Therapy at this time must be directed to:

1. Ensuring optimal filling pressures. As the compliance of the ventricles is low in infancy and reduced in all patients after cardiac surgery, high filling pressures (8–12 mmHg) will probably be required.
2. Producing an optimal cardiac rate and rhythm. This is most effectively achieved by the use of sequential pacing when necessary. Sinus rhythm (i.e., atrial contraction) significantly augments cardiac output.
3. Reducing the afterload. The use of vasodilators in patients with ventricular dysfunction increases cardiac output, with little change in cardiac work or arterial BP. When vasodilators are used, the preload must be maintained by infusion of appropriate fluids; SNP infusion is commonly used to produce vasodilation (infusion rates start at 1–2 μg/kg/min and increase up to 5 μg/kg/min. Alternatively, phenoxybenzamine may be administered to produce a long-lasting adrenergic blockade. Some patients will not tolerate LV afterload reduction well, for example, those with impaired right ventricular function, (e.g. following tetralogy repair).
4. Inotropic agents: If a low cardiac output persists despite the above measures, resorting to an inotropic agent becomes necessary:
   (a) Dopamine is infused at 5–10 μg/kg/min by infusion pump. In infants and children, dopamine has been shown effective in increasing cardiac output, *but*
      (i) Higher doses are required than in adults.

(ii) The vasodilating effect is less than in adults. Hence the concurrent infusion of a vasodilator (SNP) is usually warranted. The combined administration of dopamine and SNP may also be effective in reducing PVR in patients with pulmonary hypertension but must often be given as soon as the patient is weaned from bypass.

(b) Calcium is infused to maintain the serum Ca^{2+} at a high normal level (1–1.2 mmol/dl).

(c) If serious low output persists despite the above, an epinephrine infusion of 0.05–1 μg/kg/min may be needed.

FLUID AND ELECTROLYTE THERAPY

1. Blood should be administered to maintain the Hb level at near-normal levels (14–15 g/dl), especially when cardiac dysfunction is present.

2. Acid-base status should be monitored and acidosis corrected by sodium bicarbonate infusions.

3. Dextrose-containing electrolyte solutions should be infused at low maintenance rates:
   (a) 5% dextrose plus 0.3 N saline for older children
   (b) 10% dextrose plus 0.3 N saline for infants, to provide dextrose at 4–6 mg/kg/min

4. KCl, 2 mEq/kg/day, should be added, *provided* the urine output is >1 ml/kg/hr.

5. Magnesium sulfate, 1 mEq/kg/day, is added to the IV fluid regimen for infants after procedures under profound hypothermia.

6. If urine output falls (<1 ml/kg/hr) in the absence of hypotension, fluid orders should be reviewed to ensure an adequate intake, a "fluid challenge" may be administered, and if there is no result, a diuretic is ordered (furosemide, 1–2 mg/kg IV).

SPECIAL CONSIDERATIONS FOR ANESTHESIA OF NEONATES

Cardiac surgery in neonates should be performed only where the most expert, comprehensive medical and nursing care and all requisite facilities are available.

GENERAL PRINCIPLES

1. Assess the patient's condition carefully and ensure that the patient's status is the best that can be achieved before surgery.

2. Ventilation may be indicated preoperatively, especially if heart failure or metabolic acidosis is severe. (Respiratory care is as important preoperatively as postoperatively.)
3. Metabolic acidosis must be corrected as far as possible by infusion of $NaHCO_3$.
4. Congestive heart failure must be controlled as far as possible. The following therapy should be instituted:
   (a) Optimal digitalization.
   (b) Diuretic therapy: furosemide, 1 mg/kg IV.
   (c) Place in a neutral thermal environment.
   (d) Maintain slight head-up position.
   (e) Oxygen therapy to maintain PaO_2 at 70–90 mmHg.
   (f) Correct any acidosis.
   (g) Plus—if above measures fail:
      (i) Intubation and controlled ventilation.
      (ii) Other inotropic agents (e.g., dopamine).

Anesthetic Management in Addition to Routine Measures
Preoperative
1. Prepare all drugs and equipment before the baby is brought to the OR.
2. Ensure that epinephrine, dopamine, calcium, and atropine are at hand for immediate use.
3. Maintain the infant's body temperature and avoid cold stress during transportation and preparation for anesthesia. Patients with cyanotic CHD cool very rapidly.
4. Establish reliable IV lines as rapidly as possible, but use cutdowns if necessary.
5. If the infant is severely hypoxic or in shock, correct the acid-base status, oxygenate, and adminsiter methylprednisolone sodium succinate (25 mg/kg) very slowly at this stage.
6. Premedication: give IM atropine only 30 minutes preoperatively.

Perioperative
1. After oxygenation, give thiopental, 2–3 mg/kg, or fentanyl, 5–10 μg/kg, followed by vecuronium, 0.1 mg/kg. Ventilate with oxygen for 4 minutes and intubate.
2. Maintain anesthesia with low concentrations of isoflurane, or, if this is not tolerated, fentanyl, 10–15 μg/kg. Most patients will tolerate the addition of some nitrous oxide, but oxygenation and blood pressure must be carefully monitored.
3. Avoid hyperventilation. Physiologic $PaCO_2$ must be maintained.
4. Monitor continuously:

    (a) Ventilation and heart rate via esophageal stethoscope.

    (b) BP via Doppler or intra-arterial catheter.

    (c) Transcutaneous O_2 saturation.

    (d) End-tidal CO_2.

5. Assess frequently:

    (a) Temperature.

    (b) Blood loss.

    (c) Blood gases.

6. Particularly if cardiac output is falling, anticipate and correct acidosis—but be careful not to produce metabolic alkalosis.

7. If bradycardia occurs, assume it is due to hypoxia until proved otherwise.

    (a) Discontinue anesthetics.

    (b) Request removal of packs and retractors.

    (c) Expand lungs with 100% O_2.

    (d) If hypoxia persists, anticipate acidosis and treat it if it occurs.

9. Maintain fluid balance but avoid overhydration.

    (a) Infuse lactated Ringer solution, 4 ml/kg/hr.

    (b) Dextrose at 4–6 mg/kg/min.

    (c) Record intake; include fluid given with drugs, etc.

10. Maintain blood volume:

    (a) Replace losses, volume for volume, with lactated Ringer solution or whole blood, depending on volumes lost.

    (b) Maintain Hct at optimal level (35–45%) at all times.

Postoperative

1. *See* routine management, page 268.

2. All neonates require meticulous attention to respiratory care and constant, highest quality nursing care, including

    (a) Maintenance of body temperature at about 37°C.

    (b) Avoidance of cold stress.

3. They should be nursed with a slight head-up tilt and moved frequently from side to side. Dressings and chest drains should be located to cause minimal restriction.

4. Controlled ventilation may be required for long periods. PEEP or CPAP usually improves arterial oxygenation.

5. Atelectasis, particularly of the upper lobes, is a common complication. It is treated by aspiration of lung secretions and application of chest physiotherapy.

6. If the period of intensive care is prolonged, special attention must be paid to ensuring adequate nutrition.

SPECIFIC CLOSED HEART OPERATIONS

LIGATION OF PATENT DUCTUS ARTERIOSUS

OLDER INFANTS AND CHILDREN

1. PDA as the sole lesion in older infants and children usually presents no problems.
2. Routine anesthetic management as for thoracotomy is appropriate.
3. Monitor carefully:
   (a) For bradycardia during dissection near the vagus nerve.
   (b) For change in murmur after ligation (diastolic pressure may rise at this time).
4. Blood loss is usually minimal, seldom necessitating transfusion, but it may be sudden and massive if a major vessel is torn. Therefore, establish a reliable large-bore IV infusion line (18-gauge cannula if possible) and check that blood is immediately available in the OR.

PREMATURE INFANTS

Persistence of the ductus arteriosus may occur in preterm infants, especially those under 1,500 g. In addition to prematurity, respiratory distress syndrome (RDS), excessive fluid therapy, neonatal asphyxia, hypoxia, and acidosis predispose to this condition. PDA results in a large L → R shunt, with pulmonary vascular engorgement and congestive heart failure. Clinical signs include tachypnea, hepatomegaly, and "bounding pulses." Diagnosis is confirmed by auscultation of the typical murmur, radiographic evidence of increased vascularity, and echocardiogram findings of a large left atrium: aorta ratio. PDA may prevent weaning from ventilatory support of infants with RDS.

Therapy for Patent Ductus Arteriosus

1. *Medical therapy.* Administration of indomethacin, a prostaglandin inhibitor, 0.1–0.2 mg/kg PO, for several days may induce closure of the PDA. Indomethacin may cause renal damage and suppress bone marrow and hence is contraindicated in patients with renal failure or co-

agulopathy. Very small infants (<1,000 g) do not respond as well with closure of the PDA as do larger, less immature infants.
2. *Surgical treatment (ligation).* This is necessary if indomethacin therapy fails or is contraindicated.

Special Anesthetic Problems
Observe all special precautions for the preterm infant (*see* page 96).

Preoperative
1. Assess the patient carefully.
2. Ensure that all arrangements are made to transfer the patient to the OR in a transport incubator with a ventilator (if indicated).
3. No premedication is ordered.

Perioperative
1. Ensure that the OR is heated and that all warming devices are in position before transferring the patient to the OR table.
2. Attach monitors.
3. (a) If the patient is intubated, ensure that the tube is firmly fixed and absolutely patent and well positioned; otherwise, reintubate.
   (b) If the patient is not intubated, give atropine, 0.02 mg/kg, fentanyl, 15 μg/kg, vecuronium, 0.1 mg/kg, ventilate with O_2 for 3 minutes, and intubate.
4. Induce and maintain anesthesia with N_2O (in a concentration appropriate to ensure saturation) and isoflurane, 0.5–1.0%, or fentanyl, 10–12 μg/kg.
5. Small doses of vecuronium (0.05 mg/kg) may be used to facilitate ventilation and prevent movement.
6. Establish a reliable IV line. Blood loss is usually minimal but can be catastrophic if a vessel is torn.
7. Give minimal maintenance fluids. These patients are often overhydrated preoperatively and do not suffer "third space" losses.

Postoperative
1. Continued ventilation is necessary for most patients, with increased attention to respiratory care in view of possible post-thoracotomy complications (atelectasis, etc.).
2. Improvement in respiratory status after ligation of PDA is dictated by the relative contributions of pulmonary vascular congestion and pulmonary disease (RDS or bronchopulmonary dysplasia) to the preoperative status.

3. Rarely, the thoracic duct may be injured during PDA ligation. The resulting chylothorax may require drainage.
4. Damage to the (left) recurrent laryngeal nerve is a rare complication.

RESECTION OF AORTIC COARCTATION

Aortic coarctation is classified according to its site in relation to the ductus arteriosus (i.e., preductal or postductal). The preductal (infantile) type usually is accompanied by other anomalies (e.g., VSD or PDA) and presents as cardiac failure in an infant under 6 months of age. The postductal (adult) type may be asymptomatic; it is usually diagnosed during investigation of hypertension in the upper limbs in preschoolers.

PREDUCTAL (INFANTILE TYPE) AORTIC COARCTATION

Special Anesthetic Problems
1. Most of these infants have severe cardiac failure and are already being treated with digoxin and diuretics. Assisted ventilation is essential for some, and it benefits many others.
2. Severe associated anomalies are common.

Anesthetic Management
Preoperative
1. Blood gases should be determined and abnormalities corrected if possible.
2. Ensure that supportive drugs are at hand (e.g., epinephrine, dopamine); they may be necessary during surgery.

Perioperative
1. Maintain normothermia.
2. While the aorta is clamped, do not allow the systolic pressure to exceed 80 mmHg. In the (rare) event that a drug is necessary to lower the BP, administer low concentrations of isoflurane and titrate this against the BP.
3. Be prepared to support the circulation when the clamps are removed; infusion of small amounts of fluid and/or cardiotonic drugs may be required.

Postoperative
The course is usually stormy. Therefore:

1. Transfer the infant to the ICU with a nasotracheal tube in place.
2. Controlled ventilation is necessary for at least 48–72 hours.

POSTDUCTAL (ADULT TYPE) AORTIC COARCTATION

Special Considerations

1. Clamping the aorta could compromise the blood supply to the spinal cord; hence the need to maintain an optimal blood pressure.
2. While the aorta is clamped, severe proximal hypertension may occur and require treatment.
3. Hypertension may be troublesome postoperatively; this may be controlled by the use of β-blockers over the perioperative period.
4. Although blood must (of course) be available for transfusion, suprisingly few children require this. (Bleeding from collateral vessels is less profuse than in adults.)
5. In the very rare event that severe proximal hypertension cannot be controlled after aortic clamping, or if the distal pressure is very low, a temporary shunt must be placed to bypass the site of anastomosis.

Anesthetic Management

Preoperative

1. Apply a BP cuff and Doppler flowmeter probe to the right arm.
2. Establish a reliable IV site other than in the left arm.

Perioperative

1. Follow routine management as on page 265. Maintain anesthesia with nitrous oxide and isoflurane; use *d*-tubocurarine for relaxation.
2. Place an arterial line into the right radial artery.
3. During the period of aortic clamping, control the BP if necessary by increasing the inspired concentration of isoflurane. The BP should not be allowed to exceed 140 mmHg, but do not attempt to reduce the pressure if it remains below this. Distal aortic pressure during clamp-off varies with the proximal pressure; the former should be maintained at a mean of 50 mmHg, if possible, to perfuse the spinal cord.
4. The surgeon first removes the distal clamp and then (slowly) the proximal clamp. Watch the BP continuously: if hypotension develops, infuse fluids; if this is unsuccessful, ask the surgeon to partly reapply the proximal clamp briefly. The BP may remain slightly lower for a while but is usually back above normal levels by the end of the operation; SNP should be used to control this if necessary.
5. Blood loss is usually minimal and transfusion is unnecessary.

6. In most cases, controlled ventilation is not required postoperatively, and the patient can be extubated at the end of the operation.

Postoperative
1. The patient should be monitored continuously in the ICU, special attention being paid to signs of blood loss—measure the chest drainage and observe the clinical indices.
2. Hypertension usually persists for several days postoperatively and, if severe, may necessitate therapy with SNP and/or propranolol. Prevention of hypertension is essential to prevent arteritis (*see below*).
3. Rarely, the postoperative course is complicated by intestinal ileus owing to mesenteric arteritis. In extreme cases, bowel resection may be required.
4. Other serious postoperative complications include paraplegia owing to spinal cord ischemia during repair. This is fortunately very rare.

DIVISION OF VASCULAR RINGS AND SUSPENSION OF ANOMALOUS INNOMINATE ARTERY

Abnormalities of the great vessels may encircle or compress the trachea, bronchi, and esophagus. Severe compression by vascular rings leads to stridor and difficulty with feeding during early infancy. The infant with a vascular ring will often assume a characteristic opisthotonic position. Anomalous vessels may compress the bronchi and lead to gas trapping in an individual lobe of the lung, the resultant emphysematous lobe compressing the adjacent lung (*see* page 221).

Patients with repaired tracheoesophageal fistula are particularly prone to develop tracheal compression between the aorta and esophagus during feeding. The onset of symptoms of dyspnea and "dying spells" during feeding is usually between 2 and 4 months of age. This condition is caused by an abnormally soft trachea becoming compressed against the aorta by a dilated esophagus. Aortopexy usually relieves symptoms, but in some patients insertion of an external stent to reinforce the trachea may be necessary.

Special Anesthetic Problems
1. Respiratory failure may exist.
   (a) Chronic respiratory infection may have impaired pulmonary function.
   (b) Vascular compression may have resulted in emphysema of one or more lobes, compressing other lung tissue.

2. Airway compression may be at the level of the carina or main bronchi; if so, a normally situated endotracheal tube will not relieve the obstruction.
3. Endotracheal intubation may be required preoperatively to relieve serious symptoms. Air trapping in a lobe owing to vascular compression can often be alleviated by the application of PEEP.
4. The use of an esophageal stethoscope in infants with vascular ring has been reported to cause acute airway obstruction.

Anesthetic Management
Preoperative
1. Order intensive respiratory care to achieve optimal pulmonary status.
2. Bronchoscopy with endobronchial suction may be required.

Perioperative
1. For intubation, use a method that ensures a good airway past the obstructing lesion. If the obstruction is low:
   (a) Pass into a main bronchus a long endotracheal tube with side holes for ventilating the other bronchus, or
   (b) Ventilate the patient via a bronchoscope. (This can be placed accurately under direct vision and adjusted perioperatively if necessary.)
2. For aortopexy, a bronchoscope should be used to ensure that the compression is relieved. Compression of the trachea should always be assessed during spontaneous ventilation and coughing. If controlled ventilation is used, the trachea is held open and appears corrected in every case.
3. If it is necessary to assess the airway during surgery, use halothane and spray the larynx with lidocaine prior to inserting the bronchoscope. During the remainder of the operation, ventilation can be assisted or controlled. Do not give relaxants.
4. Operations on the great vessels may cause serious bleeding. Establish a reliable large-bore IV infusion route.

Postoperative
1. Order constant care in a humidified croup tent for at least the first 24 hours.
2. If residual obstruction persists, continue nasotracheal intubation for 24 hours and then reassess.
3. Partial obstruction may be improved by a small 1- to 2-inch-thick bolster below the shoulders.

4. Racemic epinephrine or dexamethasone may be required for postinstrumentation croup.

PALLIATIVE SURGERY TO INCREASE PULMONARY BLOOD FLOW

The operations include

1. Blalock-Taussig procedure (subclavian artery anastomosed to pulmonary artery). A modified Blalock procedure employing a synthetic graft between the vessels and preserving the continuity of the subclavian artery is most commonly performed.
2. Potts operation (pulmonary artery anastomosed to descending aorta).
3. Waterston procedure (pulmonary artery anatomosed to ascending aorta).
4. Glenn procedure (superior vena cava [SVC] anatomosed to pulmonary artery).

These operations are performed for infants and children with tetralogy of Fallot, tricuspid atresia, etc. in whom rightsided cardiac lesions have decreased the pulmonary blood flow. They are usually performed during infancy and may be followed by total correction of the defect at an older age.

Special Anesthetic Problems

1. Many of these patients are severely hypoxemic and polycythemic.
2. During surgery one pulmonary artery is partly occluded so that the anastomosis can be completed; this causes a further temporary decrease in pulmonary blood flow.
3. Patients with polycytemia may have a coagulation defect, though this is rarely a problem.
4. In small infants, the narrow lumen of the new shunt is prone to thrombose. This may be avoided by the use of a small dose of heparin and appropriate fluid therapy.

Anesthetic Management

Preoperative

1. Ensure that the respiratory system is in an optimal state for that patient, with no active infection or recent history of upper respiratory tract infection.

2. If the patient is taking digoxin, order the morning dose for the day of operation to be given at 0600 hours.
3. Order adequate sedation (including morphine for children over 1 year or weighing >10 kg).
4. If the patient is taking β-blocking agents, these should be continued up to the evening before surgery.
5. Order IV maintenance fluids for patients with a Hb of >16 g/dl during the preoperative fasting period. Do not place an IV in the arm on the side to be used for a subclavian shunt.

Perioperative

1. Follow routine management as on page 265.
2. Induce anesthesia IV (most of these patients have a R→ L shunt).
3. For the Blalock-Taussig procedure: place a BP cuff on the arm opposite the operative site.
4. Maintain anesthesia with 0.5–0.75% halothane in at least 50% oxygen.
   (a) Halothane tends to decrease the (right) ventricular contractility and hence obstruction to outflow.
   (b) If desaturation occurs intraoperatively it should be treated with propranolol, 0.05 mg/kg IV.
   (c) If hypotension occurs with the halothane (rare), it will be necessary to substitute fentanyl.
5. Immediately before the pulmonary artery is clamped, switch to 100% O_2, inflate the lungs well, and give a further dose of relaxant.
6. Once the clamps are in place, and if the patient's oxygenation appears stable, allow the surgeon to proceed with the anastomosis.
7. While the anastomosis is being performed: if there is a fall in BP or bradycardia occurs, infuse cardiotonic drugs (e.g., epinephrine, 1–5 μg/kg) until the anastomosis is completed and the clamps are removed.
8. A "modified" Blalock anatomosis is usually performed with a synthetic graft. In small infants, it is usual to give a small dose of heparin (100 units/kg) to prevent thrombosis of the shunt. A bolus of fluid after the clamps are released may enhance flow through the shunt.
9. Throughout the surgery give plasma to replace blood loss and decrease the Hct.

Postoperative

1. Check that a new murmur is audible (this indicates that the shunt is functioning).
2. Extubation in the OR is preferred. IPPV is seldom necessary, and spontaneous ventilation with low intrathoracic pressure may improve flow through the new shunt.

3. Review the digitalis dosage; the child may require a larger dose than previously (right ventricular work is now increased, myocardial perfusion may be compromised by the lower diastolic pressure, and failure could ensue).
4. If the anastomosis is small and considered likely to be blocked by thrombosis, order heparin in suitable dosage for several days postoperatively.

PALLIATIVE SURGERY TO INCREASE INTRA-ATRIAL MIXING

The Blalock-Hanlon operation is a closed operation that creates a large atrial septal defect to allow intra-atrial mixing to occur. The usual indication is transposition of the great vessels with an intact septum. Patients with this condition often deteriorate soon after birth, as the ductus arteriosus (possibly the only route for mixing of pulmonary and systemic blood) starts to close. A balloon septostomy is usually attempted initially but does not always create an adequate atrial septal defect (ASD). The patency of the ductus arteriosus can usually be maintained by a continuous infusion of PGE_1 until septostomy or the Blalock-Hanlon operation can be completed.

Special Anesthetic Problems
1. These infants may have had recent attempts at balloon septostomy and are therefore not in optimal condition.
2. Many infants are dependent on an infusion of PGE_1 to maintain the patency of the ductus arteriosus. This must be continued intraoperatively.
3. During the actual creation of the defect, the cardiac output is reduced dramatically for a short period of time (approximately 30 seconds).
4. Blood loss may be significant.

Anesthetic Management
Preoperative
1. Follow routine management as on page 265.
2. Correct acidosis, hypothermia, etc., if present.
3. Maintain prostaglandin infusion.
4. Check Hct; look for signs of hypovolemia if bleeding occurred during attempted balloon septostomy.

Perioperative

Manage as for the Blalock-Taussig operation except:

1. Before clamp is applied:
   (a) Ventilate the lungs with 100% O_2 for 3 minutes.
   (b) Give an incremental dose of d-tubocurarine to ensure paralysis and to prevent ventilation during the time the atria are open.
   (c) Infuse sodium bicarbonate, 1 mEq/kg, calcium gluconate, 10 mEq/kg, and isoproterenol, 1 μg/kg, just before clamping. (This "cocktail" gives the myocardium a boost over the critical period.)
2. As the clamp is applied to the atria to create the ASD, allow the lungs to collapse briefly.
3. During closure of the atrium, inflate the lungs with O_2.

Postoperative

1. Usually the patient can be extubated soon after the operation. This is desirable to allow increased pulmonary blood flow.
2. If IPPV is required, attempt to maintain a low mean intrathoracic pressure.
3. Prostaglandin infusion can be discontinued.
4. PaO_2 should be improved to 40 mmHg or higher.
5. Intensive respiratory care is required for several days.

PALLIATIVE SURGERY TO DECREASE PULMONARY BLOOD FLOW

Pulmonary artery banding is performed to diminish blood flow to the lungs in infants who have a large L→R shunt and thus to decrease pulmonary vascular congestion and avert the development of fixed pulmonary hypertension. This is usually performed as an emergency procedure in the newborn.

Special Anesthetic Problem

Many of these patients are in severe congestive heart failure.

Anesthetic Management

Preoperative

1. Follow routine management as on page 265.
2. Check that the congestive heart failure is under optimal control.
3. Emply all necessary measures to improve the infant's general status (e.g., IPPV for several hours may be very beneficial).

Perioperative
1. Do not administer myocardial depressants (e.g., halothane).
2. Give a muscle relaxant (vecuronium) and narcotic analgesic (fentanyl).
3. Monitor the patient closely as the band is applied. The systemic BP should rise, but the saturation should not fall (i.e., no R→L shunt should occur). It is usual to also monitor the distal pulmonary artery pressure during banding. This should fall to approximately 30–50% of systemic pressure.

Postoperative
1. Controlled ventilation may be required for several days.

OPEN HEART SURGERY

Anesthetic Management
1. Follow routine preoperation management as on page 265.
2. Perioperatively, after induction the following are placed in position:
   (a) Esophageal stethoscope.
   (b) Doppler flowmeter and BP cuff (usually in the right arm).
   (c) Esophageal and rectal thermistor probes.
   (d) A large-bore IV infusion line.
   (e) An arterial line, usually in the left radial artery, and a double-lumen central venous pressure (CVP) line, usually via the external or internal jugular vein. The second lumen can be used for vasoactive drug infusion.
   (f) Urinary catheter, for measurement of urine output perioperatively and postoperatively.
   (g) Electroencephalogram electrodes connected to a cerebral function monitor.
3. Maintain anesthesia with:
   (a) N_2O plus O_2 in suitable proportions to ensure a SaO_2 of 100%; use air plus O_2 for rare patients for whom N_2O may be contraindicated.
   (b) If tolerated, give isoflurane, 0.5–0.75%, or halothane, 0.5%, depending on the lesion, and supplement this with generous doses of fentanyl.
   (c) Patients with any failure who benefit from afterload reduction will probably do well with isoflurane (e.g., VSD). Patients who may benefit from myocardial depression will usually do well with halothane (e.g., tetralogy of Fallot).

4. Give incremental doses of relaxant drugs as needed.
5. Control ventilation with a volume-cycled ventilator, maintaining normocarbia. Confirm by end-tidal and serial arterial blood gas analysis.
6. Give maintenance fluids, for example, lactated Ringer solution, according to body weight (*see* page 88) to replace the calculated deficit during fasting (if any) and maintain urine output at >1 mg/kg/min. Additional "fluid loading" prior to bypass has not been shown to be advantageous.
7. Blood loss from sponges, suction, drapes, *and specimens* must be measured carefully, and the running totals maintained. It is seldom necessary to transfuse blood before CPB unless major blood loss occurs during dissection around the heart (e.g., during repeat operations).
   (a) Aim to maintain the Hct at near-preoperative level and the intravascular volume high enough to maintain CVP.
   (b) If the Hct was very high preoperatively, replace initial losses with plasma but beware of too much hemodilution prior to bypass.
   (c) During venous cannulation in small infants, a significant volume of blood may be lost. Be prepared to replace this.
8. During dissection around the heart, watch the BP closely; arrhythmias are common, although most are innocuous. If hypotension or arrhythmia persists, ask the surgeon to desist until the condition corrects itself.
9. Before the heart is cannulated, give the initial dose of heparin. First determine the dose by plotting a dose-response curve (Fig. 11-1).
   (a) Take a blood sample and determine the control activated clotting time (ACT).
   (b) Give heparin, 1 mg/kg.
   (c) Repeat the ACT and plot on graph (Fig. 11-1).
   (d) Give a further dose of heparin, 1 mg/kg.
   (e) Again determine and plot the ACT.
   (f) Draw the dose-response curve and determine the additional dose of heparin required to prolong the ACT to 600 seconds.
   (g) Give this dose and recheck the ACT after 2–3 minutes.
10. Advise the surgeon that the heart can now be cannulated.

Note. Hypotension may occur when the venous cannulas are inserted. If this happens, discontinue volatile agents and increase the inspired O_2 concentration until bypass has been instituted. Additional fluid infusion may also help; if the aorta is already cannulated, this can be delivered from the pump.

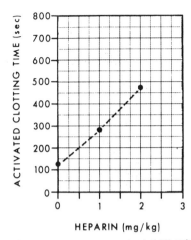

FIG. 11-1. Heparin dose-response curve. Last ACT value (after end of bypass) indicating equivalent of 3 mg heparin/kg. This is then modified according to the PNF stated on the heparin vial to determine the dose of protamine required to reverse heparinization.

11. Once on bypass, the pump flow should be increased to establish a satisfactory perfusion. Indicators of adequate perfusion are the cerebral function monitor, urine output, and repeated acid-base studies. Note that in patients with cyanotic CHD perfusion pressures may be low during early bypass. This is due to the increased vascular bed of the patient and the use of a low-viscosity perfusate. High flows may be required initially, but the systemic pressure will increase progressively, especially as cooling progresses. The use of vasoconstrictors is not necessary. When the perfusion pressure is low, it is of vital importance that the SVC pressure should be at or near zero. Any increase in SVC pressure may have a serious effect on cerebral perfusion pressure.

12. During partial bypass, ventilate the lungs with O_2. Do not give any N_2O because of the possibility of air embolism.

13. During total bypass:
    (a) Keep the lungs inflated at 5 cm H_2O pressure.
    (b) Add 0.5% isoflurane to the oxygenator to continue anesthesia and improve perfusion, or give additional doses of fentanyl. Remember that fentanyl is bound to the plastic of the CPB circuit, so blood levels fall precipitously on bypass. Do not add volatile agents to the oxygenator during hypothermic bypass as high blood

levels will result. Discontinue any volatile agents 15 minutes before the end of bypass.

14. During bypass (partial and total), repeat the ACT every 30 minutes and give additional doses of heparin as necessary to prolong the ACT to >600 seconds.

15. Take blood samples for acid-base, electrolyte, and Hct determinations every 30 minutes and just before bypass is discontinued.

16. During discontinuance of bypass, to avoid the possibility of cerebral air embolism:
    (a) Compress the carotid arteries for 20 seconds.
    (b) During the early post-bypass phase do not give N_2O (which might increase the danger if air emboli are present).

17. Commence an infusion of SNP at 1–2 μg/kg/min to reduce afterload prior to weaning from bypass. SNP is also most important for the patient with pulmonary hypertension.

18. As CPB is discontinued:
    (a) Order infusion of blood from the pump until the left atrial pressure is adequate (8–12 mmHg, depending on the cardiac lesion).
    (b) Carefully maintain the preload at this level.

19. If the patient remains hypotensive:
    (a) Commence sequential pacing if the heart rate is slow or if sinus rhythm is absent.
    (b) Commence a dopamine infusion (5–10 μg/kg/min) if hypotension still persists despite a good rate and rhythm.
    (c) Calcium infusion may improve performance in some patients, but calcium should not be given until the heart has resumed a good regular beat.
    (d) If all else fails, an infusion of epinephrine, 0.1–0.5 μg/kg/min, may be indicated.

20. When the patient's condition is stable and the cannulas have been removed, give protamine. To determine the dose, repeat the ACT and plot it on the line of the heparin dose-response curve; drop a line to determine the heparin equivalent and modify this by the protamine neutralization factor (PNF) for the vial of heparin used. (For example, if the ACT at the end of bypass represents 3 mg/kg heparin, give 3 mg/kg protamine, adjusted by the appropriate PNF) (Fig. 11-1).

21. At 20 minutes after bypass, take blood samples for coagulation studies, electrolytes, and blood gases. Repeat ACT and give more protamine if indicated.

22. If bleeding persists, give platelets (1 unit/5 kg) and/or fresh-frozen plasma (20 ml/kg), according to coagulation indices.

Note. Anticipate continued bleeding owing to platelet and other factor deficiencies:

(a) After a long pump run.

(b) In children with cyanotic CHD.

(c) In small babies—in whom the pump-priming volume is large in relation to their blood volume. All bleeding must be well controlled before the chest is closed.

23. At the end of surgery after all but the simplest procedures (e.g., closure of ASD secundum):

(a) Insert a nasotracheal tube for continuing IPPV and/or CPAP or intermittent mandatory ventilation. (This is usually continued for 12–48 hours.) Ensure that the tube allows a slight leak with 20 cm H_2O positive pressure.

(b) *Do not reverse the muscle relaxants.*

24. A chest radiograph is obtained. Examine it carefully, looking for pneumothorax, hemothorax, and atelectasis, and ensure that the tip of the endotracheal tube is well above the carina. Check placement of all other indwelling lines.

25. During transportation to the ICU (all patients):

(a) Attach a full bag of blood to the IV line to ensure immediate availability in case of sudden hemorrhage.

(b) Cover the patient with warm blankets.

(c) Give O_2 and monitor the pulse oximeter.

(d) If the patient is still intubated, continue artificial ventilation.

(e) Monitor:

   (i) Breath and heart sounds via a stethoscope.

   (ii) ECG and arterial pressure.

   (iii) Radial pulse via a Doppler flowmeter.

Postoperative

1. Follow routine management as on page 268.

Suggested Additional Reading

Textbook

Lake CL: Pediatric Cardiac Anesthesia. Norwalk, CT, Appleton & Lange, 1988.

General

Duc G: Assessment of hypoxia in the newborn: suggestions for a practical approach. Pediatrics 48:469, 1971.

Engle MA (ed): Pediatric cardiovascular disease. Cardiovasc Clin 11(2), 1981.

Jones RS, and JB Owen-Thomas (eds): Care of the Critically Ill Child. London, Arnold, 1971.

Mustard WT, P Bedard, and G Trusler: Cardiovascular surgery in the first year of life. J Thorac Surg 59:761, 1970.

Ross DN: A Surgeon's Guide to Cardiac Diagnosis. Part I. The Diagnostic Approach. Berlin, Springer-Verlag, 1962.

Rudolph AM: Congenital Diseases of the Heart. Chicago, Year Book Medical Publisher, 1974.

Werner JC, RR Fripp, and V Whitman: Evaluation of the pediatric surgical patient with congenital heart disease. Surg Clin North Am 63:1003–1015, 1983.

Young D: Pathophysiology of congenital heart disease. Int Angesthesiol Clin 18:5–26, 1980.

Anesthetic Management

Burrows FA: Physiologic dead space, venous admixture, and the arterial to end-tidal carbon dioxide difference in infants and children undergoing cardiac surgery. Anesthesiology 70:219–225, 1989.

Daley MD, WL Roy, and FA Burrows: Hypoxaemia produced by an oesophageal stethoscope: a case report. Can J Anaesth 35:500–502, 1988.

DeBock TL, RL Petrilli, PJ Davis, and EK Motoyama: Effect of premedication on preoperative arterial saturation in children with congenital heart disease. Anesthesiology 67A:492, 1987.

Drop LJ: Ionised calcium, the heart, and hemodynamic function. Anesth Analg 64:432–451, 1985.

Duncan PG: Anaesthesia for patients with congenital heart disease. Can Anaesth Soc J 30:S20–S26, 1983.

Glover WJ: Management of cardiac surgery in the neonate. Br J Anaesth 49:59–64, 1977.

Hickey PR: Anesthesia for Children with Cardiac Disease. International Anesthesia Research Society, Review Course Lectures 1988, p. 86–90.

Hickey PR, and DD Hansen: Fentanyl and sufentanil-oxygen-pancuronium anesthesia for cardiac surgery in infants. Anesth Analg 63:117–124, 1984.

Hickey PR, DD Hansen, and M Strafford: Pulmonary and systemic effects of nitrous oxide in infants with normal and elevated pulmonary vascular resistance. Anesthesiology 65:374–378, 1986.

Hickey PR, DD Hansen, GM Cramolini, et al: Pulmonary and systemic hemodynamic responses to ketamine in infants with normal and elevated pulmonary vascular resistance. Anesthesiology 62:287–293, 1985.

Hickey PR, DD Hansen, DL Wessel, et al: Blunting of stress responses in the pulmonary circulation of infants with fentanyl. Anesth Analg 64:1137–1142, 1985.

Hill JD, L Dontigny, M de Leval, and CH Mielke, Jr: A simple method of heparin management during prolonged extracorporal circulation. Ann Thorac Surg 17:129, 1974.

Jonmarker C, A Larsson, and O Werner: Changes in lung volume and lung-thorax compliance during cardiac surgery in children 11 days to 4 years of age. Anesthesiology 65:259–265, 1986.

Laishley RS, FA Burrows, J Lerman, and WL Roy: Effect of anesthetic induction regimens on oxygen saturation in cyanotic congenital heart disease. Anesthesiology 65:673–677, 1986.

Lazar HL, GD Buckberg, RP Foglia, et al: Detrimental effects of premature use of inotropic drugs to discontinue cardiopulmonary bypass. J Thorac Cardiovasc Surg 82:18–25, 1981.

Lucero VM, J Lerman, and FA Burrows: Onset of neuromuscular blockade in children with congenital heart disease. Anesth Analg 66:788–790, 1987.

Mattox KL, GA Guinn, PA Rubio, and AC Beall, Jr: Use of the activated coagulation time in intraoperative heparin reversal for cardiopulmonary operations. Ann Thorac Surg 19:634, 1975.

Morgan P, AM Lynn, C Parrott, and JP Morray: Hemodynamic and metabolic effects of two anesthetic techniques in children undergoing surgical repair of acyanotic congenital heart disease. Anesth Analg 66:1028–1030, 1987.

Neuman GG, DD Hansen: the anaesthetic management of preterm infants undergoing ligation of patent ductus arteriosus. Can Anaesth Soc J 27:248–253, 1980.

Radnay PA, and H Nagashima: Anesthetic considerations for pediatric cardiac surgery. Int Anesthesiol Clin 18:1, 1980.

Silove ED: Pharmacological manipulation of the ductus arteriosus. Arch Dis Child 61:827–829, 1986.

Steward DJ, and IAJ Sloan: Recent upper respiratory infection and pulmonary clamping in the aetiology of postoperative respiratory complications. Can Anaesth Soc J 16:57, 1969.

Stockard JJ, RB Bickford, and JF Schauble: Pressure-dependent cerebral ischemia during CPB. Neurology 23:521, 1973.

Stow PJ, FA Burrowa, J Lerman, and WL Roy: Arterial oxygen saturation following premedication in children with cyanotic congenital heart disease. Can J Anaesth 35:63–66, 1988.

Tanner GE, DG Angers, PG Barash, A Mulla, et al: Effect of left to right, mixed left to right, and right to left shunts on inhalational anesthetic induction in children: a computer model. Anesth Analg 64:101–107, 1985.

Yates AP, SGE Lindahl, and DJ Hatch: Pulmonary ventilation and gas exchange before and after correction of congenital cardiac malformations. Br J Anaesth 59:170–178, 1987.

Cardiopulmonary Bypass and Myocardial Protection

Bull C, J Cooper, J Stark: Cardioplegic protection of the child's heart. J Thorac Cardiovasc Surg 88:287–293, 1984.

Cohen JA, HL Bethea, and WJ Rush: Heparin kinetics during pediatric open heart operations. Perfusion 1:271–275, 1986.

Chu-Jeng Chiu R, and W Bindon: Why are newborn hearts vulnerable to global ischemia: Circulation 76(suppl V):146–149, 1987.

Horrow JC: Protamine: a review of its toxicity. Anesth Analg 64:348–361, 1985.

McDonald MM, LJ Jacobson, WW Hay, and WE Hathaway: Heparin clearance in the newborn. Pediatr Res 15:1015–1018, 1981.

Murkin JM, JK Farrar, WA Tweed, FN McKenzie, and G Guiraudon: Cerebral autoregulation and flow/metabolism coupling during cardiopulmonary bypass: the influence of $PaCO_2$. Anesth Analg 66:825–832, 1987.

Yamashita M, S Wakayama, A Matsuki, M Kudo, and T Oyama: Plasma catecholamine levels during extracorporeal circulation in children. Can Anaesth Soc J 29:126–129, 1982.

Postoperative Care

Braimbridge MV: Postoperative Cardiac Intensive Care, 2nd ed. Oxford, Blackwell, 1972.

Downes JJ, HF Nicodemus, WS Pierce, and JA Waldhausen: Acute respiratory failure in infants following cardiovascular surgery. J Thorac Cardiovasc Surg 59:21, 1970.

Faraci PA, HF Rheinlander, and RJ Cleveland: Use of nitroprusside for control of pulmonary hypertension in repair of ventricular septal defect. Ann Thorac Surg 29:70, 1980.

Gregory GA, LH Edmunds, Jr, JA Kitterman, RH Phibbs, and WH Tooley: Continuous positive airway pressure and pulmonary and circulatory function after cardiac surgery in infants less than three months of age. Anesthesiology 43:426, 1975.

Hickey PR, DD Hansen, WI Norwood, and AR Castaneda: Anesthetic complications in surgery for congenital heart disease. Anesth Analg 63:657–664, 1984.

Jenkins J, AM Lynn, J Edmonds, and G Barker: Effects of mechanical ventilation on cardiopulmonary function in children after open heart surgery. Crit Care Med 13:77–80, 1985.

Lang P, RG Williams, WI Norwood, and AR Castenada: The hemodynamic effects of dopamine in infants after corrective cardiac surgery. J Pediatr 96:630, 1980.

Long WA, and LJ Rubin: Prostacyclin and PGE_1 treatment of pulmonary hypertension. Am Rev Respir Dis 136:773–776, 1987.

Palmisano BW, DM Fisher, M Willis, GA Gregory, and P Ebert: The effect of paralysis on oxygen consumption in normoxic children after cardiac surgery. Anesthesiology 61:518–522, 1984.

Stephenson LW, LH Edmunds, R Raphaely, DF Morrison, WS Hoffman, and LJ Rubis: Effects of nitroprusside and dopamine on pulmonary arterial vasculature in children after cardiac surgery. Circulation 60(suppl I):104, 1979.

Winters RW (ed): The Body Fluids in Pediatrics. Boston, Little, Brown, 1973.

PROFOUND HYPOTHERMIA WITH CIRCULATORY ARREST

Profound hypothermia with circulatory arrest is used for some neonates and infants undergoing cardiac surgery. It is particularly advantageous when surgery involves the atria:

1. The heart is still and exsanguinated, making more precise surgery possible.
2. The cannulas can be removed from the operative field during repair.
3. The duration of CPB is shorter.

Hypothermia is now usually achieved by means of bloodstream cooling on CPB.

Anesthetic Management

Preoperative
1. See routine management on page 265.
2. Ensure that the operating room is cool (<20°C).

Perioperative
1. Give 100% O_2 by mask.
2. Apply monitoring devices (*see* page 283).
3. Induce anesthesia IV with a small dose of thiopental, 3 mg/kg, and/or fentanyl, 5–10 μg/kg.
4. Give vecuronium, 0.1 mg/kg, and ventilate the patient with 100% O_2 for 3 minutes. Then perform intubation.
5. Maintain anesthesia with appropriate concentrations of N_2O, adding 0.5–0.75% isoflurane if tolerated, supplemented by large doses of fentanyl.
6. Give maintenance fluids as outlined for CPB (*see* page 266) and give blood or plasma when indicated to replace losses. No dextrose-containing solutions should be given as hyperglycemia may increase the danger of cerebral damage during total circulatory arrest. Large doses of fentanyl (>50 μg/kg) may limit the increase in blood glucose that occurs during hypothermic CPB.
7. Give Solu-Medrol, 15–25 mg/kg IV slowly, and administer heparin as outlined on page 284.

8. After CPB is begun, ensure that the difference between the esophageal temperature and the temperature of the pump's output does not exceed 10°C.
9. Administer phentolamine, 0.2 mg/kg, to improve tissue perfusion, speed even cooling, and minimize acidosis on rewarming.
10. Before CPB is discontinued, give an incremental dose of relaxant. (Once circulatory arrest has occurred, no further drugs can be given.)
11. When the esophageal temperature is 16°C and the rectal temperature below 20°C, CPB is discontinued, blood is drained to the oxygenator, and the venous cannulas are removed.
12. Pack ice bags around the head; record the duration of circulatory arrest.
13. Keep the lungs inflated at 5 cm H_2O with an air-O_2 mixture.
14. When the repair is complete, the venous cannulas are replaced and the patient is rewarmed until the esophageal temperature is 37°C. The temperature of the blood from the pump should never exceed 39°C, and the patient's temperature should not be raised above 37°C.
15. Do not correct the metabolic acidosis that is seen during rewarming. This will be corrected as the patient's metabolism resumes. Administration of sodium bicarbonate results in postoperative metabolic alkalosis.
16. The rest of the procedure is as described for CPB management (*see* page 268).

Postoperative

1. A nasotracheal tube and controlled ventilation may be necessary for 24–48 hours.
2. Apply measures as for routine postoperative cardiac care (*see* page 268).
3. Order magnesium sulfate (1 mEq/kg/24 hr) with KCl (2–4 mEq/kg/24 hr) to be added to the maintenance fluid, which is given at a constant rate over each 24 hours.

Suggested Additional Reading

Abbott TR: Oxygen uptake following deep hypothermia. Anaesthesia 32:524, 1977.
Bridges KG, GA Richard, H MacVaugh, et al: Effect of phentolamine in controlling temperature and acidosis associated with cardiopulmonary bypass. Crit Care Med 13:72–76, 1985.
Ellis RJ, E Hoover, WA Gay, and PA Ebert: Metabolic alterations with profound hypothermia. Arch Surg 109:659, 1974.
Ellis DJ, TF Flegel, and DJ Steward: Fentanyl reduces hyperglycemia in

pediatric patients undergoing hypothermic cardiopulmonary bypass. Anesthesiology 69A:740, 1988.

Johnston AE, IC Radde, DJ Steward, and J Taylor: Acid-base and electrolyte changes in infants undergoing profound hypothermia for surgical correction of congenital heart defects. Can Anaesth Soc J 21:23, 1974.

Rittenhouse EA, H Mohri, DH Dillard, and KA Merendino: Deep hypothermia in cardiovascular surgery. Ann Thorac Surg 17:63, 1974.

Steward DJ, IA Sloan, and AE Johnston: Anaesthetic management of infants undergoing profound hypothermia for surgical correction of congenital heart defects. Can Anaesth Soc J 21:15, 1974.

Steward DJ, CA Da Silva, and T Flegel: Elevated blood glucose levels may increase the danger of neurologic deficit following profoundly hypothermic cardiac arrest. Anesthesiology 68:653, 1988.

Tharion MS, DC Johnson, JM Celermajer, et al: Profound hypothermia with circulatory arrest. J Thorac Cardiovasc Surg 84:66–72, 1982.

CARDIOLOGIC PROCEDURES

CARDIAC CATHETERIZATION

This is usually an elective procedure, and older children will benefit from preoperative teaching, a visit to the catheter laboratory, and familiarization with the process to be performed.

Cardiac catheterization may be performed under general anesthesia or with a combination of sedation plus local or regional analgesia. The important prerequisites for gathering reliable catheter data are

1. Hemodynamic parameters should be maintained as constant and unchanged as possible.
2. The inspired oxygen concentration should remain constant throughout the procedure: Room air is preferred if this is safe for the patient, otherwise a constant optimum inspired oxygen concentration should be selected.
3. The patient should be maintained in an optimal physiologic state (Normothermic, well hydrated, euglycemic etc.)

Special Anesthetic Problems

1. The patient may be seriously ill and in cardiac failure.
2. The condition may further deteriorate during cardiac catheterization, especially if arrhythmias occur.
3. Contrast media used for angiograms may cause adverse effects.

When the procedure is to be performed under sedation, the following technique has proved satisfactory:

1. An IV route is established with local analgesia.
2. Monitors are applied (ECG, pulse oximeter, BP cuff and Doppler, temperature probe).
3. Intravenous sedation is administered. A mixture containing 25 mg of meperidine, 6.25 mg of chlorpromazine, and 6.25 mg of Phenergan (promethazine) per milliliter ("CM3") is commonly used. The dose is 0.05 ml/kg IV (equal to 1.25 mg/kg of meperidine, with 0.3 mg/kg each of chlorpromazine and Phenergan); maximal dose is 2 ml. If given undiluted, this mixture causes pain along the vein; therefore, mix it with saline or administer into a freely flowing IV infusion. The child usually settles well and sleeps once the regional or local analgesia is established.
4. Small infants may be offered a brandy soother and will often settle with this alone.
5. Caudal analgesia may be useful for some children, especially if bilateral femoral catheterization is necessary or if large catheters are to be inserted (e.g., Gruntzig catheters).

If general anesthesia is preferred, the patient should be carefully monitored as above. A technique employing endotracheal nitrous oxide and low concentrations of halothane in 30% oxygen with spontaneous ventilation has been found satisfactory.

Some forms of CHD are now being treated by therapeutic-interventional cardiac catheterization, for example, by balloon dilation of the stenotic valve or "umbrella" closure of the ASD or PDA. General anesthesia is usually preferred as the patient must be absolutely immobile, and the need for urgent open operation if complications occur is a real possibility. A large-bore IV route suitable for rapid transfusion should be in place.

CARDIOVERSION

Cardioversion is usually an emergency. The arrhythmia may be severe, markedly reducing cardiac output and producing shock.

Anesthetic Management
Preoperative
1. Give 100% O_2 by mask.
2. Ascertain whether the child has eaten recently (*see below*).
3. Prepare and check all equipment.

4. Apply monitors:
   (a) Precordial stethoscope.
   (b) BP cuff.
   (c) ECG.

Perioperative
1. Tape needle in vein.
2. Give 100% O_2 by mask.
3. Induce anesthesia. If you suspect that the patient has a full stomach:
   (a) Continue 100% O_2.
   (b) Give atropine, 0.015 mg/kg IV.
   (c) Inject methohexital, 2 mg/kg, and succinylcholine, 1 mg/kg.
   (d) Have an assistant apply cricoid pressure until you have completed the intubation.

If the patient has fasted:
   (a) Continue 100% O_2.
   (b) Inject methohexital, 2 mg/kg.
4. As soon as anesthesia has been induced and good oxygenation achieved, countershock can be applied.
   (a) Repeat methohexital, 1 mg/kg, if necessary.

Postoperative
1. The period of recovery is short, but the patient should be closely monitored (including ECG) for several hours afterward.

Suggested Additional Reading

Manners JM: Anesthesia for diagnostic procedures in cardiac disease. Br J Anaesth 43:276, 1971.

Manners JM, and VA Codman: General anaesthesia for cardiac catheterisation in children. The effects of spontaneous and controlled ventilation. Anaesthesia 24:541, 1969.

Naylor D, TJ Coates, and J Kan: Reducing distress in pediatric cardiac catherization. Am J Dis Child 138:726–729, 1984.

Smith C, RD Rowe, and P Vlad: Sedation of children for cardiac catheterization with an ataractic mixture. Can Anaesth Soc J 5:35, 1958.

Soyka LF: Pediatric clinical pharmacology of digoxin. Pediatr Clin North Am 28:203, 1981.

Topkins MJ: Anesthetic management of cardiac catheterisation. Int Anesthesiol Clin 18:59–69, 1980.

12

Urologic Investigation and Surgery

SURGICAL PROCEDURES

Anesthesia is administered for:

1. Urologic investigation.
    (a) Cystoscopy, cystogram, retrograde pyelogram.
    (b) Renal biopsy.
        (i) Open.
        (ii) Closed (needle biopsy).
    (c) Urethral pressure profile.
2. Urologic surgery.
    (a) Upper urinary tract.
        (i) Nephrectomy, heminephrectomy.
        (ii) Ureterostomy, ureterectomy, ureteroplasty.
        (iii) Reimplantation of ureters.
    (b) Lower urinary tract.
        (i) Hypospadias, epispadias.
        (ii) Circumcision.
3. Patients with renal failure:
    (a) Insertion of a peritoneal catheter.
    (b) Creation of an arteriovenous (AV) fistula or shunt.
    (c) Open renal biopsy.
    (d) Nephrectomy.
    (e) Renal transplantation.

GENERAL PRINCIPLES

The anesthetic risk depends on the state of the patient's renal function.

1. Most children who come for investigation or surgery of the lower urinary tract have good renal function.
2. Many of those who require renal biopsy have mild renal dysfunction (usually insufficient to pose an anesthetic risk).
3. All children in renal failure are seriously ill and present multiple problems for the anesthesiologist (as well as the nephrologist).
4. Renal disease may be part of a syndrome and therefore requires consideration of all aspects of the condition (*see* Appendix I).

CHILDREN WITH GOOD RENAL FUNCTION

Anesthetic Management

For minor procedures (e.g., cystoscopy, retrograde pyelography, circumcision, hypospadias repair): always use general anesthesia, with agents appropriate for the procedure. Healthy children having short investigative procedures or operations are admitted and discharged the same day. Others are admitted the day before surgery.

Preoperative
1. Sedatives are omitted for day patients but may be given to inpatients.

Perioperative
1. Induce anesthesia with intravenous (IV), rectal, or inhalational agents.
2. Maintain anesthesia with N_2O, O_2, and halothane, by mask.
3. Provide for analgesia postoperatively when indicated (e.g., circumcision, *see* page 100).

Postoperative
1. Order little or no analgesic. (Day patients are discharged after 1 hour.)

For major genitourinary surgical procedures: Apply anesthetic management as for minor procedures (above) plus:

1. Use general endotracheal anesthesia with muscle relaxants and controlled ventilation.
2. Be prepared for major hemorrhage: Measure blood losses carefully and replace as indicated.
3. Children who have dilated ureters may develop hypertension postoperatively. This may require treatment with hydralazine.

CHILDREN WITH POOR RENAL FUNCTION OR IN RENAL FAILURE

Many children with disturbed renal function are undergoing hemodialysis regularly and therefore have a shunt or fistula in place. Special care must be taken to ensure that this device is kept functioning at all times—the patient must not lie on that limb (which also cannot be used for blood pressure [BP] recordings) during the operative procedure, transport to the intensive care unit or postanesthesia room, or during the postoperative period.

Special Anesthetic Problems

1. Anemia (usually normochromic, normocytic) caused by:
   (a) Decreased erythropoietin production. (If erythropoietin is absent, the hemoglobin [Hb] cannot rise above 7–9 g/dl.)
   (b) Increased hemolysis.
   (c) Increased bruising and bleeding from increased capillary fragility.
   (d) Iron and/or folic acid deficiency.
   (e) Bone marrow depression owing to an increase in blood urea nitrogen.
   Usually the anemia leads to compensatory changes, for example:
      (i) Increased red blood cell (RBC) 2,3-diphosophoglycerate.
      (ii) Increased cardiac output (via increased heart rate).
   After successful renal transplantation, the Hb rises rapidly.
   N.B. Arterial oxygen desaturation cannot be detected clinically in the very anemic patient, but the pulse oximeter will measure this accurately—hence, it is an invaluable monitor.
2. Coagulopathies resulting from:
   (a) Increased capillary fragility.
   (b) Functional platelet defect (decreased adhesiveness), possibly owing to retention of guanidinosuccinic acid.
   (c) Thrombocytopenia owing to bone marrow depression.
   (d) Drugs: heparin, acetylsalicylic acid, etc.
3. Acid-base imbalance.
   (a) Metabolic acidosis predominates, though compensated to a variable degree by respiratory alkalosis; plasma bicarbonate falls to 12–15 mEq/L.
   (b) In longstanding stable renal failure, H^+ displaces Ca^{2+} from bone and K^+ from intracellular fluid.
4. Fluid and electrolyte changes. Children on dialysis (particularly hemodialysis) are likely to be hypovolemic.
   (a) "Sodium losers"—children with polycystic kidneys or severe pyelonephritis (tubular damage is disproportionately greater than glomerular injury):
      (i) Normotension or slight hypotension.
      (ii) Edema (uncommon).
      (iii) Hypokalemia (in some).
      (iv) Renal function is improved by increasing intake of sodium and water.

    (b) "Sodium retainers"—children with glomerulonephritis (salt retention, hypertension, and edema predispose them to cardiac failure).

    (c) Potassium shifts owing to displacement of K^+ from the cells by H^+:

        (i) High serum K^+ levels.

        (ii) Depressed excitability of muscles and nerves. This is particularly significant if cardiac muscle is affected—further sudden rises in K^+ (e.g., with succinylcholine or increased acidosis) may precipitate cardiac arrest.

    (d) Calcium shifts.

        (i) If displacement of Ca^{2+} by H^+ is prolonged, osteoporosis may develop.

    (e) Anion changes.

        (i) Plasma HCO_3^- is decreased.

        (ii) Plasma SO_4^{2-} is increased.

        (iii) Plasma HPO_4^{2-} is increased.

        (iv) Plasma Cl^- is increased.

5. Cardiovascular problems.

    (a) Hypertension.

        (i) In most patients (those with hypertension secondary to sodium and water retention), this can be controlled conservatively.

        (ii) In some patients, the BP can be titrated against sodium and water content during dialysis.

        (iii) In others, even large doses of antihypertensive agents fail to control the hypertension (which is probably due to overproduction of renin). Retinopathy and/or encephalopathy may develop, and bilateral nephrectomy may become necessary.

    (b) Incipient heart failure.

        (i) Increased cardiac output to meet O_2 transport requirements in the presence of anemia or an AV fistula can predispose the heart to failure.

        (ii) Hypertension further stresses the left ventricle.

    (c) Fatty degeneration of myocardium owing to chronic renal failure.

6. Pulmonary congestion.

    (a) The A-aPO$_2$ difference may be large.

    (b) Sodium and water retention, left ventricular failure, and hypoproteinemia contribute to the development of "uremic lung."

7. Gastrointestinal (GI) disturbances.

    (a) Nausea and vomiting (owing to bacterial breakdown of urea to ammonia in the GI tract) may aggravate the water, electrolyte, and acid-base imbalance.

8. Multiple medications.
   (a) Many of these patients are receiving long-term steroid therapy with resultant osteodystrophy, cushinoid state, and glycosuria.
      (i) Continue steroid therapy preoperatively.
      (ii) Observe aseptic techniques meticulously.
   (b) Antihypertensive polypharmacy: potential cardiovascular instability under anesthesia must be anticipated. (The drugs are not discontinued before surgery.)
   (c) Digitalis and diuretic therapy: may lead to K^+ depletion and therefore increased susceptibility to cardiac arrhythmias.
   (d) Antibiotics (e.g., gentamicin): may prolong the effect of nondepolarizing muscle relaxants.
   (e) Antimetabolites (e.g., azathioprine) that are highly protein-bound may increase the bioavailability of other protein-bound drugs by displacing them on the protein molecule.
9. Reduced immunity: risk of infection.
10. Poor quality of life and potentially major psychological disturbances:
   (a) Resulting from chronic debilitating disease.
   (b) Heightened by the uremic state and knowledge of a life-threatening condition.

In summary, these children have:

1. Low O_2-carrying capacity.
2. Increased tendency to bleeding (in an already anemic state).
3. Incipient or apparent cardiac failure:
   (a) Left ventricular failure if hypertensive, hypervolemic, and anemic.
   (b) Right ventricular failure (late).
4. High risk of cardiac arrest owing to increased K^+ and acidosis.
5. Intolerance of inaccurate administration of blood, other fluids, and electrolytes.
6. Cardiovascular instability owing to long-term administration of antihypertensive drugs.
7. Low resistance to infection.
8. Very low tolerance to further discomfort, however minor (e.g., finger prick, movement from one bed to another).

Preoperative Assessment and Preparation

Pay careful attention to the following physical and psychological aspects.

1. Do not use a limb with a shunt or fistula in situ for:

(a) BP readings.
(b) Intra-arterial or IV lines.
2. Patients in dialysis program: usually dialyzed 12–18 hours before surgery.
3. Plan ahead so that the child's discomfort is not increased and any necessary disturbances are minimized.
4. Psychological preparation and support are of special benefit to these patients—and are safer than depressant medication.
5. Check results of laboratory tests.
   (a) Hb: chronic anemia is surprisingly well tolerated by these patients.
       (i) Take into account the patient's usual Hb level and what the patient can do at that level. (Some children are active even at 4 g/dl).
       (ii) A level of 5 g/dl is acceptable if there is no recent or sudden fall.
       (iii) Do not give transfusion unless it is absolutely essential, in which case washed RBCs may be preferable. Transfusion:
       Depresses the bone marrow further.
       May produce antibodies.
       Is of temporary benefit only.
       Tends to increase serum K^+.
   (b) Serum potassium: below 5 mEq/L is acceptable. (Even in an emergency, levels over 6 mEq/L are unacceptable—but remember that higher levels are normal in very small and preterm infants.)
       (i) If the serum K^+ level is elevated, surgery is usually delayed until hemodialysis has been performed.
       (ii) In an emergency, K^+ can be lowered rapidly by giving 50% glucose with insulin (dose according to body weight, proportional to 50 ml of glucose with 20 units of regular insulin in an adult). If at all possible, consult a nephrologist first.
   (c) Acid-base balance.
       (i) pH above 7.32 is acceptable: if necessary, employ $NaHCO_3$ correction, even if Na^+ levels are elevated.
       (ii) Correction must be cautious and gradual. (If the serum Ca level is low, sudden correction may precipitate tentany or convulsions.)

Anesthetic Management

1. Pay meticulous attention to details of asepsis.
2. For short procedures (e.g., insertion of a peritoneal catheter) in poor-risk patients who are cooperative and emotionally suited, use local anesthesia (1–2% lidocaine without epinephrine; maximum 3 mg/kg).

3. For all other cases, and if in doubt, use general anesthesia.

Preoperative

1. Use smaller doses of drugs than for "healthy" patients.
2. Do not discontinue antihypertensive drugs.
3. Premedicate only when required, with one-third to one-half the standard dose of sedative (e.g., diazepam orally 1.5 hours preoperatively).
4. Check all medications and their last expected dose before surgery.
5. Check the location of a shunt or fistula.
6. Ensure that all supportive drugs are available in the operating room (OR).
7. Ensure that adequate supplies of blood and other fluids are available (including washed cells when indicated).

Perioperative

1. Give 100% O_2 by mask.
2. Apply monitors:
   (a) Precordial stethoscope.
   (b) Electrocardiogram and pulse oximeter.
   (c) Doppler flowmeter (for BP)—do not use a limb with a shunt or fistula.
3. Ensure that the limb with the shunt or fistula is easily accessible. Monitor function continually throughout the procedure.
4. Induce anesthesia with thiopental, 2–3 mg/kg (more may be required), followed by N_2O-O_2-halothane.
5. For intubation:
   (a) Do not give succinylcholine unless serum K^+ is less than 4.5 mEq/L—and always pretreat with curare (0.005 mg/kg).
   (b) Otherwise give atracurium.
6. Maintain anesthesia with:
   (a) N_2O-O_2 and isoflurane with atracurium.
7. Control the ventilation in all cases that last more than 45 minutes. Use moderate hyperventilation to compensate for metabolic acidosis and to encourage K^+ movement back into the cells.
8. Administer fluids to ensure adequate blood volume for satisfactory BP, good peripheral perfusion, and function of an AV fistula or shunt.
   (a) Give 5% glucose with 0.2% N saline to replace the preoperative deficit and for perioperative maintenance.
   (b) For small blood losses: replace with maintenance solution.
   (c) For significant blood losses: replace with washed RBCs and salt-poor albumin.
   (i) Check Hb and hematocrit (Hct); keep Hct below 30%.

(ii) Avoid overtransfusion.
9. Reverse muscle relaxants at end of surgery.

Postoperative
1. Ensure good ventilation and oxygenation.
2. Order analgesics in one-third to one-half the usual doses; monitor the effect and give supplements if necessary.
3. Ensure that the shunt or fistula is functioning; record this.
4. Check Hb, Hct, electrolytes, and blood gases.
5. Consult a nephrologist for continuing care.

RENAL TRANSPLANTATION

Anesthetic Management
Preoperative
Recipient
1. General management is as for patients in renal failure (*see* page 299). Discuss with the nephrologist and urologist to ascertain exact present status (state of hydration, etc.).
2. Check the nephrologist's reports about the patient's renal status, special problems, etc.
3. If the patient is not in optimal condition, surgery should be postponed until after dialysis.
4. Review the immunosuppressive therapy plan for the child: drug dosage, timing, etc.

Donor
1. If the kidney has already been removed from the donor, it will arrive in the OR perfused or cooled and ready for implantation.
2. If the donor is brought to the OR for removal of a kidney:
   (a) In the case of a brain-dead donor, maintain full respiratory and cardiovascular support to ensure good urinary output until the kidneys have been removed (*see* page 254).
   (b) Ensure that preservation of the kidneys (cooling, perfusion) is started immediately and continued until implantation into the recipient.

Perioperative
1. General management is as for patients in renal failure (*see* page 299).
2. After induction of anesthesia:

    (a) Insert a central venous line.

    (b) Check its position with a pressure tracing and/or radiograph.

    (c) Maintain the central venous pressure (CVP) at an acceptably high level to ensure diuresis (see below). Dextrose 5% with 0.2N saline is the preferred maintenance fluid (cf. lactated Ringer solution, which contains K^+).

3. Insert an arterial line (to monitor blood gases, Hb, Hct, and electrolytes).

    (a) If an external shunt is available, place a T-piece aseptically into the shunt. Clamp the venous end before withdrawing arterial samples.

4. Note the time for implantation anastomosis (i.e., time between removal from preservation container to reperfusion by the recipient).

5. Give diuretics and immunosuppressives according to a predecided schedule.

6. Maintain the CVP at a level that produces a good urine output. If the CVP is adequate but urine flow is low:

    (a) Give furosemide, 2–4 mg/kg IV.

    (b) If necessary, add 20% mannitol, 1 g/kg.

7. Anticipate the need to infuse large volumes of fluid (three to five times the normal) to compensate for "third space losses."

8. At the end of surgery, determine serum electrolytes:

    (a) If urine output is adequate, serum K^+ should be within the normal range.

    (b) If the serum K^+ is greater than 6 mEq/L and urine output is poor, continue to hyperventilate the patient, plan to arrange for dialysis or therapy with glucose and insulin.

Postoperative

1. General management is as for patients in renal failure (*see* page 305).

2. Check the pulmonary status. The need to "push fluids" to ensure diuresis may result in pulmonary edema, and occasionally therapy may be needed for this.

3. Transfer care of the patient to a nephrologist.

Note. Renal function in the transplanted kidney is as follows:

1. Glomerular function is initially normal but falls during the first 48 hours as the kidney swells. Increased IV fluids are required to maintain diuresis at this time.

2. Some degree of tubular damage is always present. Therefore, diuresis and loss of sodium results and requires sodium and water replacement. Other electrolytes must be infused as indicated by serum studies.

3. Declining urine flow after 48 hours despite fluid loading is indicative of mechanical problems (vascular) or rejection of the transplant.

Suggested Additional Reading

Basrton RD, and S Deutsch: Anesthesia and the Kidney. Orlando, FL, Grune & Stratton, 1976.

Don HF, RA Dieppa, and P Taylor: Narcotic analgesics in anuric patients. Anesthesiology 42:745, 1975.

Geha DG, CD Blitt, and BJ Moon: Prolonged neuromuscular blockade with pancuronium in the presence of acute renal failure: a case report. Anesth Analg 55:343, 1976.

Ghoneim MM, and H Pandya: Plasma protein binding of thiopental in patients with impaired renal or hepatic function. Anesthesiology 42:545, 1975.

*Gradus D, and RB Ettenger: Renal transplantation in children. Pediatr Clin North Am 29:1013, 1982.

Hunter JM, RS Jones, and JE Utting: Use of atracurium in patients with no renal function. Br J Anaesth 54:1251, 1982.

Koide M, and BE Waud: Serum potassium concentrations after succinylcholine in patients with renal failure. Anesthesiology 36:142, 1972.

Logan DA, HB Howie, and J Crawford: Anaesthesia and renal transplantation: an analysis of fifty-six cases. Br J Anaesth 46:69, 1974.

Miller RD, WL Way, WK Hamilton, and RB Layzer: Succinylcholine-induced hyperkalemia in patients with renal failure? Anesthesiology 36:138, 1972.

Symposium on the kidney and the anaesthetist. Br J Anaesth 44:236, 1972.

---

* Key article

13

Orthopedic Surgery

A considerable proportion of children who undergo elective orthopedic surgery have multiple congenital anomalies and/or neuromuscular disease (*see* Appendix I). Underlying disease, particularly with muscle weakness, requires special anesthetic care, and minor surgery may be fraught with major anesthetic complications.

GENERAL PRINCIPLES

1. Children with orthopedic deformities may require repeated surgery and spend much time in the hospital. Their sympathetic management is particularly important, and preoperative sedation should be chosen carefully.
2. Drug selection is influenced by the underlying disease; therefore, check the history carefully. Neuromuscular disease is particularly relevant; in general, muscle relaxants should not be given to patients with myopathies (*see* Appendix I). Succinylcholine particularly should not be given to patients with muscle disease.
3. Major surgery of the vertebral column deserves special consideration.
4. Malignant hyperpyrexia, though very rare, is more common in patients with orthopedic diseases. Maintain vigilance for the early signs (*see* page 133).
5. Many surgical procedures are performed with a tourniquet. One important index of patient well-being, the color of the blood in the surgical wound, is then lost. Be extra cautious in monitoring when a tourniquet is in use.
6. When a tourniquet is used, blood loss is negligible. In other cases, surgery of bone may result in significant losses (e.g., innominate osteotomy). Therefore, establish a reliable intravenous (IV) route and check that blood is available.
7. When a tourniquet is inflated, there usually follows a progressive increase in the heart rate and the blood pressure (BP). The exact cause of this is unknown, but it has been suggested to be due to stimulation of sympathetic nerves. The danger of this is that, on release of the tourniquet, a quite abrupt fall in pressure may occur. If the anesthesiologist has been "chasing" the tourniquet-induced hypertension by giving high levels of volatile agents, serious hypotension may now ensue. Therefore, use caution with dosage of potent volatile agents while a tourniquet is used, and reduce the concentration in anticipation of tourniquet release.

8. Hemodynamic responses to tourniquet release in children are usually not clinically significant. A transient decrease in arterial pH associated with an increase in base deficit and PCO_2 does occur; this is most marked after long tourniquet times (>75 minutes) or with the use of double tourniquets. General recommendations include:

(a) Attempt to limit tourniquet times to under 75 minuutes.

(b) Do not release bilateral tourniquets simultaneously.

(c) Use controlled ventilation before and after tourniquet release to remove the respiratory component of the acidosis.

(d) In children who might have difficulty compensating for the metabolic or respiratory acidosis (renal disease, pulmonary disease), consider determining blood gases 5 minutes after tourniquet release.

KYPHOSCOLIOSIS

Kyphoscoliosis may be congenital (15% of cases) but more commonly is acquired. It is idiopathic in 65% of cases and secondary to neuromuscular disease in 20%. More than 80% of patients with idiopathic scoliosis are female.

Pulmonary function is usually impaired.

PULMONARY FUNCTION

Changes in pulmonary function are related to the underlying cause, the speed of development of the scoliosis, and the severity of the curvature. The cardiorespiratory effects of scoliosis are summarized in Figure 13-1.

The pulmonary abnormality is restrictive rather than obstructive. Lung compliance is reduced. The vital capacity (VC) and total lung capacity may be greatly reduced, and the functional residual capacity somewhat less so. The respiratory volume tends to be maintained. The elastic resistance of the chest wall may be high, increasing the work and energy cost of breathing. Severe and prolonged lung compression impairs gas exchange, but that becomes evident only in later stages of the disease in the untreated patient.

The principal concern of young patients with idiopathic scoliosis is the cosmetic effect of the spinal and pelvic or chest wall deformity, especially when the curvature increases during the years of rapid body growth. At this stage, respiratory symptoms are uncommon, but pulmo-

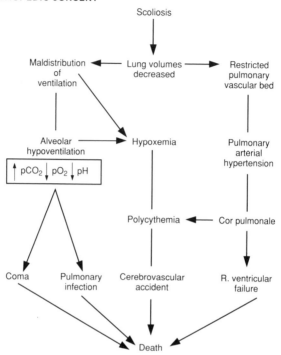

FIG. 13-1. Pathophysiology of the cardiorespiratory effects of kyphoscoliosis. (By kind permission of Henry Levison, MD, FRCP(C), Director of Respiratory Physiology, The Hospital for Sick Children, Toronto.)
Progressive alveolar hypoventilation, leading to hypoxia, may be accompanied by pulmonary hypertension and right ventricular failure.

nary function studies may reveal an abnormality. Although lung volumes may be normal, exercise tolerance may be reduced. In severe cases, the mechanical effects of scoliosis on respiratory function are apparent even at rest.

It must be emphasized that pulmonary function is relatively normal in most children who present for correction of idiopathic scoliosis with a curvature of less than 65%. Respiratory disability is more likely in association with congenital scoliosis or curvature of paralytic etiology.

Special Anesthetic Problems

1. Anesthetic management must take into account.
   (a) Etiology and severity of the curvature.
   (b) Degree of respiratory and cardiovascular impairment.

(c) Type of corrective procedure proposed.
2. If the scoliosis is secondary to neuromuscular disease, special consideration of drug selection is necessary. (The pulmonary function impairment resulting from the mechanical effects of the spinal curvature may be compounded by involvement of respiratory muscles in the disease process.) Postoperatively, hypoventilation, secretion retention, and atelectasis are likely in response to pain, analgesic drugs, and immobilization.
3. Preoperative assessment must include
(a) Detailed history and examination for an indication of abilities and stamina.
(b) Pulmonary function studies, including blood gas analysis.
4. Be alert for signs of significant respiratory impairment (e.g., tachypnea at rest, severely reduced VC, abnormal blood gas values, inability to cough effectively).
5. Severe impairment of respiratory function is not a contraindication to surgery provided resources are available for postoperative intensive respiratory care (including controlled ventilation if necessary). Fixation of the spinal deformity is essential to prevent further deterioration of respiratory function (but usually does not result in significant improvement).
6. Children with a VC <35% of normal can be expected to have major respiratory complications. Those with a VC <30–40% of normal will probably require postoperative ventilation.

CORRECTIVE SURGERY BY THE POSTERIOR APPROACH

Special Anesthetic Problems

1. Because the patient must be prone, endotracheal intubation is essential. If preoperative correction of the spinal curvature has been achieved with an exoskeletal apparatus, intubation will probably be difficult—fixation of the head and neck may render adequate laryngoscopy impossible.
2. Blood loss may be severe (in excess of 50% of the expected blood volume [EBV]). Most bleeding originates from the vertebral veins, which become engorged if there is any pressure on the anterior abdomen. Blood loss is also related to the extent of the surgery (length of spine to be fused) and to the surgeon's speed and expertise. Patients with scoliosis secondary to a recognized neuromuscular disorder generally have a larger blood loss than those with idiopathic scoliosis.

3. Spinal cord function should be monitored during the operation: the use of somatosensory evoked responses (SSEPs) from the posterior tibial nerve has become a standard technique. However, SSEPs only monitor sensory pathways in the spinal cord. Alternatively the "wake up test" has been used, but this is not without risk and mainly tests the motor pathways. Motor evoked potentials stimulating the cord above the level of the surgery and recording from a peripheral nerve have been experimentally performed but are not routinely available. I monitor SSEPs routinely but also use a wake-up test for very severe deformities. Every patient should be awake at the end of the operation so that both sensory and motor function can be tested immediately.

4. Pulmonary function may be severely impaired. The anesthesiologist must check that the present state is optimal and exclude superimposed acute respiratory distress.

5. Postoperative pain may be considerable; the use of caudal morphine has been demonstrated to be effective if administered intraoperatively. This can readily be given in the prone patient positioned for surgery.

Anesthetic Management

Preoperative

1. Premedication with oral diazepam is usually adequate if combined with reassurance and a full explanation of procedures to be performed.

2. Do not give respiratory depressant drugs to patients whose respiratory function is impaired.

3. Ensure that all equipment and drugs are at hand in case of emergency.

4. Check that an adequate supply of blood and other fluid replacements is at hand.

5. If the patient is to be wakened perioperatively (see item 7 in next section), explain this and reassure the patient that he or she will feel no pain at that time—and in fact will not remember the event postoperatively.

Perioperative

1. If halo-loop traction is in place, check that instruments to release the connecting rods are at hand.

2. If a body cast has been applied:
   (a) The cast is cut to the manubrium to facilitate intubation and provide access if tracheotomy is required.
   (b) A precordial window is cut to allow external cardiac massage if this becomes necessary.

3. Intubation:

(a) Uncomplicated cases (no exoskeletal apparatus in place). Induce anesthesia with thiopental followed by succinylcholine.* Intubate. If monitoring of SSEPs is planned, it is necessary to allow the patient to recover from the succinylcholine and to check the positioning of the stimulating electrodes over the posterior tibial nerve before giving further relaxants.

(b) If the exoskeletal apparatus is present, adequate laryngoscopy may not be possible.

(i) Do not give muscle relaxant drugs until airway control by intubation has been accomplished.

(ii) Select a suitable intubation technique:
Blind nasal intubation under general anesthesia.
Laryngoscopy under deep general anesthesia. If the epiglottis is visible, a curved stylet is invaluable.
Local anesthesia of the nose, pharynx, and upper respiratory tract. (This is a difficult technique at best and is unacceptable in younger age groups.)

4. Maintenance: Use N_2O plus O_2 controlled hyperventilation and a long-acting muscle relaxant (d-tubocurarine preferred as it does not increase the BP). A loading dose of 5 μg/kg of fentanyl followed by an infusion of fentanyl at 2 μg/kg/hr is commonly used. Low concentrations of isoflurane (0.5–1%) can be added to control the BP as necessary. This technique does not interfere with SSEP monitoring and does allow for the possibility of a wake-up test.

5. Position the patient on a scoliosis operating frame that prevents external pressure on the anterior abdominal wall (e.g., the Relton frame). (Perioperative maintenance of the correct prone-suspended position is essential to ensure minimal blood loss—if the patient is malpositioned so that vertebral venous engorgement is present, heavy blood loss is inevitable.)

6. Monitor:

(a) Ventilation—esophageal stethoscope, airway pressure.

(b) Circulation—arterial line, BP cuff with Doppler flowmeter, and electrocardiogram.

(c) Temperature—rectal or esophageal probe.

(d) Acid-base status—blood gas analysis.

(e) Neuromuscular blockade—peripheral nerve stimulator.

(f) Blood loss—gravimetric method.

(g) Urine output—indwelling catheter.

---

* Do not use succinylcholine for patients with Duchenne-type muscular dystrophy.

(h) SSEPs—before, during, and after correction.
7. If the SSEPs show any changes or if the surgeon requests confirmation of spinal cord integrity after application of the distraction and compression apparatus: perform a wake-up test.
  (a) Anticipate this request by withholding relaxant increments for 1 hour before awakening if possible. Discontinue isoflurane.
  (b) Discontinue N_2O. Administer 5% CO_2 in O_2 for 3 minutes to return the PCO_2 to normal levels. Ask the patient to move the toes. (Voluntary movement of the feet confirms spinal cord integrity.) Re-anesthetize the patient with a small dose of thiopental (1 mg/kg).
8. Blood loss is minimized by:
  (a) Proper posture (see item 5, above) and complete muscle relaxation.
  (b) Deep infiltration of the wound site (by the surgeon) with a large volume of dilute epinephrine-saline solution (up to 500 ml of 1:500,000 may be used).
  (c) Controlled hyperventilation, maintaining $PaCO_2$ at 25–30 mmHg (to cause peripheral vasoconstriction).
  (d) Surgical technique (firm packing and meticulous subperiosteal plane dissection).
  (e) Avoiding high concentrations of anesthetic agents that cause vasodilation (halothane, isoflurane, etc.).

Note. Induction of arterial hypotension is not recommended. This technique may reduce blood loss but incurs great potential hazards with the patient prone, for example, ischemia of the spinal cord while it is being manipulated or stretched, leading to paraplegia.

Alternative methods of blood conservation have been used, including staging of complex procedures, autotransfusion by extracorporeal pump, or acute normovolemic hemodilution with blood withdrawal and reinfusion (using lactated Ringer solution). The latter procedure is carried out as follows:

1. When the patient is anesthetized and lines inserted, a volume of blood is withdrawn into chronic peritoneal dialysis bags for storage.
2. A calculated volume of blood is withdrawn to reduce the hematocrit (Hct) to 30. Calculate by using the formula:

$$\text{Volume withdrawn} = \frac{(\text{preoperative Hct} - 30) \times \text{EBV (ml)}}{100}$$

3. During blood withdrawal, a volume of warmed lactated Ringer solution equal to twice the blood volume withdrawn is infused.

4. As surgery progresses, the blood that has been withdrawn is reinfused.

This method results in loss of lower-Hct blood during surgery and conservation of the patient's cells for reinfusion.

Postoperative
1. Insert a nasogastric suction tube.
2. Patient must be awake before leaving the operating room.
   (a) Check for movement of legs and feet.
   (b) Check air entry throughout lungs. (Pneumothorax is a possible complication of spinal surgery.)
3. On arrival in the postanesthesia room:
   (a) Give 40% O_2 by mask.
   (b) Supplement analgesia as necessary (e.g., morphine infusion)
   (c) Obtain plain radiographs of the chest and vertebral column. Check the lung fields, looking especially for pneumothorax.
   (d) Obtain hemoglobin and Hct values, and order blood transfusion accordingly.
4. The patient must remain supine for at least 12 hours. Order physiotherapy; encourage breathing exercises.
5. Ensure that the child is nursed in a warm environment. (Body temperature usually falls 1–2°C during surgery because of large wound exposure, hyperventilation, air-conditioning, etc.)

POSTOPERATIVE PULMONARY INSUFFICIENCY

Clinical observation and serial blood gas analyses during the postoperative period indicate the patient's ability to ventilate adequately. Pulmonary insufficiency postoperatively may result from:

1. Severe pulmonary neuromuscular disease.
2. Pneumothorax; hemothorax; pleural effusion.
3. Secretion retention and atelectasis (owing to pain, analgesics, and/or immobilization, especially in patients with neuromuscular disease).
4. Aspiration of gastric contents.
5. Fat embolism syndrome.
6. Alteration in thoracic mechanics and/or persistent effects of muscle relaxants.

Management
1. Continue to monitor arterial blood gases.
2. Insert a nasotracheal tube and institute intermittent positive-pressure ventilation.

3. A decision to establish a tracheotomy can be deferred depending on the patient's progress.
4. Bear in mind that weaning from assisted ventilation may take days or weeks.

CORRECTIVE SURGERY BY THE ANTERIOR APPROACH

ZILKIE INSTRUMENTATION

For the treatment of a curve in the lumbar region, the vertebral column is approached laterally on the convex side of the curvature. Thoracotomy is performed, and the diaphragm is divided at its peripheral attachments to provide access to the vertebrae.

Note. This surgical trauma to the diaphragm and chest wall increases the risk of postoperative respiratory insufficiency.

Anesthetic management is as for the posterior approach (N_2O plus O_2, controlled hyperventilation, muscle relaxation, and supplementary analgesia), with the following modifications:

1. Selective endobronchial intubation of the dependent lung may be advantageous, permitting easier access to upper thoracic curvatures. (Serial blood gas measurements dictate the feasibility of continuing this technique throughout the procedure.)
2. If bilateral ventilation is selected, ventilation of the exposed lung will be impeded by surgical packing and retractors. Periodically, expand the lung fully (to avoid prolonged atelectasis).

SPINAL OSTEOTOMY

Spinal osteotomy with wedge excision consists of local resection of deformed vertebrae. This procedure may result in excessive blood loss owing to the proximity of the vertebral and epidural venous plexuses. It may be difficult to control the hemorrhage.

Monitor blood loss by:

1. Gravimetric method (weigh sponges and measure suction losses).
2. Continuous central venous pressure (CVP) measurement and direct BP readings via an arterial line.
3. Clinical observation (skin temperature, etc.)

If massive transfusion is required:

1. Use packed cells in recently thawed fresh frozen plasma.

2. Warm all blood to 40°C.
3. Monitor coagulation indices, especially platelets.
4. Order platelet concentrates (1 unit/5 kg) if the platelet count is <100,000/mm³.
5. Monitor the acid-base status and correct acidosis.
6. If citrate toxicity is suspected (hypotension despite volume replacement), inject calcium gluconate IV (2 ml of 10% solution slowly; repeat as indicated).

ELECTROSPINAL INSTRUMENTATION

Electrospinal instrumentation is performed for the correction of minor curvature. It consists of the implantation of stimulating electrodes into the paravertebral muscles and placement of a subcutaneous receiving unit. The patient uses an external generator to induce a current in the electrodes and thus produce a contracture in the paravertebral muscles to correct the developing deformity.

Special Anesthetic Problem

The electrodes are tested during surgery, and therefore muscle relaxant drugs must be avoided.

Anesthetic Management

Preoperative

1. The patient is usually healthy, with a minor degree of idiopathic scoliosis.
2. Premedication with oral diazepam is usually adequate.

Perioperative

1. Position basic monitors and induce anesthesia with thiopentone.
2. Intubate with succinylcholine.
3. Maintain anesthesia with N_2O plus O_2 and 1% halothane. Control ventilation.
4. Establish a secure IV route.
5. Position as for posterior spinal fusion.
6. Blood loss is usually minimal. No arterial line or CVP line is necessary.

Postoperative

1. Check ventilation and extubate.
2. Order analgesics as required.

FRACTURES

See Trauma (page 336).

See also Plastic and Reconstructive Surgery (page 209) for mandibular fractures.

Suggested Additional Reading

Grundy BL, PB Nelson, E Doyle, and PT Procopio: Intraoperative loss of somatosensory evoked potentials predicts loss of spinal cord function. Anesthesiology 57:321–322, 1982.

Jenkins JD, D Bohn, JF Edmonds, H Levison, and GA Barker: Evaluation of pulmonary function in muscular dystrophy patients requiring spinal surgery. Crit Care Med 10:645, 1982.

Lynn AM, T Fischer, HG Brandford, and TW Pendergrass: Systemic responses to tourniquet release in children. Anesth Analg 65:865–872, 1986.

*Relton JES: Anesthesia in the surgical correction of scoliosis. *In*: Scoliosis and Other Deformities of the Axial Skeleton (EJ Riseborough and JH Herndon, eds). Boston, Little, Brown, 1975, p. 309.

Relton JES, and AW Conn: Anaesthesia for the surgical correction of scoliosis by the Harrington method in children. Can Anaesth Soc J 10:603, 1963.

Reston JES, and JE Hall: An operation frame for spinal fusion: a new apparatus designed to reduce hemorrhage during operation. J Bone Joint Surg 49B:327, 1967.

Rosenberg H, and T Heiman Patterson: Duchenne's muscular dystrophy and malignant hyperthermia: another warning. Anesthesiology 59:362, 1983.

Shannon DC, EJ Riseborough, and H Kazemi: Ventilation perfusion relationships following correction of kyphoscoliosis. JAMA 217:579, 1971.

---

* Key article

14

Management of Trauma Including Acute Burns and Scalds

Children are commonly involved in accidents. Even if the injury is relatively minor, some of these patients require emergency anesthesia— in which case the anesthesia may pose the greater threat to life and health.

Most children injured in accidents were previously healthy. Therefore, considerations of past health are usually less significant than in an adult. However, a complete medical history must be obtained as soon as appropriate.

From the arrival of the child with major trauma in the emergency department, the anesthesiologist must be included in the treatment team. The anesthesiologist can thereby contribute to immediate care while evaluating the patient's condition for anesthesia and the need for further continuing care.

MAJOR TRAUMA

Diagnosis and treatment must proceed rapidly and simultaneously. Vigorous resuscitative measures must be continued without interruption during anesthesia. The two common major problems for the anesthesiologist are

1. To secure and maintain a safe, reliable airway and ensure optimal ventilation.
2. To achieve adequate blood and fluid replacement.

Note. Although injuries may appear to be limited to a single anatomic site or body system, the possibility of serious injuries elsewhere must be constantly kept in mind. The fractured femur may be the obvious injury, but the as yet undiagnosed ruptured spleen could be the greater threat to life.

INITIAL URGENT PROCEDURES

1. Ensure a safe airway, optimal ventilation, and oxygenation.
2. The cardiovascular status must be determined.
   (a) If hypovolemia is present, it must be corrected.
   (b) Effective cardiac action must be maintained or restored.
3. Blood is withdrawn without delay for typing and cross-matching. The blood bank should be advised if massive transfusion seems to be a possible requirement.

ESTABLISHING THE AIRWAY

Airway obstruction is common in head and facial injuries and may have a disastrous effect on the outcome.

1. All children with head injury should be given oxygen by mask immediately upon admission.
2. For patients with depressed consciousness, if simple positioning does not provide a clear airway, perform endotracheal intubation without delay.
3. Do not use an oropharyngeal airway for unconscious patients. This has more resistance to ventilation than an endotracheal tube and does not protect against aspiration of gastric contents.
4. If injury of the cervical spine is suspected, do not move the child's neck. Use sandbags, a plaster shell, or a bean bag* to immobilize the neck. Note, however, that cervical spinal injury is much less common in small children than in adults, so, if difficulties arise, optimal airway management must be the first priority.
5. Be alert to the possibility of foreign bodies (e.g., teeth, bone fragments) in the mouth, pharynx, or trachea, especially if there are facial injuries.
6. "Awake" laryngoscopy and intubation causes a marked increase in intracranial pressure (ICP), which may be detrimental in the head-injured child. Such children should preferably be given intravenous (IV) lidocaine, 1–2 mg/kg, thiopental, 5 mg/kg, atropine, 0.02 mg/kg, and succinylcholine, 1 mg/kg, prior to intubation. This procedure cannot, however, be safely followed if the patient is also hypovolemic; in such instances, either ketamine should be substituted for thiopental or IV lidocaine alone should be given. Cricoid pressure should be used to prevent regurgitation during induction. Succinylcholine does not increase intragastric pressure in young children.
7. Vomiting and aspiration commonly occur following an accident. Immediately after intubation, check air entry to all lung regions and suction via the endotracheal tube if necessary.
8. A nasogastric tube should be passed in all children with chest or abdominal injuries, as acute gastric dilation is common.
9. Be alert to the possibility of pneumothorax or hemothorax (*see* page 331).

---

* Vac-Pac surgical positioning system, VenTech Healthcare Inc., Toronto.

TABLE 14-1. BLOOD REPLACEMENT AFTER ABDOMINAL TRAUMA IN CHILDREN

Trauma	No.	Volume Transfused (% of EBV)	
		Average	Range
Ruptured spleen	9	52	20–100
Lacerated liver	5	119	14–285

INTRAVENOUS THERAPY

Large-bore IV lines must be established. These must be placed in the upper limbs or neck in children with abdominal (Table 14-1) or thoracic injuries. All fluids should be warmed.

Clues to blood volume status are as follows:

1. Cardiovascular indices:
   (a) In infants, the systolic blood pressure (BP) varies in parallel with the intravascular volume.
   (b) In older children, as in adults, hypovolemia results in vasoconstriction. Therefore, the systolic BP may be near normal, despite a loss of up to 20% of the blood volume. The central venous pressure (CVP) also may be maintained initially. When vasoconstriction can no longer compensate and maintain venous return to the heart, the CVP falls and becomes a more reliable guide to the adequacy of the blood volume.
2. General appearance: pallor and sweating are signs of hypovolemia, as is coolness of the skin, especially if the extremities. This can be quantified by simultaneous measurement of skin and body temperatures; a large difference indicates vasoconstriction, and lessening of the difference indicates improving skin perfusion as blood volume increases toward normal.
3. Confusion and irrational behavior often occur with hypovolemia.
4. Urine output: the severely injured patient should be catheterized and the urine output monitored. A urine flow of >1 mg/kg/hr indicates adequate renal perfusion and hence adequate volume replacement.

SELECTION OF FLUIDS FOR INFUSION

The types of fluid given depend on (1) what is indicated and (2) what is available.

Frequently, initial replacement is necessarily with fluids other than blood. If at all possible, do not transfuse noncross-matched universal donor blood. (A rapid cross-match can be performed in 20 minutes.) If blood loss is massive, consider the possibility of autotransfusion (*see* page 327).

A crystalloid solution (e.g., lactated Ringer solution) and/or plasma substitute (e.g., dextran 70) can be used initially to expand the circulating blood volume but if used in excess may contribute to pulmonary insufficiency later. Dextran may also impair coagulability and interfere with cross-matching: do not exceed 7 ml/kg.

Expansion of the blood volume with albumin or plasma is longer-lasting than with clear fluids. Infusion of recently thawed, warmed, fresh-frozen plasma also provides coagulation factors that are essential in the event of massive transfusion (*see below*).

INDICATIONS FOR BLOOD TRANSFUSION

Unfortunately, one can seldom measure the volume of blood lost after trauma. Large volumes may be lost from the intravascular volume but remain within hematomas (e.g., following fracture of the femur). Volume replacement must therefore be judged on the basis of the clues listed above. We recommend that the fluid replacement be sufficient to correct clinical signs of hypovolemia and that blood be given in volumes sufficient to maintain the hematocrit (Hct) at or above 30%.

The young child who is showing obvious signs of hypovolemia (pallor, sweating, hypotension) must be assumed to have lost at least 25% of the blood volume. Estimate the weight of the child, assume the normal blood volume to be 75–85 ml/kg, and 25% of this total is the initial volume to be replaced rapidly. The situation can then be reassessed. The need for continuous infusion to maintain the BP or a deterioration after an apparently stable period indicates persistent bleeding.

Children who have lost large volumes of blood require transfusion of whole blood. The trend toward blood component therapy has made it difficult to obtain whole blood. Packed cells resuspended in plasma (preferably recently thawed fresh-frozen plasma) must be substituted.

MASSIVE BLOOD TRANSFUSION

Loss of an amount of blood that would be negligible in an adult (500 ml) may constitute a major loss in a child. Therefore, massive blood transfusion is required for many severely injured children. For example, after thoracoabdominal injury, one may need to replace over 250% of the estimated blood volume (EBV).

Serious problems may be expected after the rapid infusion of 150% of the EBV (transfusion of 120 mg/kg). These problems include

1. Hypothermia and accompanying cardiac arrhythmias.
   (a) Warm all blood and fluids to 40°C.
2. Coagulation problems.
   (a) Thrombocytopenia and impaired platelet function.
      (i) Check platelet count after each 50% blood volume replacement.
      (ii) If platelets are <100,000/cm³, order platelet concentrates (1 unit/5 kg).
   (b) Deficiency of coagulation factors.
      (i) Measure prothrombin time (PT) and partial thromboplastin time (PTT).
      (ii) If these times are prolonged, give recently thawed fresh-frozen plasma (20 ml/kg).
   (c) Disseminated intravascular coagulation (DIC).
      (i) Bleeding increases at all sites (e.g., old venipuncture sites).
      (ii) Measure PT, PTT, clot lysis time, fibrinogen, and fibrin split product levels.
      (iii) Prolonged PT and PTT, low fibrinogen level, and presence of fibrin split products suggests DIC.
      (iv) If DIC is suspected, enlist the aid of a hematologist if possible. Treatment must include removal of the cause (e.g., correction of hypovolemic shock), replacement of coagulation factors, and possibly heparinization.
3. Acidosis.
   (a) Check acid-base determinations frequently.
   (b) Correct metabolic acidosis with sodium bicarbonate.
4. Citrate toxicity (owing to infusion of citrated blood or plasma).
   (a) Results in hypotension that persists despite adequate volume replacement.
   (b) May be diagnosed by prolonged rate-corrected Q-T interval on the electrocardiogram (ECG).
   (c) Correct by administering 10% calcium gluconate (10 mg/kg) slowly under ECG control.
      N.B. Volume for volume, plasma contains more citrate than does whole blood.
5. Serum potassium disturbances.
   (a) Monitor serum K^+ levels periodically. (Hypokalemia may occur, but also serious hyperkalemia is possible, especially in low cardiac output states.)

6. Post-traumatic pulmonary insufficiency. This is characterized by falling compliance, impaired gas exchange, and radiographic findings of diffuse infiltrates. The following factors may contribute:
   (a) Too liberal use of clear fluids.
       (i) Give diuretics (furosemide, 1 mg/kg) if indicated.
   (b) Microembolization of the pulmonary vessels by infused particulate matter (platelet or leukocyte clumps).
       (i) Filter all blood given through a micropore (20–40 μm) filter.
   (c) Damage to alveolar-capillary membrane.
       (i) This results in low-pressure pulmonary edema.
       (ii) Large doses of steroids may help prevent this.

AUTOTRANSFUSION

Autotransfusion may be life-saving for some trauma patients. Advantages are the ready availability of absolutely compatible warm blood and possible prevention of some coagulation problems. In the extreme emergency, autotransfusion can be performed by using only a large syringe and an in-line filter in the IV line. A collection of freshly shed uncontaminated blood in an accessible body cavity is the main requirement.

HEAD INJURY

Head injury is extremely common during childhood and a cause of very significant mortality and morbidity—much of which might be reduced by early and efficient medical intervention. If consciousness is depressed, airway obstruction is very common and seriously compromises the prognosis. The first priority of the anesthesiologist must be to ensure an absolutely clear airway, excellent oxygenation, and optimal ventilation. Therefore, in serious head injury:

1. Give oxygen and intubate the patient without delay (*see* page 323). Use an oral tube. Nasal tubes (or nasogastric tubes) are contraindicated in patients with fractures of the base of the skull; perforation of the cribniform plate may occur.
2. Apply controlled ventilation to produce mild hypocapnia ($PaCO_2$ 25–30 mmHg) pending further evaluation of the patient's injuries.
3. Continue anesthesia (if required) with N_2O, O_2, fentanyl, and relaxant drugs.

The use of computed tomographic (CT) scans has been a major advance in the diagnosis of intracranial injuries of childhood. Accurate anatomic mapping of lesions has removed the need for exploratory burr holes. The characteristic appearance of diffuse cerebral damage on the CT scan can obviate the need for craniotomy and permit early specific therapeutic measures, that is

1. Continued artificial ventilation as above.
2. Intracranial pressure monitoring—most commonly by using an extradural bolt connected to an external transducer.
3. Therapy to control ICP:
    (a) Optimal positioning, slightly head up and face central.
    (b) Diuretics, preferably furosemide (1 mg/kg).
    (c) Barbiturates; these appear more effective in children than adults.
    (d) Adrenocortical steroid hormones; the use is controversial but is continued in many centers.
4. Maintenance of optimal perfusion pressure and arterial oxygenation.

When anesthetizing or caring for patients with a head injury, be alert for evidence of other injuries. Do not ascribe signs of hypovolemic shock (e.g., tachycardia or hypotension) to the head injury. If such signs are present, an exhaustive search must be made for bleeding from wounds in the scalp and/or other sites (intra-abdominal, intrathoracic, or in the limbs). Be constantly aware that hemorrhage at another site may have been overlooked. While anesthetizing a patient for emergency neurosurgery, monitor the cardiovascular system closely and continue measurements (e.g., abdominal girth) to detect hemorrhage.

THORACOABDOMINAL INJURY

Special Anesthetic Problems
1. Major hemorrhage requiring massive blood transfusion.
2. The patient may have a full stomach (food or blood).
3. Impaired cardiorespiratory function (in patients with diaphragmatic or thoracic trauma).

Immediate Management
1. Prepare for transfusion.
    (a) Insert a wide-bore plastic cannula into an upper limb or neck vein, by cutdown if necessary.
    (b) Send a blood sample for typing and cross-matching.
    (c) Insert a central venous cannula via a second upper limb or neck vein for measurement of CVP and to provide an alternative route for transfusion if necessary.

2. Assess the extent of hypovolemic shock.
3. Infuse appropriate solutions with a blood warmer from the outset.
4. Do not infuse large volumes of cold fluids or administer drugs via a central vein.

Anesthetic Management

During anesthesia the anesthesiologist is responsible for continuing vigorous blood volume replacement and other resuscitative measures.

Preoperative

1. Before induction, make every effort to restore the blood volume to near-normal levels. (This may not be possible until the source of bleeding has been controlled surgically.)
2. Order adequate supplies of blood for transfusion and have them available in the operating room (OR).
3. Premedication is not usually required.
4. If the patient is hypovolemic, given any necessary drugs in minimal dose, slowly, and only by the IV route.

Perioperative

Induction

1. Prepare and check all necessary equipment and drugs.
2. In the OR, reexamine the patient rapidly to ascertain current status.
3. Give 100% O_2 by mask for at least 4 minutes.
4. Check IV lines.
5. Connect monitoring equipment.
6. Give atropine IV immediately before induction.
7.
   (a) If hypovolemia has been corrected, induce anesthesia IV with thiopental (up to 4 mg/kg) and succinylcholine, 1 mg/kg. Inject these agents directly into a wide-bore venous cannula (to avoid the delayed transit through IV lines).
   (b) If the hypovolemia cannot be corrected and anesthesia is urgently required, do not give thiopental; instead, give ketamine 2 mg/kg IV, followed immediately by succinylcholine.
8. Position the patient supine and horizontally for intubation (to facilitate rapid insertion of the tube).
9. Do not inflate the lungs before intubation (ventilation may precipitate vomiting). Have an assistant apply cricoid pressure until an endotracheal tube of suitable size is in place and the cuff (if any) is inflated.

10. Do not give any drugs (except atropine) to moribund patients before intubation.

Maintenance

1. Give N_2O with a nondepolarizing neuromuscular blocking agent. (Pancuronium or vecuronium is preferred.)
2. Control the ventilation to produce near-normal $PaCO_2$. If the hypovolemia is still uncorrected, avoid positive end-expiratory pressure and adjust the inspiratory:expiratory ratio to give a low mean intrathoracic pressure.
3. Insert an arterial cannula for direct BP monitoring and for repeated blood sampling for serial determination of the acid-base status, blood gases, Hct, and coagulation studies.
4. Monitor ventilation, heart rate and rhythm, BP, CVP, pulse oximeter, and urine output.
5. Once the bleeding is controlled and the hypovolemia is corrected, give small doses of narcotic analgesics IV (e.g., fentanyl, 2 μg/kg).

Postoperative

1. In the absence of chest injury or significant impairment of pulmonary function, remove the endotracheal tube after full reversal of relaxant drugs and with the patient awake, responding, and in the lateral position.
2. If the patient has thoracic injuries of impaired pulmonary function, is still unconscious, or the condition is otherwise labile, continue ventilatory support and reevaluate the patient's condition later in the intensive care unit.

Special Considerations

During initial assessment of the child with thoracoabdominal trauma, one must consider possible physiologic consequences of the injury and the additional effect of anesthesia on the patient's condition. In patients with intra-abdominal injuries, the anesthesiologist's prime concerns are the amount of blood lost and the problem of securing a safe endotracheal airway. Some injuries demand special considerations.

1. Overt or suspected hepatic injury. Do not give drugs that are metabolized by the liver (e.g., barbiturates, narcotic analgesics). Substitute those that are excreted relatively unchanged by the lungs or kidneys (e.g., N_2O, isoflurane, pancuronium).

2. Overt or suspected renal injury or if acute renal failure is likely as a complication of prolonged hypovolemia and hypotension. Do not give drugs that are excreted through the kidneys (e.g., pancuronium, gallamine).

3. Ruptured diaphragm. Rupture of the diaphragm, leading to traumatic diaphragmatic hernia as a consequence of blunt abdominal trauma, is commoner in children than in adults. This condition requires thoracoabdominal repair. Respiratory distress is usually not severe.

   (a) Insert a gastric tube to decompress the upper gastrointestinal tract.

   (b) If the chest cavity contains a large volume of bowel, do not give N_2O until the herniation has been corrected.

4. Injury to chest wall and lungs.

   (a) Chest wall injuries may produce flailing and lead to hypoventilation. In young children, the ribs are relatively soft and less likely to fracture at two points, but the injury may have separated the costochondral junctions; this, in association with fractures of posterior ribs, may lead to "flail chest."

      (i) If it results in hypoventilation, intubate the patient and control the ventilation without delay.

   (b) Injuries to the chest wall are usually accompanied by contusion of underlying lung. This increases the shunting of blood through damaged lung, necessitating a higher inspired O_2 concentration.

      (i) Pneumothorax, hemothorax, or both may be present. If these are suspected, request insertion of a chest drain with a suitable valve or underwater seal before you anesthetize the patient. Pneumothorax should be suspected in the patient with grunting respiration and may occur without rib fractures in children.

5. Overt or suspected tracheal or bronchial injury.

   (a) If there is any evidence of such injury or if there is subcutaneous emphysema of the face, neck, or chest, bronchoscopy is required to define the extent of damage.

   (b) Induce anesthesia with halothane in O_2 (very smoothly and deeply, avoiding coughing and straining. Maintain spontaneous ventilation and avoid positive pressure, which may increase any air leak. Do not use nitrous oxide. For a penetrating wound, cover this with a sterile polyethyelene dressing (e.g., Opsite).

   (c) Give lidocaine, 1.5 mg/kg IV, wait 3 minutes, and then perform laryngoscopy and spray the larynx with lidocaine. The bronchoscope can then be inserted.

   (d) During bronchoscopy, give halothane in O_2 via the bronchoscope.

(e) If thoracotomy is required and damage is limited to one bronchus, intubate the uninjured main bronchus with a long endotracheal tube. During one-lung ventilation, add O_2 in high concentration.

(f) If a tracheal injury is present, tracheostomy may be required, though immediate surgical repair is sometimes possible. During such repair the endotracheal tube may be passed almost to the carina. Check bilateral ventilation and allow spontaneous respiration.

6. Injury to the heart and pericardium is rare in children but usually necessitates immediate exploration. If cardiac tamponade develops secondary to hemopericardium, induction of anesthesia may be very hazardous (because the fixed low cardiac output cannot compensate for drug-induced alterations in systemic vascular resistance).

(a) In hypotensive patients with hemopericardium, the surgeon should drain the pericardium (under local analgesia) before inducing general anesthesia.

(b) If tamponade is less severe, induction with ketamine may be possible. (**Note:** until the pericardium is open, controlled ventilation is poorly tolerated.)

ACUTE BURNS AND SCALDS

Children are unfortunately often the victims of burns and scalds. Their treatment demands a great deal of skill. Extensive burns have widespread systemic effects; massive fluid shifts occur, plasma protein is lost, and all the major organ systems are affected. The lungs may be directly damaged or their function affected by subsequent pulmonary vascular changes. The cardiovascular system is affected by changes in blood volume and possibly by a circulating myocardial depressant factor. The kidneys are subject to damage by myoglobinuria, hemoglobinuria, and hypovolemia. The liver may be damaged as a result of hypotension, hypoxemia, inhaled toxins, or sepsis. Anemia and disordered coagulation occur. Gastric distension, intestinal ileus, and stress ulcers may develop.

The anesthesiologist may become involved in the early treatment:
1. Airway management and fluid resuscitation.
2. Fasciotomy.
3. Early debridement and grafting.

Special Anesthetic Problems
1. Airway and pulmonary involvement, leading to airway obstruction and respiratory failure. Edema of the tissues surrounding the upper airway may occur very rapidly and make intubation extremely difficult.

2. Maintenance of fluid balance and renal function. There are several formulas used to calculate fluid regimens for the burned patient. These are based on the burn area (excluding erythema). The Parkland formula prescribes 4 ml/kg of lactated Ringer solution for each 1% burn area to be added to normal maintenance requirements. One-half of this is given in the first 8 hours and the other half over the next 16 hours. In practice, fluid therapy should be frequently adjusted as dictated by the clinical and biochemical status of the patient. The urine output is an essential guide.
3. Acute gastric dilation commonly occurs, adding to the danger of regurgitation. The stomach should be decompressed and special care taken during induction and emergence from anesthesia.
4. Management of body temperature. Loss of normal skin severely impairs the patient's ability to conserve heat.
5. In patients with extensive burns:
   (a) Monitoring may be difficult.
   (b) Sites for IV infusions may be limited.
6. Possibility of carbon monoxide and other gaseous poisoning (e.g., cyanide) caused by burning plastics.
7. The danger of infection. Extreme care must be taken to observe strict asepsis with invasive procedures.

Anesthetic Management
Preoperative
1. If the fire occurred in a close space or involved burning hydrocarbons, suspect respiratory tract burns.
   (a) Look for burning around the face (singed eyebrows, etc.).
   (b) Assess the airway very carefully. (Patients with airway burns may have considerable swelling of the pharyngeal and laryngeal tissues, making intubation difficult.)
   (c) Endotracheal intubation should be performed before massive edema forms if possible. Otherwise, the technique for the "difficult airway" should be adopted (*see* page 68).
2. Give humidified oxygen by mask. This is especially important if there are signs of possible carbon monoxide poisoning (impaired consciousness). Severe respiratory impairment dictates immediate intubation and ventilation.
3. Check the blood carbon monoxide level if indicated. Suspect carbon monoxide poisoning in the child who has unexplained confusion or coma plus cherry red discoloration of the mucosa.
4. Check the adequacy of fluid and blood replacement:

(a) Hct should be >30% and the serum albumin should be >2 g/dl.
(b) Patient should be catheterized and urine output should be at least 1 ml/kg/hr.

Beware of the excessive use of glucose-containing solutions for fluid resuscitation; hyperosmolar, hyperglycemic nonketotic coma may occur in association with burns.

5. Ensure that the OR temperature is at least 24°C and that heating blankets and lamps are ready for use. Humidify all anesthetic gases. All blood and IV fluids should be warmed.
6. Check whether the child has been given narcotic analgesics. (In many cases, these are not necessary in the early stages of severe burns.) Analgesics should be given to prevent pain during transportation to the OR.

Perioperative

General endotracheal anesthesia may be used, but:

1. The dose requirement for thiopental may be increased by 40% in children with burns.
2. Succinylcholine is contraindicated as it may cause cardiac arrest secondary to massive potassium release from muscle.
3. The dose requirements for nondepolarizing muscle relaxant drugs are increased in proportion to the burn area. The drug must be titrated to achieve the desired effect. Reversal of high doses is not a problem.
4. Potent volatile agents may not be tolerated by the patient with extensive burns. Fentanyl in high doses is, however, usually satisfactory.

Alternatively, ketamine has been used to greatly simplify the anesthetic management of burned or scalded children.

1. Give atropine, 0.02 mg/kg, followed by ketamine, 2 mg/kg, both IV.
2. Maintain anesthesia with ketamine, 8 mg/kg intramuscularly or incremental doses of 2 mg/kg IV.

For all patients

1. Monitor carefully:
   (a) Cardiac rate—via an esophageal stethoscope and the ECG (peripheral or esophageal leads) plus pulse oximeter (the probe can be placed on the tongue if no other site is available).
   (b) Blood pressure—if possible place cuff at any available site and use a Doppler flowmeter. For severe burns, insert an arterial line.
   (c) Temperature—esophageal and/or rectal.

(d) Blood loss—it is often difficult to estimate losses. Replacement must then be dictated by cardiovascular parameters and urine output.

(e) CVP—consider necessity versus danger of introducing infection. (If BP can be measured, CVP measurement may be unnecessary.)

2. Replace blood losses carefully; large volumes may be required. Anticipate coagulation problems with massive transfusions (see page 325).

3. Beware of hypocalcemia. Chronic low levels of ionized calcium have been described in burn patients. Give calcium chloride if unexpected hypotension cocurs. If large volumes of blood or plasma are given, give calcium chloride prophylactically (100–150 mg/unit.)

Postoperative

1. Order maintenance fluids:
   (a) Clear fluids to maintain urine output at >1 ml/kg/hr.
   (b) Blood to maintain Hct at >30%.
   (c) Plasma to maintain total serum protein at >3 g/dl.
   (d) Electrolyte supplements as indicated by serial determinations.

2. Order analgesics as required. Burn patients should be provided with constant nursing supervision so that generous dosage of analgesics can be safely administered.

3. Watch closely for developing respiratory insufficiency. (This may occur during the first 24 hours, even if the chest appears clear initially.) Rhonchi and a falling level of arterial oxygenation are the usual first signs of trouble. In severe airway burns, beware of the possibility of sudden airway obstruction owing to sloughed mucosa.

4. Cimetidine and antacids should be administered to protect against stress ulcer. Burn patients may require larger than usual doses of cimetidine to reduce acid secretion.

CHRONIC BURNS

See Chapter 9.

GUNSHOT WOUNDS

Children may become victims of gunshot wounds. The free access to military-style weapons in the United States (with the frequent choice of children as targets by the deranged) plus the universal problems of terrorism and firearm accidents contribute to this toll.

Anesthesiologists should be particularly aware of the tissue damage that is caused by modern high-velocity bullets. Tissue over an extensive area surrounding the path of the bullet will be damaged or destroyed by the energy of the projectile. This is of particular importance when such wounds occur in the upper chest or neck region. Tissue swelling can be expected to spread to involve a wide surrounding area. Therefore, the airway may be jeopardized, and it should be secured as early as possible, before distortion of the anatomy progresses further.

Very aggressive fluid resuscitation (guided by invasive monitoring) will be required for any major wound.

MINOR TRAUMA

Children with minor trauma must be provided with anesthesia that is safe, as pleasant as possible, and suitable for a young patient who may be ready to go home in an hour or so. Usually, there is no extreme urgency in these cases, permitting a considered approach to the selection of both the anesthetic and the optimal time for surgery. However, fractures with vascular compression may require immediate intervention.

Keep in mind the "full stomach": gastric emptying may be considerably delayed after even minor injury. Hence, even if one can wait for a full fasting period (6 hours), it is advisable to use a regional technique or to induce general anesthesia and secure the airway rapidly with an endotracheal tube. Although metoclopramide (Maxeran) may help to speed gastric emptying, neither regional analgesia nor general anesthesia should be administered without fasting unless surgery is needed urgently: The need to convert unsatisfactory regional anesthesia to general anesthesia is more frequent in children than in adults.

CLOSED LIMB FRACTURES

Injuries to upper limbs constitute the largest group for emergency anesthesia. Many of these patients are older children; therefore, regional analgesia can be used. If so:

1. Use sufficient local analgesia to produce a profound block.
2. Perform the block well in advance of the scheduled surgery.
3. If supplementary analgesia or sedation is required, give a small dose of Innovar (0.04 ml/kg IV).

FRACTURES OF THE FOREARM

1. Perform a block of the brachial plexus via the axillary route, using 1% lidocaine (maximum 5 mg/kg).
2. Do not use IV blocks before reduction of fractures. It is more difficult to apply an optimally tight cast to an exsanguinated limb.

Anesthetic Management

Do not give a general anesthetic in an emergency room unless the room is well equipped and is staffed with nurses experienced in the care of anesthetized patients. An adequately staffed recovery area must be available.

Preoperative

1. Give 100% O_2 by mask.

Perioperative

1. In ambulatory patients: immediately before induction give d-tubocurarine, 0.05 mg/kg IV (to prevent muscle pains caused by succinylcholine), and increase the dose of succinylcholine by 70% to produce a similar degree of relaxation.
2. Induce anesthesia with thiopental and succinylcholine IV.
3. Have an assistant apply cricoid pressure until endotracheal intubation is completed.
4. Maintain anesthesia with N_2O-halothane-O_2. Allow spontaneous ventilation.

Postoperative

1. Extubate when the patient is awake and lying laterally.

FRACTURED MANDIBLE

See Chapter 9.

Suggested Additional Reading

Trauma

Birch AA, Jr, GD Mitchell, GA Playford, and CA Lang: Changes in serum potassium response to succinylcholine following trauma. JAMA 210:490, 1969.

Brock-Utne JG, GE Dimopoulos, JW Downing, and MG Moshal: Effect of metochlopramide given before atropine sulphate on lower oesophageal sphincter tone. S Afr Med J 61:465, 1982.

Feuer H: Early management of pediatric head injury: physiologic aspects. Pediatr Clin North Am 22:425, 1975.

*Giesecke AH Jr (ed): Anesthesia for the surgery of trauma. Clin Anesth 11:3, 1976.

Hamilton Farrell MR, L Edmondson, and WDJ Cantrell: Penetrating tracheal injury in a child. Anaesthesia 43:123–125, 1988.

* Key article

Howells TH, T Khanam, L Kreel, C Seymour, B Oliver, and JAH Davies: Pharmacological emptying of the stomach with metoclopramide. Br Med J 2:558, 1971.

Ivan LP, SH Choo, and ECG Ventureya: Head injuries in childhood: a 2-year survey. Can Med Assoc J 128:281, 1983.

Miller RD: Complications of massive blood transfusions. Anesthesiology 39:82, 1973.

Moss E, JS Gibson, DG McDowall, and RM Gibson: Intensive management of severe head injuries. Anaesthesia 38:214, 1983.

Olsson GK, and B Hallen: Pharmacological evacuation of the stomach with metoclopramide. Acta Anaesth Scand 26:417, 1982.

Peters WJ: Inhalation injury caused by the products of combustion. Can Med Assoc J 125:249, 1981.

Raphaely RC, DB Swedlow, JJ Downes, and DA Bruce: Management of severe pediatric head trauma. Pediatr Clin North Am 27:715–727, 1980.

Salem MR, AY Wong, and VJ Collins: The pediatric patient with a full stomach. Anesthesiology 39:435, 1973.

Stehling LC, HL Zauder, and W Rogers: Intraoperative autotransfusion. Anesthesiology 43:337, 1975.

Steward DJ, and RE Creighton: Anesthetic management of the injured child. *In*: Care for the Injured Child (The Hospital for Sick Children, Surgical Staff). Baltimore, Williams & Wilkins, 1975, p. 26.

Burns

Belin RP, and CI Karleen: Cardiac arrest in the burned patient following succinylcholine administration. Anesthesiology 27:516, 1966.

Charnock EL, and JJ Meehan: Postburn respiratory injuries in children. Pediatr Clin North Am 27:661–676, 1980.

Cote CJ, and AJ Petkau: Thiopental requirements may be increased in children reanesthetized at least one year after recovery from extensive thermal injury. Anesth Analg 64:1156–1160, 1985.

Hickerson W, M Morrell, and RS Cicala: Glossal pulse oximetry. Anesth Analg 69:73, 1989.

Martyn JAJ, SK Szyfelbein, and HH Ali: Increased *d*-tubocurarine requirement following major thermal injury. Anesthesiology 52:352–355, 1980.

Moncrief JA: Burns. N Engl J Med 288:444–454, 1973.

Overton JH, and HA Kilham: Aspects of management of the burned child. Anaesthe Intensive Care 1:535, 1973.

Peters WJ: Inhalation injury caused by the products of combustion. Can Med Assoc J 125:249–251, 1981.

Raine PA, and A Azmy: A review of thermal injuries in young children. J Pediatr Surg 18:21–26, 1983.

Szyfelbein SK, LJ Drop, and JAJ Martyn: Persistent ionized hypocalcemia during resuscitation and recovery phases of body burns. Crit Care Med 9:454–458, 1981.

APPENDIX I

Anesthetic Implications of Syndromes and Unusual Disorders

This appendix contains brief descriptions of most of the syndromes encountered in pediatric anesthetic practice and describes important considerations for the anesthesiologist. The reader should consider all the information given in the description (and if in doubt consult the literature) before choosing an anesthetic technique.

Inevitably, this list is incomplete. "New" syndromes are being reported and "old" ones redefined, and anesthesiologists may experience unreported difficulties and complications.

Invaluable sources of information are the latest editions of *Syndromes of the Head and Neck,*[1] *Mendelian Inheritance in Man,*[2] and *The Metabolic Basis of Inherited Disease* (the end-of-chapter summaries are especially useful for quick reference).[3] However, anesthesiologists must bear in mind constantly the possibility of overlap of syndromes and the confusion over their nomenclature.

When in doubt as to the identity and implications of a syndrome—a feeling we experience frequently—the anesthesiologist should make preparations that take into account all possible associated disorders.

NAME	DESCRIPTION	ANESTHETIC IMPLICATIONS
Achondroplasia[10]	Most common form of dwarfism. Decreased rate of endochondreal ossification leads to shorter tubular bones. Foramen magnum or spinal stenosis may occur. Sleep apnea may be related to brain stem compression. May need suboccipital craniectomy, laminectomy, or CSF shunts.	Intubation may be difficult but is usually not. Endotracheal tube size best judged by weight (not age). Intravenous access difficult owing to excess lax skin. High incidence of complications when operated on in the sitting position.
Acrocephalopolysyndactyly	See Carpenter's syndrome.	
Acrocephalosyndactyly	See Apert's syndrome.	
Adrenogenital syndrome[2,3]	Inability to synthesize hydrocortisone; virilization of female.	All need hydrocortisone, even if not salt-losing. Check electrolytes preoperatively.[11]
Albers-Schönberg disease (marble bone disease; osteopetrosis)[2]	Brittle bones: pathologic fractures. Anemia from marrow sclerosis; hepatosplenomegaly.	Care in positioning and use of restraints.[6]
Albright–Butler syndrome	Renal tubular acidosis, hypokalemia, renal calculi.	Renal impairment. Correct electrolytes to within normal limits.[12]

Albright's hereditary osteodystrophy (pseudohypoparathyroidism)[1,2]	Ectopic bone formation, mental retardation. Hypocalcemia: possible ECG conduction defects, neuromuscular problems, convulsions.	Check electrolytes, monitor ECG. Do not use muscle relaxants.[13]
Aldrich's syndrome	*See* Wiskott–Aldrich syndrome.	
Alexander's disease	Severe mental retardation; megalocephaly. Death in infancy.	No reports of anesthesia.
Alport's syndrome[2]	Nephritis and nerve deafness; renal pathology variable. Renal failure in 2nd–3rd decade.	Use caution with drugs excreted by kidneys.[14]
Alström's syndrome[2]	Obesity, blindness by 7 years, hearing loss, diabetes after puberty, glomerulosclerosis. Renal impairment.	Diabetes and obesity require special consideration. Use caution with drugs excreted by kidneys.
Amaurotic familial idiocy	*See* Gangliosidosis GM$_2$ (Tay–Sachs disease).	
Amyotonia congenita (infantile muscular atrophy)[2]	Anterior horn cell degeneration.	Sensitive to thiopental (due to reduced muscle mass) and respiratory depressants. Do not use muscle relaxants.[15–18]

NAME	DESCRIPTION	ANESTHETIC IMPLICATIONS
Amyotrophic lateral sclerosis[2,3]	Degeneration of motor neurons.	Do not use succinylcholine—possible K^+ release and cardiac arrest. Use minimal doses of thiopental and curare; do not use respiratory depressants.[19]
Analbuminemia[2,3]	Extremely low level of serum albumin (4–100 mg/dl).	Very sensitive to drugs that bind to protein (e.g., thiopental, curare, pancuronium).
Analphalipoproteinemia	*See Tangier disease.*	
Andersen's disease (glycogen storage disease type IV)[1–3]	Deficiency of glucosyl transferase (brancher enzyme). Early severe hepatic cirrhosis; liver failure; splenomegaly; hemorrhagic tendency.	Check coagulation factors preoperatively; treat excessive bleeding with fresh-frozen plasma. Possibility of hypoglycemia under anesthesia.
Anderson's syndrome[1]	Severe midfacial hypoplasia → relative mandibular prognathism; abnormal structure and angle of mandible (triangular facies), kyphoscoliosis.	Possible airway problems, and intubation may be difficult. Assess respiratory status.
Angioedema (angioneurotic edema), hereditary[1,2,20,21,22]	Episodic brawny edema of extremities, face, trunk, airway abdominal viscera, usually for 24–72 hr (4 hr to 1 wk). Onset in	Check results of complement assay.[20,21] Hct, fluid status, treatment history, previous drug reactions. Observe for voice

childhood differentiates this from idiopathic form. Etiology: abnormal levels of C1 and C4 esterase inhibitor → accumulation of vasoactive substances → increased vascular permeability → edema. Usually painless; may have prodromal focal tingling or "tightness." Often induced by trauma or vibration. May have bouts of abdominal pain, diarrhea; hemoconcentration leading to hypotension, shock, pharyngeal edema (usually develops slowly). Most deaths from laryngeal edema; mortality rate up to 33%.[20] Long-term treatment is with antifibrinolytic and hormonal agents: **N.B.** adverse side effects of long-term ε-aminocaproic acid (EACA).[20]

change or dysphasia. *Prophylaxis* (especially in cases for dental or oropharyngeal manipulation): EACA for 2–3 days, and/or fresh-frozen plasma for 1 day pre-operatively. Continue EACA IV peri- and postoperatively. Danazol (androgen) may be useful.[23] *Acute attack*: give epinephrine, steroids, antihistamine; possibly fresh-frozen plasma. *If pharyngeal edema is imminent/ develops*: endotracheal or nasotracheal intubation (leave in place for 24–72 hr); if this is not possible, perform tracheotomy.[20–25]

Anesthesia: regional when possible. Otherwise, extreme care when instrumenting airway. *Peri- and postoperatively*: monitor vital signs closely.

Angiokeratoma corporis diffusum	*See Fabry's disease.*	
Angioosteohypertrophy	*See Klippel–Trénaunay–Weber syndrome.*	

NAME	DESCRIPTION	ANESTHETIC IMPLICATIONS
Anhidrotic ectodermal dysplasia	*See* Christ–Siemens–Touraine syndrome.	
Aper's syndrome (acrocephalosyndactyly)[1,2]	Hypoplastic maxilla and exophthalmos. Craniosynostosis, possibly with increased ICP; mental retardation, syndactyly. CHD may be present.	If CHD present: antibiotic prophylaxis preoperatively. Intubation may be difficult.[26,27]
Arachnodactyly	*See* Marfan's syndrome.	
Arthrogryposis multiplex[1,2]	Multiple congenital contractures; CHD in about 10% of cases.	If CHD present: antibiotic prophylaxis preoperatively. Minimal thiopental required— muscles replaced by fat. Possible airway problem due to limitation of mandibular movement.[28]
Asplenia syndrome[2]	Absent spleen; malposition of abdominal organs. Very complex cardiovascular anomalies; cyanosis and heart failure in many cases. Heightened susceptibility to overwhelming infection.	Antibiotic prophylaxis preoperatively; reverse isolation. Assess cardiovascular status carefully. Do not use cardiac depressants.[6]
Ataxia telangiectasia[1–3]	Cerebellar ataxia, skin and conjunctival telangiectasia; decreased serum IgA or IgE. Defective immunity → recurrent	Check Hb and Hct levels and pulmonary function if indicated. Treat anemia. Use sterile technique (reverse isolation).

Syndrome	Description	Considerations
	pulmonary and sinus infections; bronchiectasis. Severe anemia may be present. RES malignancy in about 10% of cases.[29]	
Bardet–Biedl syndrome[1,2]	Mental retardation, pigmentary retinopathy, polydactyly, obesity, hypogenitalism. (Spastic paraplegia, typical in Laurence–Moon syndrome [q.v.], is absent.) May have renal abnormalities and congenital heart defects.	Assess cardiac, renal, and fluid status.[30] If CHD present: antibiotic prophylaxis preoperatively.
Bartter's syndrome[31,32]	Hypokelamic, hypochloremic metabolic alkalosis; hyper-reninemia, hyperaldosteronism, and juxtaglomerular hyperplasia—but normotension. Etiology: overproduction of prostaglandin E. Growth retardation likely in prepubertal patients.	Subnormal response to norepinephrine. Abnormal acid-base and serum Na and K values.
Beckwith's syndrome (Beckwith–Wiedemann syndrome; "infantile gigantism")[1,2]	Birth weight >4,000 g; macroglossia and exophthalmos; visceromegaly and umbilical hernia common. Persistent severe neonatal hypoglycemia due to hyperinsulinism. (*See also* Neonatal hypoglycemia)	Airway problems due to large tongue. Monitor blood glucose carefully and treat hypoglycemia.[33,34]

NAME	DESCRIPTION	ANESTHETIC IMPLICATIONS
Behçet's syndrome[35,36]	Gross ulceration of mouth (usually first sign; may extend to esophagus) and genital area; uveitis, iritis, conjunctivitis, skin lesions, nonerosive arthritis. May have vasculitis, myocardial, and CNS involvement; risk of sepsis at sites of skin punctures, etc.	Use sterile technique. May have history of steroid therapy; nutritional status may be very poor. Intubation may be very difficult due to scarring in pharynx.[35,36]
Binder's syndrome[37]	Maxillonasal dysplasia; if severe, may be corrected surgically.	Advancement of maxilla and wiring of maxilla and mandible may cause airway problems peri- and postoperatively.
Blackfan–Diamond syndrome[2]	Congenital idiopathic RBC aplasia. Liver and spleen enlarged: hypersplenism, thrombocytopenia.	Do coagulation studies preoperatively; treat anemia and have platelets available for transfusion if necessary. Give additional steroids.[38]
Bowen's syndrome	*See* Cerebrohepatorenal syndrome.	
Capillary angioma with thrombocytopenic purpura syndrome	*See* Kasabach–Merritt syndrome.	
Cardioauditory syndrome	*See* Jervell–Lange-Nielsen syndrome.	

Carpenter's syndrome (acrocephalopolysynd-actyly)[1,2]	Mental retardation, oxycephaly, peculiar facies, syndactyly, deformed extremities, CHD, hypogenitalism.	If CHD present: antibiotic prophylaxis preoperatively. Hypoplastic mandible may make intubation difficult.[26,27] Problems associated with heart disease.
Central core disease[2]	Muscular dystrophy; hypotonia without muscle wasting. Increased risk of malignant hyperpyrexia.[39]	Preoperatively, assess respiratory status carefully. Sensitive to thiopental and respiratory depressants: do not use muscle relaxants (postoperative ventilation may be required).[15–18] **Do not give** drugs that might trigger malignant hyperpyrexia (see page 133).
Cerebrohepatorenal syndrome[1,2]	Hepatomegaly, neonatal jaundice, polycystic kidneys, muscular hypotonia. CHD may be present.	If CHD present: antibiotic prophylaxis preoperatively. Treat hypoprothrombinemia. Extreme care with muscle relaxants and other drugs excreted by kidneys.[40]
Charge association	An association of coloboma, congenital heart disease, choanal atresia, ear defects, genitourinary abnormalities, and genital hypoplasia.	Airway considerations, congenital heart disease, possible impaired renal function.

NAME	DESCRIPTION	ANESTHETIC IMPLICATIONS
Chédiak–Higashi syndrome[1–3]	Disorder of neutrophil function. Partial albinism, immunodeficiency, hepatosplenomegaly, recurrent bacterial infections. Neurologic disorders and mental retardation. Steroid therapy and cytotoxic drugs may be given to induce remission.	Use sterile technique (reverse isolation). Use disposable equipment. Repeated pulmonary infections may have impaired pulmonary function. Aggressive therapy to prevent postoperative complications required. Give supplemental steroids. Thrombocytopenia may require platelet transfusions.[41]
Cherubism[1,2]	Fibrous dysplasia of mandibles and maxillae with intraoral masses may cause respiratory distress.	Intubation may be extremely difficult; if there is acute respiratory distress tracheotomy may be required. Profuse bleeding may occur during surgery.[42]
Chondroectodermal dysplasia	*See Ellis–van Creveld syndrome*	
Chotzen's syndrome[1,2]	Craniosynostosis; associated renal anomalies.	Intubation may be difficult. Renal excretion of drugs may be impaired.[26]
Christ–Siemens–Touraine syndrome (anhidrotic ectodermal dysplasia)[1,2]	Absence of sweating and tearing. Heat intolerance due to inability to control temperature by sweating. Poor mucous formation → persistent respiratory infections.	Hypoplastic mandible may make intubation difficult; monitor body temperature carefully and be prepared to institute cooling. Tape eyes closed. Chest physiotherapy pre- and postoperatively.[43]

Condition		
Chronic granulomatous disease[2]	Inherited disorder of leukocyte function: recurrent infections with nonpathogenic organisms; hepatomegaly in 95% of cases.	Poor pulmonary function. Use sterile technique (reverse isolation).[44]
Chubby puffer syndrome	Obesity, upper airway obstruction, daytime somnolence, and respiratory distress when sleeping. May be hyperactive and aggressive. Blood gases may show hypoxemia and hypercapnia. Cor pulmonale may develop.	May present for tonsillectomy. Avoid preoperative sedation. Monitor carefully postoperatively for airway obstruction. Avoid narcotic analgesics. Patients with severe obstruction may require tracheostomy.[45]
Cleft syndromes	See Ch. 29 in ref. 1.	
Collagen disease: dermatomyositis; polyarteritis nodosa; rheumatoid arthritis; systemic lupus erythematosus[2]	Systemic connective tissue diseases with variable systemic involvement. Osteoporosis, fatty infiltration of muscle, anemia, pulmonary infiltration or fibrosis.	Temporomandibular or cricoarytenoid arthritis may cause airway and intubation difficulties. Risk of fat embolism after osteotomy, fracture, or minor trauma. Supplement steroid therapy.[46,47]
Congenital heart block	Comprises <1% of congenital heart disease. Defect of conduction between AV node and bundle of His, or within bundle of His. Supraventricular arrhythmias may occur, and up to 20% progress to congestive heart failure and Adams–Stokes attacks.	Because of possibility of arrhythmia or increased AV block, preoperative insertion of a temporary transvenous pacemaker is recommended.[48,49]

NAME	DESCRIPTION	ANESTHETIC IMPLICATIONS
Conradi's syndrome (chondrodysplasia epiphysealis punctata; ch. calcificans congenita; koala bear syndrome)[1,2]	Chondrodystrophy with contractures, saddle nose, macro- or microcephaly, mental retardation; dwarfing, congenital cataracts. CHD and renal anomalies in some other cases.	If CHD present: antibiotic prophylaxis preoperatively. Do not use drugs excreted by kidneys; assess cardiac status carefully.[50]
Cori's disease	*See* von Gierke's disease.	
Cornelia de Lange syndrome.[51]	Short stature, mental retardation, microcephalic and hirsute. Short or dysmorphic extremities, hypoplastic nipples, rib and sternal defects.	Intubation may be difficult.
Cretinism (congenital hypothyroidism)[2,3]	Goiter; hypothyroidism secondary to defective synthesis of thyroxine. Large tongue. Respiratory center very sensitive to depression; CO_2 retention common. Hypoglycemia, hyponatremia, hypotension, low cardiac output.	Correct hypothyroidism and anemia preoperatively if possible. Airway problems due to large tongue. Monitor body temperature carefully. Use warming blankets if necessary. Do not use myocardial depressants. Transfuse carefully: overtransfusion is poorly tolerated because of myocardial flaccidity.[8]
Cri-du-chat syndrome[1,3]	Mental retardation, abnormal (catlike) cry, microcephaly, round face, hypertelorism. In some, ears abnormal, micrognathia, epiglottis	If CHD present: antibiotic prophylaxis preoperatively. Airway problems: stridor, laryngomalacia. Intubation may be difficult.[9]

	and larynx small. CHD may be present.	Intubation may be difficult.[26]
Crouzon's disease[1,2]	Craniosynostosis, hypertelorism, parrot beak nose, hypoplastic maxilla.	
Cutis laxa[1-3]	Elastic fiber degeneration: pendulous skin, frequent hernias. Recurrent pulmonary infections, emphysema and cor pulmonale, arterial fragility.	Assess pulmonary status carefully. Use sterile technique. Difficulty maintaining IV line due to poor tissues. Excess soft tissues around larynx may cause respiratory obstruction.[5,52]
Dandy–Walker syndrome	*See* Hydrocephalus (page 149).	
Dermatomyositis	*See* Collagen disease.	
DiGeorge's syndrome (3rd & 4th brachial arch/ pharyngeal pouch syndrome)[1-3]	Thymus and parathyroids absent— hypoparathyroidism, low serum Ca, tetany; stridor. Immune deficiency: susceptibility to fungal and viral infections; recurrent chest infections. Treated by thymic transplants. Aortic arch abnormalities.	Use sterile technique (reverse isolation). Donor blood must be previously irradiated (3,000 rads) to prevent graft-vs-host reaction.[53,54]
Donohue's syndrome	*See* Leprechaunism.	

NAME	DESCRIPTION	ANESTHETIC IMPLICATIONS
Down syndrome (mongolism; trisomy 21)[1-3] (*see also* p. 130)	Mental retardation, small nasopharynx, hypotonia. High incidence of CHD; duodenal atresia in some.	If CHD present: antibiotic prophylaxis preoperatively. Do not use barbiturate premedication but give usual doses of atropine. Airway problems: large tongue, small mouth. Risk of laryngeal spasm, especially on extubation. Problems of cardiac anomalies. These patients tolerate extensive surgery very well.[55,56]
Duchenne's muscular dystrophy.[2,3,57]	Progressive pseudohypertrophy of muscles, with cardiac muscle involvement in many cases. Most die in the 2nd decade. Succinylchloline may cause rhabdomyolysis, cardiac arrest due to hyperkalemia, and possibly malignant hyperpyrexia.	Use minimal drug dosage. Avoid respiratory depressants or muscle relaxants if possible. Do not give succinylcholine. Use caution with myocardial depressants (e.g., halothane). Monitor cardiac status carefully. Assess carefully postoperatively; IPPV may be required (if preoperative vital capacity is <50% of predicted, plan for postoperative ventilation).

Edward's syndrome (trisomy 18[E])[1]	CHD in 95%, micrognathia in 80%, renal malformations in 50–80%. Most die in infancy.	Antibiotic prophylaxis preoperatively. Intubation may be difficult; use caution with drugs excreted by kidneys; assess cardiac status carefully.[9]
Ehlers–Danlos syndrome[1–3]	Collagen abnormality— hyperelasticity and fragile tissues; dissecting aneurysm of aorta, fragility of other blood vessels; ECG conduction abnormalities. Bleeding diathesis; hernias. May have heart, lung, and GI malformations.	Difficult to maintain IV line; poor tissues and clotting defect may lead to hemorrhage. Spontaneous pneumothorax may occur.[5,52,58]
Elfin facies syndrome	*See* Williams' syndrome.	
Ellis–van Creveld syndrome (chondroectodermal/mesoectodermal dysplasia)[1,2]	Ectodermal defects and skeletal anomalies; 50% have CHD, usually septal defects. Chest wall anomalies cause poor lung function. May have abnormal maxilla, cleft lip, cleft palate; hepatosplenomegaly. Many die before 6 months of age.	If CHD present: antibiotic prophylaxis preoperatively. problems of associated heart disease: assess cardiorespiratory function carefully. Airway problems: intubation may be difficult.[59]
Eosinophilic granuloma	*See* Histiocytosis X.	

NAME	DESCRIPTION	ANESTHETIC IMPLICATIONS
Epidermolysis bullosa (Herlitz's syndrome)[1,2,60,61]	Skin cleavage at dermal–epidermal junction, resulting in erosions and blisters from minor trauma to skin or mucous membrane. The disease occurs in several forms: epidermolysis bullosa simplex is relatively mild with rapid healing and little scarring. Junctional epidermolysis bullosa (letalis) is severe, presents at birth, leads to extensive scarring and death (often from sepsis) usually by age 2. Dystrophic epidermolysis bullosa is very rare but severe; lesions heal slowly with extensive scarring. Strictures may form and involve the pharynx, larynx, and esophagus. Digital fusion occurs ("mitten-hand") Nutritional deprivation leads to growth retardation and anemia. Infections are common.	Antibiotic prophylaxis preoperatively. Check history of steroid therapy. Use sterile technique (reverse isolation). Airway difficulty: oral lesions, adhesion of tongue. Avoid trauma to skin or mucous membranes; avoid intubation and/or instrumentation of the airway if possible; otherwise, lubricate tube and laryngoscope generously. Use insufflation or a well-padded and lubricated mask for inhalation anesthesia or use ketamine. **Do not use adhesive tape.** Regional analgesia may be considered.[62]
Erythema multiforme	*See* Stevens–Johnson syndrome.	
Eulenberg's periodic paralysis	*See* Paramyotonia congenita.	

Fabry's disease (angiokeratoma corporis diffusum)[1-3]	X-linked lipid storage disorder. Lipid deposition in blood vessels causes periodic very severe pain and fever crises. Dark telangiectasia, particularly around genitals and buttocks; hypertension, myocardial ischemia, renal failure.	Assess cardiorespiratory and renal function carefully; monitor ECG. Do not use drugs excreted by the kidneys.[63]
Familial dysautonomia	See Riley–Day syndrome.	
Familial osteodysplasia	See Anderson's syndrome.	
Familial periodic paralysis	Periodic muscle weakness secondary to serum K$^+$ disturbance (hypo- or hyperkalemia). Muscle weakness in the hypokalemic variety is due to massive uptake of K into muscles and thus decreased serum K.	Monitor serum K and ECG; prevent hyper- or hypoglycemia. Do not use muscle relaxants; maintain body temperature. Avoid excessive glucose solutions.[64]
Fanconi's syndrome (anemia with renal tubular acidosis)[2,3]	Usually secondary to cystinosis. Proximal tubular defect: impaired renal function; acidosis, K loss, dehydration.	Treat electrolyte and acid-base abnormalities: do not use drugs excreted by kidneys. Be aware of possibility of other metabolic defects.[2,3,12]
Farber's disease (lipogranulomatosis)[2,3]	Sphingomyelin deposition; widespread visceral lipogranulomas, especially in CNS. General systemic involvement leading to cardiac, renal failure.	Assess cardiorespiratory and renal status carefully. Deposits in larynx—care with intubation.[5,65]

355

NAME	DESCRIPTION	ANESTHETIC IMPLICATIONS
Favism [glucose-6-phosphate dehydrogenase (G-6-PD) deficiency][2,3]	Diathesis for spontaneous/induced (drugs, fava beans, infection) hemolytic anemia.	Do not give drugs that cause hemolysis (e.g., ASA, phenacetin, sulfonamides, quinidine, methylene blue). Anemia: transfuse if necessary.[65]
Fetal alcohol syndrome	Abnormalities of the infant due to maternal heavy alcohol consumption: growth retardation, intellectual impairment, craniofacial abnormalities (microcephaly, microphthalmia, hypoplastic upper lip, flat maxilla), cardiac defects (especially VSD), renal abnormalities, and inguinal hernia.	If CHD present: antibiotic prophylaxis preoperatively. Difficult intubation. Problems of associated cardiac disease.[66-68]
Fibrodysplasia ossificans progressiva	*See* Myositis ossificans.	
Focal dermal hypoplasia (Goltz's syndrome)[1,2]	Multifarious features,[2] including multiple papillomas of mucous membranes, skin.	Airway may contain papillomas.
Forbes' disease (glycogen storage disease type III)	*See* von Gierke's disease.	
Freeman–Sheldon ("Whistling face") syndrome[69]	Congenital myopathy and dysplasia. Increased tone and fibrosis of facial	Very difficult intubation, tight facial musles will not relax with

	muscles. Hyperteorism, microstomia, and micrognathia. Myopathy leads to flexion contractures of limbs. Strabismus and inguinal hernia common. Later, kyphoscoliosis may lead to restrictive lung disease.	neuromuscular blockade. IV access limited by limb flexion contractures and/or splints. Pulmonary function may be impaired (late). Regional analgesia may be useful for postoperative pain.[70]
Friedreich's ataxia[2,3]	Progressive degeneration of cerebellum, lateral and posterior column of spinal cord; scoliosis; myocardial degeneration and fibrosis, leading to failure and arrhythmias.	Care with cardiac depressant drugs.
Gangliosidoses[3]		Progressive neurologic loss leads to respiratory complications.[71]
GM1, type 1	Invariably fatal. Supportive measures only treatment. *Acute onset in infancy.* Rapid neurologic decline, severe bone abnormalities; pulmonary infiltration common. Death by 2 yr.	
GM1, type 2	*Onset in early childhood.* Few somatic changes. Death from cardiopulmonary causes by 10 yr.	
GM2 (Tay–Sachs disease: Sandhoff's disease)	*Onset in infancy.* Progressive psychomotor deterioration; blindness, seizures. Death by 5 yr (by 2 yr in most cases). *Rare juvenile variants:* same features; longer survival.	

NAME	DESCRIPTION	ANESTHETIC IMPLICATIONS
Gardner's syndrome[1-3]	Familial polyposis of colon; bone tumors, sebaceous cysts, fibromas.	No specific anesthesia problems described.[72]
Gaucher's disease[2,3]	Cerebroside accumulation in CNS, liver, spleen, etc. Serum acid phosphatase increased. Pulmonary disease from aspiration (pseudobulbar palsy); hepatosplenomegaly. Hypersplenism may cause platelet deficiency. If obvious neurologic signs: usually fatal in infancy. If more chronic: bone pain, fractures.	Treat coagulation disorders and correct anemia.[71]
Glanzmann's disease (thromboasthenia)[2,3]	Abnormal platelet function, leading to mild thrombocytopenic purpura; abnormality of high-energy phosphate mechanisms.	No specific therapy for bleeding; platelet transfusion disappointing. May have history of steroid therapy.[73]
Glucose-6-phosphate dehydrogenase (G-6-PD) deficiency	See Favism	
Glycogen storage disease[2,3] Type I Type II Type III (Cori's disease; Forbes' disease) Type IV Type V	See von Gierke's disease. See Pompe's disease. See von Gierke's disease. See Andersen's disease. See McArdle's disease.	

Type VI (Hers' disease) Type VII Type VIII	See von Gierke's disease. See Muscle phosphofructokinase deficiency. See Hepatic phosphorylase kinase deficiency.
Goldenhar's syndrome (oculoauriculovertebral syndrome)[1,2]	Unilateral hypoplasia with mandibular hypoplasia; CHD in 20%.	If CHD present: antibiotic prophylaxis preoperatively. Airway problems and intubation may be difficult. Problems of associated cardiac disease.[7]
Goltz's syndrome	See Focal dermal hypoplasia. See also Gorlin–Goltz syndrome.	
Gonadal dysgenesis	See Turner's syndrome.	
Gorlin–Chaudhry–Moss syndrome[1,2]	Craniofacial dysostosis, PDA, hypertrichosis, hypoplasia of labia majora, dental and eye anomalies. Normal intelligence.	If CHD present: antibiotic prophylaxis preoperatively. Asymmetry of head—difficult airway. Problems associated with PDA.[1]
Gorlin–Goltz syndrome (basal cell nevus syndrome)[1,2]	Multiple nevoid basal cell carcinomas, hypertelorism, mandibular prognathism, multiple jaw cysts and fibrosarcomas, kyphoscoliosis, incomplete segmentation of cervical and thoracic vertebrae; congenital hydrocephalus, mental retardation, etc.	Extreme care in positioning and intubating—cervical movement may be limited. Increased ICP may be unrecognized.

NAME	DESCRIPTION	ANESTHETIC IMPLICATIONS
Groenblad–Strandberg syndrome (pseudoxanthoma elasticum)[1,2]	Degeneration of elastic tissue in skin, eye, and CVS: rupture of arteries, especially in GI tract; hypertension; arterial calcification; occlusion of cerebral and coronary arteries.	Assess cardiovascular status carefully. Difficult to maintain IV cannula.[5]
Guillain–Barré syndrome (acute [idiopathic] polyneuritis)	Acute polyneuropathy; progressive peripheral neuritis, usually involving cranial nerves; bulbar palsy with hypoventilation and hypotension. May require tracheotomy and IPPV.	Do not use succinylcholine for at least 3 months after onset of polyneuritis (K$^+$ release).[74,75]
Hallervorden–Spatz disease	Autosomal recessive disorder of basal ganglia: dementia and dystonia with torticollis, scoliosis, and trismus.	Assess pulmonary status carefully. Inhalation induction of anesthesia leads to relaxation of abnormal posturing and trismus, and facilitates intubation. Avoid succinylcholine (? hyperkalemic response [76]—may intensify rigidity) or rapid-sequence induction (in case of difficult intubation).
Hand–Schüller–Christian syndrome	*See* Histiocytosis X.	
Hemangioma with thrombocytopenia	*See* Kasabach–Merritt syndrome.	

Hepatic phosphorylase kinase deficiency (glycogen storage disease type VIII)[2,3]	Hepatomegaly; increased liver glycogen concentration.	No anesthetic complications reported.
Herlitz's syndrome	*See* Epidermolysis bullosa.	
Hermansky–Pudlak syndrome[2,3]	Albinism; bleeding diathesis due to platelet abnormality.	May require platelet transfusion during surgery.
Hers' disease	*See* von Gierke's disease.	
Histiocytosis X (eosinophilic granuloma: Hand–Schüller–Christian disease; Letterer–Siwe disease)[2]	Lesions in bones and viscera (larynx, lungs, liver, and spleen). Clinical course similar to acute leukemia. Hypersplenism, pancytopenia, anemia, purpura, hemorrhage; hepatic involvement. Pulmonary—diffuse hilar infiltration; respiratory failure, cor pulmonale. Gingival inflammation and necrosis, with loss of teeth. Diabetes insipidus if sella turcica involved. Many die in first year of life.	Correct anemia and coagulation defects. Assess cardiorespiratory status carefully (and, if indicated, fluid balance). May have history of steroid therapy. Laryngeal fibrosis; intubation may be difficult.[77]
Holt–Oram syndrome (heart–hand syndrome)[2]	Upper limb abnormalities; CHD (usually ASD); possibility of sudden death from pumonary embolus, coronary occlusion.	Antibiotic prophylaxis preoperatively. Problems of cardiac defect. No other anesthetic problem.[78]

NAME	DESCRIPTION	ANESTHETIC IMPLICATIONS
Homocystinuria[1–3]	Thromboembolic phenomena due to intimal thickening; ectopia lentis, osteoporosis, kyphoscoliosis. Angiography may precipitate thrombosis, especially cerebral.	Give fluids to maintain urine output. Give dextran 40 to reduce viscosity and platelet adhesiveness and increase peripheral perfusion.[79]
Hunter's syndrome (mucopolysaccharidosis type II)[1–3]	Similar to but less severe than Hurler's syndrome, *q.v.*	As for Hurler's syndrome.
Hurler's syndrome (mucopolysaccharidosis type 1 H; formerly classed as type I)[1–3]	Mental retardation, gargoyle facies, deafness, stiff joints, dwarfing, pectus excavatum, and kyphoscoliosis. Abnormal tracheobronchial cartilages; severe coronary artery disease at early age, valvar and myocardial involvement. Hepatosplenomegaly. Most die from respiratory and cardiac failure before 10 yr; sudden death common after 7 yr.	*See* Mucopolysaccharidoses. Antibiotic prophylaxis and chest physiotherapy preoperatively. Give large doses of atropine preoperatively. Upper airway obstruction and difficult intubation due to infiltration of lymphoid tissue and larynx and profuse thick secretions. Give adequate fluids perioperatively and humidify anesthetic gases.[65]
Hurler–Scheie compound syndrome (type I HS)	*See* Scheie's syndrome.	
Hutchinson–Gilford syndrome	*See* Progeria.	

Hyalinosis, cutaneous-mucosal	*See* Urbach–Wiethe disease.
Hyperpyrexia/hyperthermia, malignant	*See* Chapter 4 (page 133).
I-cell disease (mucolipidoses)	Mental retardation, Hurler-type bone changes, severe joint limitation, chronic pulmonary disease; valvar insufficiency common. Death in early childhood (most by 1 yr).	Intubation and airway maintenance difficult—limited jaw movement, stiffness of neck and rib cage.
Ivemark syndrome	*See* Asplenia syndrome.
Jervell–Lange–Nielsen syndrome (cardioauditory syndrome; Romano–Ward syndrome)[2]	Congenital deafness and cardiac conduction defects; arrhythmias, syncope. ECG: large T waves, prolonged Q-T interval. Death may occur suddenly.	Assess cardiac status carefully; may need digoxin and/or propranolol, or pacemaker.[80] Stellate ganglion block may be life-saving.[81]
Jeune's syndrome (asphyxiating thoracic dystrophy)[1,2]	Severe thoracic malformation; asphyxia. Cystic renal changes, progressing to failure.	Surgery to enlarge thorax may necessitate prolonged periods of assisted ventilation.[82] Care with drugs excreted by kidneys.
Kartagener's syndrome[1,2]	Dextrocardia, sinusitis, bronchiectasis, defective immunity.	Order physiotherapy preoperatively. Use sterile technique (reverse isolation). Assess respiratory status carefully.[83]

NAME	DESCRIPTION	ANESTHETIC IMPLICATIONS
Kasabach–Merritt syndrome[1,2,84–86]	Hemangioma, thrombocytopenia, hypofibrinogenemia → purpura, bleeding, anemia, increased fibrinolytic activity. Treated by radiotherapy (surgery may precipitate disseminated intravascular coagulation). Recovery follows destruction of tumor.	Correct anemia and coagulation defects (to prevent severe hemorrhage during surgery).
Kawasaki syndrome (mucocutaneous lymph node syndrome)	Acute febrile exanthematous disease secondary to vasculitis with cardiac involvement (pancarditis, valvular dysfunction, arrhythmias, and coronary artery vasculitis). Signs include fever, conjunctivitis, oral erythema, erythroedema of hands and feet, erythematous rash, and lymphadenopathy. Cardiac involvement in >20% of cases: ranges from asymptomatic ECG changes to severe congestive failure and massive myocardial infarction. Salicylates are used in treatment and may reduce coronary artery lesions. Biliary tract and bowel complications may require laparotomy. Hepatic involvement in 10% of patients.	Related to associated cardiac lesions. Assess cardiac status carefully. Avoid myocardial depressants and anesthetize as for patient with coronary artery disease. Monitor carefully for cardial ischemic changes (V_5 and lead II). Be prepared with vasoactive and antiarrhythmic drugs.[87,88]

Ketonuria, branched chain	*See Maple syrup urine disease.*	
Klinefelter's syndrome (gonosomal aneuploidy with tubular dysgenesis)[1,3]	Tall; reduced intelligence; vertebral collapse due to osteoporosis. May have diabetes mellitus.	No anesthetia problem reported, except in diabetics. Position carefully to avoid spinal cord damage.[9]
Klippel–Feil syndrome[1,2]	Congenital fusion of two or more cervical vertebrae, causing neck rigidity.	Intubation may be very difficult: should be done awake if possible; otherwise inhalation induction without muscle relaxant. Do not extubate until fully awake.
Klippel–Trénaunay–Weber syndrome (angioosteohypertrophy)[1,2]	Hemangiomas with hypertrophy of adjacent bone; thrombocytopenia. AV fistulas and anemia lead to high cardiac output, with possible cardiac failure; thrombocytopenia in association with visceral hemangiomas.	Check cardiac status carefully, correct bleeding disorders.[1]
Krabbe's disease (globoid cell leukodystrophy)[2,3]	Rapidly progressive inherited metabolic disorder of the nervous system. Symptoms usually become apparent at 3–6 months (irritability, screaming). Later: blindness, deafness, retarded development, etc. Most die by 2 yr.	No known anesthetic complications.

NAME	DESCRIPTION	ANESTHETIC IMPLICATIONS
Larsen's syndrome[1,2]	Multiple congenital dislocations, hydrocephalus, cleft palate, connective tissue defect (poor cartilage in rib cage, epiglottis, arytenoids). Chronic respiratory problems.[5]	Intubation may be difficult.[52] ICP may be increased.
Laurence–Moon syndrome[2]	Mental retardation, pigmentary retinopathy, hypogenitalism, and spastic paraplegia. (Polydactyly and obesity, typical in Bardet–Biedl syndrome [q.v.], are absent.) May have renal abnormalities and CHD.	Assess cardiac, renal, and fluid status.[89] If CHD present: Antibiotic prophylaxis preoperatively.
Leigh disease (subacute necrotizing encephalomyelopathy)[90]	May occur in infancy or childhood. Infants develop hypotonia, somnolance, optic atrophy, deafness, and pyramidal tract signs. Altered respiratory patterns may occur and may lead to SIDS. Older children present with acute neurologic deterioration and respiratory failure.	Monitor ventilation carefully in the perioperative period.
Leopard syndrome[1,2]	Multiple large freckles; hypertelorism, eyelid ptosis, etc. CHD (PS in 95%); ECG anomalies	If CHD present: antibiotic prophylaxis preoperatively. Assess cardiac status, lung function.

	include aberrant conduction. Growth retardation common; pectus carinatum, kyphosis, etc., in some. GU anomalies (hypospadias, cryptorchidism, ovarian hypoplasia, etc.).	Intubation may be difficult. Problems of associated cardiac disease.
Leprechaunism[1,2] (Donohue's syndrome)	Failure to thrive, endocrine disorders, severe mental retardation. Hypoglycemia due to hyperinsulinism from hyperplastic islets of Langerhans; renal tubular defects → impaired renal function. Most die before 1 yr.	Check metabolic status. Do not use drugs excreted by kidneys.[91]
Lesch–Nyhan syndrome[1,2]	Disorder of purine metabolism, occurs in males. Mental and growth retardation, malnutrition, choreoathetosis. Very aggressive with compulsive self-destructive behavior. Hyperuricemia leads to renal calculi, RBC damage, hypertension, and coronary artery disease. Renal failure by age 20 yr.	Avoid drugs excreted by the kidney. Beware of regurgitation, give metoclopramide. Diazepam, thiopental, isoflurane, and atracurium are recommended.[92] Caution with catecholamines.
Letterer–Siwe disease	*See* Histiocytosis X.	

367

NAME	DESCRIPTION	ANESTHETIC IMPLICATIONS
Lipoatrophy with diabetes (Seip's syndrome)[1-3]	Generalized loss of all body fat, fibrotic liver leading to failure, portal hypertension; splenomegaly, nephropathy, diabetes. May have renal failure.	Do not use drugs metabolized by liver. Check coagulation and renal function preoperatively. Take precautions as for diabetes.[71]
Lipogranulomatosis	See Farber's disease.	
Lowe's syndrome (oculocerebrorenal syndrome)[2,3]	Affects males. Cataract, glaucoma, mental retardation; hypotonia, renal acidosis, proteinuria, osteoporosis, and rickets.	Check electrolyte and acid-base balance, and serum Ca (treated with vitamin D and Ca^{2+}). Care with drugs excreted by kidneys.[12,93]
Lupus erythematosus disseminatus	See Collagen disease.	
Maffucci's syndrome[1,2]	Enchondromatosis and hemangiomas with malignant change. Pathologic fractures, GI bleeding from hemangiomas, orthostatic hypotension.	Position carefully. May be sensitive to vasodilator drugs.
Malignant hyperpyrexia/ hyperthermia	See Chapter 4 (page 133).	

Mandibulofacial dysostosis	*See Treacher Collins syndrome.*
Mannosidosis[1-3,94]	Primary metabolic deficiency of α-mannosidases A & B → lysosomal accumulation of mannose-rich substrates. Abnormal neutrophil immunologic function.	Be alert for hepatic dysfunction, and for hypoventilation peri- and postoperatively.
Type I (severe)	Hepatosplenomegaly, severe recurrent infections, and early death.	
Type II (milder)	Hearing loss, mental retardation, Hurler-like skeletal changes, gargoyle-like facies, clumsy motor function, weak connective tissues.	
Maple syrup urine disease (MSUD; branched-chain ketonuria)[2,3]	Inability to metabolize leucine, isoleucine, and valine. Severe neurologic damage and respiratory disturbances. Episodes of hypoglycemia. Treated by diet only, from birth; many die within 2 months. Acute, life-threatening episodes may require peritoneal dialysis or exchange transfusion.	Check acid-base balance, plasma amino acids preoperatively. Check serum glucose pre-, peri-, and postoperatively. Start glucose infusion (at least 10–15 mg/kg/min) preoperatively and continue until diet is reestablished.[95]

NAME	DESCRIPTION	ANESTHETIC IMPLICATIONS
Marfan's syndrome (arachnodactyly)[1-3]	Tall thin patients with long fingers, long face, and high arched palate. Connective tissue disorder leading to joint instability and dislocation (including cervical spine), dislocation of lens, kyphoscoliosis, hernia, pectus excavatum, lung cysts. Aortic root dilation may lead to AI or aneurysm; pulmonary artery or mitral valve may be diseased.	Antibiotic prophylaxis preoperatively. Intubation may be difficult. Laryngoscopy should be gentle to avoid cervical spine or temporomandibular joint damage. Position carefully to avoid dislocations. Avoid myocardial depressants, but do not allow the patient to become hypertensive (danger of aortic dissection). Beware of pneumothorax with controlled ventilation.
Maroteaux–Lamy syndrome (mucopolysaccharidosis type VI)[1-3]	Normal intellect. Kyphoscoliosis with poor lung reserve; chronic respiratory infections; hypersplenism, anemia, thrombocytopenia. Myocardial involvement; heart failure by 20 yr.	*See Mucopolysaccharidoses.* Check cardiac status, coagulation, respiratory function. Care with cardiac depressant drugs.[5,65] May require ventilation postoperatively.
Mastocystosis syndrome (urticaria pigmentosa)	Abnormal aggregates of histamine- and heparin-containing mast cells; skin lesion is a brownish-red maculopapular rash mainly on trunk. Mast cell degranulation with	Avoid stimuli and drugs known to cause mast cell degranulation. Premedicate with an antihistamine. Inhalation anesthetics may be safely used, as

	systemic histamine and heparin release may occur with trauma, temperature changes, alcohol, and drugs (including salicylates, opiates, curare, gallamine, papaverine, polymyxin, and atropine). Minor surgical procedures may lead to generalized anaphylaxis and death.	may succinylcholine. Meperidine (Demerol) can be used as an analgesic. Bleeding secondary to heparin release may require protamine therapy.[96]
McArdle's myopathy (glycogen storage disease type V)[2,3]	Muscle phosphorylase deficiency; serum lactate not increased by exercise. Initially, increased fatigability; progresses to muscle cramps and weakness (all skeletal muscles affected), myoglobinuria. Myocardium may be involved; ECG abnormalities have been reported.[3]	Do not use tourniquets; maintain infusion of dextrose during surgery; do not use succinylcholine.[97] Care with cardiac depressant drugs; monitor ECG.
Meckel's syndrome (dysencephalia splanchnocystica)[1,2]	Microcephaly, micrognathia, and cleft epiglottis; CHD; renal dysplasia. Most die in infancy.	Antibiotic prophylaxis preoperatively. Assess cardiac status. Intubation may be difficult. Care with drugs excreted by kidneys.
Median cleft face syndrome[1]	Various degrees of cleft face; lipomas and dermoids over frontal bone.	Cleft nose, lip, and palate may cause intubation difficulties.

NAME	DESCRIPTION	ANESTHETIC IMPLICATIONS
Moebius's syndrome (congenital oculofacial paralysis)[1,2]	Congenital paralyses of VIth & VIIth cranial nerves. Limb deformities, micrognathia. Feeding difficulties and aspiration may cause chronic pulmonary problems.	Assess respiratory status carefully. Intubation may be difficult.
Morquio's syndrome (mucopolysaccharidosis type IV)[1–3]	*Normal intellect.* Severe dwarfing; aortic incompetence; kyphoscoliosis with poor lung function (cardiorespiratory symptoms by 2nd decade). Unstable atlantoaxial joint leading to spinal cord compression; deafness. Inguinal hernia common.	*See Mucopolysaccharidoses.* Antibiotic prophylaxis preoperatively. Assess cardiorespiratory status; care with cardiac depressant drugs. Care with positioning and avoid excessive neck manipulation. [5,65,98]
Mucopolysaccharidosis VII: (β-glucuronidase deficiency)[1,3]	*Severe mental retardation.* Skeletal anomalies similar to type IV.	
Moschcowitz's disease (thrombotic thrombocytopenic purpura)[3]	Hemolytic anemia and thrombocytopenia; arteriolar and capillary disease, neurologic damage, renal disease. Treatment: splenectomy and steroids.	Check coagulation studies and history of steroid therapy. Care with drugs excreted by kidneys.[73]
Moya Moya disease[99,100]	Severe carotid artery stenosis with a fine network of vessels around the basal ganglia. Cerebral	Hypocapnia leads to severe cerebral ischemia: avoid hyperventilation. Halothane may

ischemia leads to paroxysmal hemiplegia. Treatment is by surgical revascularization using scalp vessels.

be useful as a cerebral vasodilator. Avoid hypocapnia or hypothermia.

Mucolipidoses   *See* I-cell disease.

Mucopolysaccharidoses[1–3]

The current classification of these disorders[3] is as follows. (The original classification I to VII was applied as each type was described.) For practical help in recognition, see the table below. Details are given under the eponyms.

I H: Hurler's syndrome
I S: Scheie's syndrome; formerly classified as type V
I HS: Hurler–Scheie compound; *see* Scheie's syndrome
II: Hunter's syndrome
III: Sanfilippo's syndrome
IV: Morquio's syndrome
V: (Vacant; formerly Scheie's syndrome)
VI: Maroteaux–Lamy syndrome
VII: β-Glucuronidase deficiency; *see under* Morquio's syndrome

Type	Affects bones	Affects intellect
I H, I HS, II, VII	+	+
III	–	+
I S, IV, VI	+	–

NAME	DESCRIPTION	ANESTHETIC IMPLICATIONS
Multiple endocrine adenomatoses Type I Type II	*See* Wermer's syndrome. *See* Sipple's syndrome.	
Muscle, eye, brain disease (MEB)	Muscle dystrophy, eye disease (glaucoma, strabismus, nystagmus), and mental retardation. Severe muscle weakness, secretion retention, bedridden.	Caution with muscle relaxants: succinylcholine results in very high CK levels and is contraindicated.[101]
Muscle phosphofructokinase deficiency (glycogen storage disease type VII)[2,3]	Reduced RBC life span (13–16 days).	No anesthetic complications have been reported.
Myasthenia congenita	Similar to myasthenia gravis in adults.[3] *See also* p. 242.	Do not use respiratory depressants or muscle relaxants: IPPV may be required postoperatively. Possibility of cholinergic crisis with anticholinesterase therapy.[102–104]
Myositis ossificans (fibrodysplasia ossificans progressiva)[2]	Bony infiltration of tendons, fascia, aponeuroses, and muscle. Thoracic involvement greatly reduces thoracic compliance; progressive respiratory failure.	Check respiratory function, history of steroid therapy. Airway and intubation problems if neck rigid and mouth fixed.[5]

Myotonia congenita (Thomsen's disease)[2,3]	Decreased ability to relax muscles after contraction; diffuse hypertrophy of muscle. (Similar to myotonia dystrophica but more benign and nonprogressive.)	Do not use muscle relaxants or respiratory depressants.[15–18]
Myotonia dystrophica (myotonic dystrophy)[1–3]	Weakness and myotonia; eyelid ptosis, cataracts, frontal baldness; cardiac conduction defects and arrhythmias; impaired ventilation; other systems may be involved. Has been reported in infancy.[1]	Check respiratory function. Do not use succinylcholine (which causes myotonia in 50%). Nondepolarizing drugs do not produce good relaxation; neostigmine induces myotonia; halothane may cause shivering and myotonia postoperatively. Extremely sensitive to respiratory depressants—use regional or inhalational agents with IPPV postoperatively if necessary. Monitor ECG carefully. Anticipate postoperative pulmonary complications.[15–18,105]
Nail–patella syndrome (arthrosteoonychondysplasia)[2,3]	Dysplasia of nails and absent or hypoplastic patellas. May have iliac horns, abnormality of elbows, nephropathy, increased mucopolysaccharide excretion.	Care with drugs excreted by kidneys.

NAME	DESCRIPTION	ANESTHETIC IMPLICATIONS
Neonatal hypoglycemia, symptomatic	Symptomatic hypoglycemia in infants: (1) SGA, (2) of diabetic mothers, (3) premature. If untreated—convulsions, lethargy, and mental retardation; no ketosis. Rarely, insulinoma or pancreatic hypertrophy requiring subtotal pancreatectomy. *See also* Beckwith's syndrome.[1]	Start IV glucose infusion (5–10 mg/kg/min—**no bolus**) preoperatively and monitor blood glucose until condition stable postoperatively. (Boluses would precipitate rebound hyperglycemia.) Patient may be receiving steroids, diazoxide, and glucagon.[33]
Nevoid basal cell carcinoma syndrome	*See Gorlin–Goltz syndrome.*	
Niemann–Pick disease[2,3]	Hepatosplenomegaly and accumulation of sphingomyelin and other lipids throughout body. (*See also* Wolman's disease.) Marrow, liver, and spleen involvement lead to anemia and thrombocytopenia. Diffuse foam cell infiltration of lungs leads to pulmonary insufficiency, pneumonia.	Check coagulation studies and cardiorespiratory function.[71]
Types A, C, D, (onset in infancy)	Mental retardation. Epilepsy, ataxia. Death usually by 3rd yr (type A) to 15th yr (type C).	
Type B	Normal intellect. Pulmonary disease (foam cells in alveoli). Not fatal.	

Noack's syndrome[1,2]	Craniosynostosis and digital anomalies; obesity.	Intubation may be difficult because of skull deformity.[26]
Noonan's syndrome[1,2]	Short stature, mental retardation, CHD (usually PS), micrognathia; hydronephrosis or hypoplasia of kidneys; may have platelet dysfunction.	Antibiotic prophylaxis preoperatively. Intubation may be difficult. Care with cardiac depressant drugs and those excreted by kidneys.[5]
Oculoauriculovertebral syndrome	*See* Goldenhar's syndrome.	
Oculocerebrorenal syndrome	*See* Lowe's syndrome.	
Oculofacial paralysis, congenital	*See* Moebius's syndrome.	
Ollier's syndrome (enchondromatosis)[1,2] with cavernous hemangioma	Multiple chondromas within bones, usually unilateral; pathologic fractures. *See* Maffucci's syndrome.	Position carefully.
Opitz–Frias syndrome (G syndrome, hypospadius dysphagia syndrome)[106]	X-linked or autosomal dominant, affects males more than females. Craniofacial and genital abnormalities. Dysphagia and recurrent aspiration, achalasia, hiatus hernia. Hypertelorism, micrognathia, and a high arched palate. Laryngeal malformations (including laryngotracheal cleft) and pulmonary hypoplasia. Bifid scrotum.	Difficult airway, small larynx (prepare small endotracheal tubes). Danger of regurgitation—empty stomach before induction.

NAME	DESCRIPTION	ANESTHETIC IMPLICATIONS
Oral–facial–digital syndrome[1,2]	Cleft lip and palate, lobed tongue, hypoplastic mandible and maxilla, digital anomalies; hydrocephalus, polycystic kidneys.	Airway problems and intubation may be difficult; possible renal impairment—do not use drugs excreted by the kidneys.
Osler–Rendu–Weber syndrome (hemorrhagic telangiectasia)[1–3]	Multiple capillary and venous dilation, most commonly of skin and nasal mucosa, but any organ may be affected. High incidence of pulmonary and hepatic AV fistula.	Anemia; internal hemorrhage may occur perioperatively.[73]
Osteogenesis imperfecta (fragilitas ossium)[1–3]	I. Congenita—Usually stillbirth or rapidly fatal. II. Tarda—Pathologic fractures, blue sclera, deafness. Osteoporosis → kyphoscoliosis → lung pathology. Fragility of vessels results in subcutaneous hemorrhage. Dentine deficiency results in carious, fragile teeth.	Use extreme care in positioning and intubating. Teeth are easily broken.[107]
Osteopetrosis	See Albers-Schönberg disease.	
Paramyotonia congenita (Eulenberg's periodic paralysis)[2,3]	Myotonia on exposure to cold; paroxysmal weakness; serum K may be high or low.	As for myotonic dystrophy; check serum K level.[15–18]
Patau's syndrome (trisomy 13)[1,3]	Mental retardation, microcephaly, micrognathia; cleft lip or palate;	If CHD present: antibiotic prophylaxis preoperatively.

	CHD (usually VSD and/or dextrocardia). Most die by 3 yr.	Intubation may be difficult. Problems associated with heart disease.[9]
Pendred's syndrome[2,3]	Deafness and goiter; incomplete block of thyroxine production. May be euthyroid or hypothyroid.	Preoperatively ensure that patient is euthyroid; otherwise as for cretinism.[108]
Periodic paralysis	See Familial periodic paralysis *and* Paramyotonia congenita.	
Phenylketonuria[2,3]	Phenylalanine hydroxylase deficiency. Vomiting, CNS irritability, mental retardation, hypertonia, convulsions. Phenylalanine-deficient diet must be maintained.	Induction and maintenance by inhalation technique. Control ventilation. Give 10% dextrose infusion (tendency to hypoglycemia). Hypersensitive to narcotics and other CNS depressants. Do not use ketamine or enflurane; monitor body temperature carefully.[3] If epilepsy, continue drugs.
Pierre Robin syndrome[1,3]	Cleft palate, micrognathia, glossoptosis; CHD in some. Neonates: respiratory obstruction may occur and can lead to cor pulmonale; maintain airway by nursing prone on a frame; may require tongue suture, intubation, or tracheotomy.	If CHD present: antibiotic preoperatively. Intubation may be very difficult: use awake technique. Patient should be fully awake before extubation.[109]

NAME	DESCRIPTION	ANESTHETIC IMPLICATIONS
Polyarteritis nodosa	See Collagen disease.	
Polycystic kidneys[2]	Associated cysts in liver, pancreas, spleen, lungs, bladder, thyroid in one-third; cerebral aneurysm in 15%.	Check renal status. Do not use drugs excreted by kidneys if renal function impaired. Lung cysts may lead to pneumothorax. Prevent hypertension (possible cerebral aneurysm).[110]
Polyneuritis, acute	See Guillain–Barré syndrome.	
Polysplenia (bilateral visceral left-sidedness)	Complex cardiac anomalies are common: ASD and endocardial cushion defects, usually not so complex as in asplenia.	If CHD present: antibiotic prophylaxis preoperatively. Do not use cardiac depressants.[50]
Pompe's disease (glycogen storage disease type II)[2,3]	Deposits of glycogen in muscles—severe hypotonicity: large tongue; massive cardiomegaly. Death from cardiorespiratory failure before 2 yr of age.	**Extreme care:** do not use respiratory or cardiac depressants or muscle relaxants. Large tongue may cause airway problem.[97]
Porphyrias[2,3]	Paralyses, psychiatric disorder; autonomic imbalance—hypertension, tachycardia; abdominal pain precipitated by drugs, infection, etc. High incidence of diabetes.	**Do not give:** barbiturates (including thiopental), sedatives (including meprobamate, Librium, glutethimide, carbromal), hydroxydione (steroid anesthetic), nikethamide, hydantoin

Syndrome	Clinical features	Anesthetic considerations
		derivatives, sulfonamides, antipyretics, or hypoglycemic agents. *The following have been used safely:* atropine, chloral, chlorpromazine, *d*-tubocurarine, ether, gallamine, morphine, N_2O, neostigmine, pentolium, pethidine, procaine, promazine, promethazine, propanidid, succinylcholine.[64]
Prader–Labhart–Willi syndrome[1-3,111]	*Neonate:* hypotonia, poor feeding, reflexes absent. *2nd phase:* hyperactive, uncontrollable polyphagia, mental retardation. Extreme obesity leading to cardiopulmonary failures.	Danger of hypoglycemia developing: monitor blood sugar carefully and infuse glucose solution IV pre-, peri, and postoperatively.[112] Assisted or controlled ventilation may be necessary peri- and postoperatively.
Progeria (Hutchinson–Gilford syndrome)[1-3]	Premature aging starts at 6 mo to 3 yr; cardiac disease—ischemia, hypertension, cardiomegaly. Death from coronary artery disease may occur before 10 yr of age.	Anesthesia as for adults with myocardial ischemia.[113]
Prune-belly syndrome[2]	Agenesis of abdominal musculature with renal anomalies (respiration requires use of accessory muscles). Poor cough mechanism, respiratory infections. May have renal insufficiency.	Check renal status. Treat as for full stomach; intubate and assist or control ventilation. Do not use muscle relaxants. Care with drugs excreted by kidneys.[114]

NAME	DESCRIPTION	ANESTHETIC IMPLICATIONS
Pseudohypoparathyroidism	*See* Albright's osteodystrophy.	
Pseudoxanthoma elasticum	*See* Groenblad–Strandberg syndrome.	
Pyle's disease (metaphyseal dysplasia)[1,2]	Craniofacial abnormalities; enlarged mandible; cranial nerve paralyses.	Assess airway carefully.
Reye's syndrome[2,3,115]	Severe encephalopathy and fatty degeneration of viscera (especially liver): hyperaminoacidemia; increased prothrombin time, blood ammonia, serum transaminases. Most reliable diagnosis by liver biopsy. If untreated, increased ICP usually fatal.	Anesthetized for investigation of and decompression for increased ICP. May be on steroids and controlled hypothermia. Care with drugs metabolized by liver. Do not give halothane (increased ICP; hepatic dysfunction). Control ventilation and continue hypothermia.
Rheumatoid arthritis	*See* Collagen disease.	
Rieger's syndrome[1,2]	Hypodontia, malformations of anterior chamber of eye, myotonic dystrophy. May have other developmental abnormalities, including maxillary hypoplasia.	Anesthetic requirements dictated by muscle disease: *see* Amyotonia congenita; Myotonia congenita; Myotonia dystrophica.[15–18]

Riley–Day syndrome[1,2,118]	Deficiency of dopamine-β-hydroxylase: autonomic dysfunction and decreased sensation, hyper- and hypotensive attacks, emotional lability, absent lacrimation, abnormal sweating, poor sucking and swallowing. Recurrent aspiration pneumonia and chronic lung disease.	Premedicate with diazepam and cimetidine. Atropine can be given. Give IV fluids to maintain hydration. Replace fluid losses carefully to maintain volume status. Titrate anesthetic agents carefully; inhalation agents, barbiturates, narcotics, and relaxants may be used. Respiratory center insensitive to CO_2—IPPV necessary postoperatively if narcotics given. Beware of aspiration postoperatively. Diazepam is useful for dysautonomic crises.[116,117]
Robin Pierre syndrome	See Pierre Robin syndrome.	
Romano–Ward syndrome	See Jervell–Lange-Nielsen syndrome.	
Rubinstein–Taybi syndrome	Broad thumb and great toes, mental retardation, microcephaly. May have CHD (usually PS), frequent chest infections, repeated aspiration leading to pneumonia and chronic lung disease.[6] Estimated frequency: 1/500 institutionalized mentally retarded persons.[2]	If CHD present: antibiotic prophylaxis preoperatively. Do not use respiratory depressants. Problems associated with heart disease.[6]

NAME	DESCRIPTION	ANESTHETIC IMPLICATIONS
Sandhoff's disease	*See* Gangliosidosis GM$_2$.	
Sanfilippo's syndrome (mucopolysaccharidosis type III)[1-3]	CNS malfunction in childhood progresses to mental retardation and dementia. Emotional disturbance and agitation. No hepatosplenomegaly, cardiac problems, or major bone problems.	*See* Mucopolysaccharidoses. No anesthetic problems described.[5,64]
Scheie's syndrome (mucopolysaccharidosis type IS, formerly classified as type V)[1-3]	Normal or almost normal intellect. Corneal clouding, hernias; joint stiffness, especially of hands and feet; aortic insufficiency. Sleep apnea may occur.	*See* Mucopolysaccharidoses. Monitor carefully for apnea. Antibiotic prophylaxis preoperatively. Position with care. Problems associated with heart disease.[5,64,119]
Scleroderma	Diffuse cutaneous stiffening. May have hemifacial atrophy.[1] Plastic surgery required for contractures and constrictions. May have cardiac fibrosis or cor pulmonale.	Scarring of face and mouth—difficult airway and intubation. Chest restriction—poor compliance. Diffuse pulmonary fibrosis—hypoxia. Veins may be invisible, impalpable. Check history of steroid therapy.[120]

Sebaceous nevi, linear[2]	Linear nevi from forehead to nose; hydrocephalus, mental retardation; may have coarctation and hypoplasia of aorta.	If CHD present: antibiotic prophylaxis preoperatively. Problems associated with heart disease. May have increased ICP.[1]
Seip's syndrome	*See* Lipoatrophy with diabetes.	
Shy–Drager syndrome[2]	Orthostatic hypotension; diffuse degeneration of central and autonomic nervous systems; lability of pulse and BP possibly due to defective baroreceptor response; decreased sweating; hypersensitivity to catecholamines and angiotensin.	**Do not use** potent inhalation anesthetics; use halothane cautiously; accurate fluid balance important; treat hypotension with IV fluids and phenylephrine. Use muscle relaxants with caution.[121,122]
Silver–Russel dwarfism[1,2]	Short stature, skeletal asymmetry, micrognathia, low birth weight. May have anomalous sexual development.	Intubation may be difficult.[7]
Sipple's syndrome (multiple endocrine adenomatosis type II)[1,2]	Pheochromocytoma (bilateral in 75% of cases), medullary thyroid carcinoma, parathyroid adenoma, multiple endocrine neoplasia.	*See* Pheochromocytoma (page 244). Problem of multiple endocrine disorders.[123]

NAME	DESCRIPTION	ANESTHETIC IMPLICATIONS
Sleep apnea syndromes (*See also* Chubby puffer syndrome)	Disorders of breathing during sleep, including: (a) central sleep apnea, due to CNS immaturity (? SIDS), trauma, infections, or neoplasms, and primary central alveolar hypoventilation (Ondine's curse). Apnea occurs without evidence of respiratory muscle activity. (b) Obstructive sleep apnea due to obesity, adenoid hypertrophy, Pierre Robin syndrome, or any other condition causing chronic airway obstruction. Apnea occurs because of obstruction and is accompanied by increased respiratory muscle activity. (c) Mixed forms may occur. Medical history may include daytime somnolence, loud snoring, restless sleep, insomnia, fatigue. Children may be hyperactive and aggressive.	Assess airway carefully. Avoid preoperative sedation. Intubate and ventilate during anesthesia. Beware of acute obstruction during induction of anesthesia. Intubation may be difficult. Avoid narcotic analgesics during and after anesthesia. Awaken patient completely during transfer to PAR. Monitor closely for apnea postoperatively.[124,125]
Smith–Lemli–Opitz syndrome[1,2]	Microcephaly, mental retardation, genital and skeletal anomalies (including micrognathia), thymic hypoplasia, hypotonia; may have increased susceptibility to infection.	Use sterile technique. Airway and intubation problems.[7] Care with muscle relaxants. Assisted or controlled ventilation may be necessary peri- and postoperatively.

Syndrome	Features	Anesthetic considerations
Sotos's syndrome (cerebral gigantism)[1,2]	Acromegalic features, dilated cerebral ventricles but normal ICP. Nonprogressive.	Possible airway problems due to acromegalic skull. No other problems reported.[7]
Stevens–Johnson syndrome (erythema multiforme)[1]	Urticarial lesions; erosions of mouth, eyes, genitalia. Possible hypersensitivity to exogenous agents (drugs, infections, etc.). If pleural blebs, pneumothorax may occur. Dehydration and malnutrition common. May have myocarditis, pericarditis.	Antibiotic prophylaxis preoperatively. Check cardiac and pulmonary function. Use sterile technique (reverse isolation). Oral lesions—avoid intubation and insertion of esophageal stethoscope. **Monitoring is difficult** (because of skin lesions) **but essential**: danger of ventricular fibrillation; temperature control—febrile episodes: IV infusion essential but do not use cutdown (possibility of infection). Ketamine is probably the best anesthetic agent.[126]
Stiff baby syndrome[127] (hyperexplexia, "startle disease")	Rare, genetic syndrome. Severe muscle rigidity appears at birth and persists for several years. Exaggerated startle response is present. Choking, vomiting, and difficulty swallowing may occur. EMG shows continuous muscle activity.	Caution with relaxant drugs, monitor effects carefully. May be resistant to succinylcholine, but respond normally to pancuronium. Effect of neostigmine is normal.[128]

NAME	DESCRIPTION	ANESTHETIC IMPLICATIONS
Sturge—Weber syndrome[1,2]	Cavernous angioma over 1st—3rd divisions of Vth cranial nerve. Intracranial calcification → convulsions. May have progressive neurologic deficit → mental retardation. Possibility that larynx and trachea may be involved.	No specific anesthetic problems.[129] Care with lower airway—undiagnosed angioma may be present.
Supravalvar aortic stenosis with idiopathic infantile hypercalcemia	*See* Williams' syndrome.	
Tangier disease (analphalipoproteinemia)[2,3]	Low plasma cholesterol; large orange tonsils; anemia and thrombocytopenia due to hypersplenism; peripheral neuropathy and abnormal EMG; premature coronary disease.	Check Hb and platelet count preoperatively. Do not use muscle relaxants. Be alert for premature ischemic heart disease.[71]
Tay—Sachs disease	*See* Gangliosidosis GM$_2$.	
Telangiectasis, hemorrhagic	*See* Osler—Rendu—Weber syndrome.	
Thomsen's disease	*See* Myotonia congenita.	
Thromboasthenia	*See* Glanzmann's disease.	

Thrombocytopenia with absent radius[2]	Episodic thrombocytopenia precipitated by stress, infection, surgery, etc. Platelets increase to normal by adulthood. CHD in 30% of cases.	If CHD present: antibiotic prophylaxis preoperatively. Platelet transfusion for surgery or bleeding. Avoid elective surgery in 1st yr (35–40% die in 1st year of intracranial hemorrhage).[130]
Thrombocytopenia with eczema and repeated infections	*See Wiskott–Aldrich syndrome.*	
Thrombotic thrombocytopenic purpura	*See Moschcowitz's disease.*	
Treacher Collins syndrome (mandibulofacial dysostosis)[1,2]	Micrognathia, aplastic zygomatic arches, microstomia, choanal atresia. CHD may be present.	If CHD present: antibiotic prophylaxis preoperatively. Possible airway and intubation difficulties (less severe than with Pierre Robin deformity).[5]
Trismus-pseudocamptodactyl (Dutch–Kentucky syndrome)[131]	Autosomal dominant condition. Decreased mouth opening due to enlarged coronoid process of the mandible and/or abnormal ligaments plus flexion deformity of the fingers when wrist extended. Short stature and foot deformities may occur. May present for surgery to mandible.	Extremely difficult intubation. May require blind nasal or fiberoptic method.

389

NAME	DESCRIPTION	ANESTHETIC IMPLICATIONS
Trisomies[1-3]		
Trisomy 13	See Patau's syndrome.	
Trisomy 18[E]	See Edwards syndrome.	
Trisomy 21	See Down syndrome.	
Tuberous sclerosis[1,2]	Adenoma sebaceum of skin; epilepsy, mental retardation. Intracranial calcification in 50%. May have tumors in lungs, heart, kidneys. Pyelonephritis and renal failure.	Care with drugs excreted by kidneys. Possible cardiac arrhythmia and rupture of lung cysts.[132]
Turner's syndrome (gonadal dysgenesis)[1-3]	XO females. Short stature, infantile genitalia, webbed neck; possible micrognathia, coarctation, dissecting aneurysm of aorta or PS. Renal anomalies in more than 50% of cases.	If CHD present: antibiotic prophylaxis preoperatively. Intubation may be difficult. Assess cardiovascular status. Care with drugs excreted by kidneys.[133]
Umbilical hernia in infancy		Be alert to possibility of Beckwith's syndrome.
Urbach–Wiethe disease (cutaneous mucosal hyalinosis)[1,2]	Hoarseness or aphonia (hyaline deposits in larynx and pharynx) and skin eruption.	Establishing and maintaining airway may be difficult.[77]
Vater association	A nonrandom association of defects: V = vertebral, A = anal	Those of the individual lesions. Examine patient carefully for

	atresia, T = tracheoesophageal fistula, E = esophageal atresia, R = radial dysplasia.	other congenital lesions, especially renal and cardiac abnormalities.[134]
Velocardiofacial syndrome	Speech difficulties due to velopharyngeal anomalies, learning disability (mild), congenital heart disease (especially VSD), and characteristic faces: large nose with broad nasal bridge, vertically long face, narrow palpebral fissures, and retruded mandible.	May present for pharyngoplasty, considerations of CHD. Obstructive sleep apnea may occur after pharyngoplasty and may cause death.[135,136]
von Gierke's disease Type I glycogen storage disease[2,3]	Hepatomegaly, renal hyperplasia; fasting causes severe hypoglycemia. Severe biochemical disturbances; unresponsive to epinephrine and glucagon. May have Fanconi's syndrome also.	Continuous IV glucose infusion pre- and perioperatively. Monitor blood sugar and acid-base balance.[97] Bleeding problems reported.[3]
Type III (Cori's disease; Forbes' disease) *and* Type VI (Hers' disease)[2,3]	Similar to but milder than type I.	
Von Hippel–Lindau syndrome[2]	Retinal angiomas and cerebellar hemangioblastomas; pheochromocytoma in some; may have pulmonary, pancreatic, hepatic, adrenal, renal cysts. Paroxysmal hypertension due to cerebellar tumor or pheochromocytoma.	Assess renal and hepatic function and investigate for pheochromocytoma (urinary VMA). Hypertensive crises may occur.[123]

NAME	DESCRIPTION	ANESTHETIC IMPLICATIONS
von Recklinghausen's disease (neurofibromatosis)[1,2]	Café au lait spots; tumors in all parts of the CNS (may be in larynx and right ventricular outflow tract); peripheral tumors associated with nerve trunks. Kyphoscoliosis in 50%. May have "honeycomb (cystic) lung." Pheochromocytoma and renal artery dysplasia (hypertension) common.	All these patients should be investigated for pheochromocytoma (urinary VMA). Test response to neuromuscular drugs—effects of depolarizing and nondepolarizing muscle relaxants may be prolonged.[137] Check pulmonary, renal function. If kidneys involved, care with drugs excreted by kidneys.[138,139]
Von Willebrand's disease (pseudohemophilia)[2,3]	Prolonged bleeding time (decreased factor VIII activity leading to defective platelet adhesiveness) and capillary abnormality.	Bleeding can be controlled by transfusions of fresh blood or fresh-frozen plasma and/or cryoprecipitate. Do not use salicylates (effect on platelets, possible GI bleeding).[73] Monitor factor VIII and bleeding time, maintain factor VIII at >50% activity.
Weber–Christian disease (chronic nonsuppurative panniculitis)	Necrosis of fat—in any situation, including: *retroperitoneal tissue*: may cause acute or chronic adrenal insufficiency;	Check cardiac and renal function. Avoid trauma to fat by heat, cold, or pressure. Maintain blood volume; do not use cardiac depressants.[140]

pericardium: leads to restrictive pericarditis; *meninges*: causes convulsions.

Welander's muscular atrophy (late distal hereditary myopathy)	Initially involves distal muscles. Prognosis: for life good, for ambulation poor. See also Werdnig–Hoffman disease.	May require spinal fusion. **Use extreme care** with thiopental and muscle relaxants; do not use respiratory depressant drugs.[15–18]
Werdnig–Hoffman disease (infantile muscular atrophy)[2]	Earlier onset and more severe than Welander's muscular atrophy. Feeding difficulties; aspiration of stomach contents. Chronic respiratory problems. Most die before puberty.	Minimal anesthesia required. Do not use muscle relaxants or respiratory depressant drugs. Ventilatory support may be required, and weaning from this may be difficult.[15–18]
Wermer's syndrome (multiple endocrine adenomatosis type I)[141]	Hyperparathyroidism, tumors of pituitary and pancreatic islet cells (hypoglycemia), gastric ulcer. Carcinoid tumors of bronchial tree are common. Renal failure due to stones.	Control blood sugar carefully. Care with drugs excreted by kidneys.[141]
Werner's syndrome[1,3]	Premature aging; diabetes in 50%, mental retardation in 50%, early cataracts, osteomyelitis-like bone lesions, cardiac infarction and failure.	Anesthesia as for adult with myocardial ischemia and diabetes.[5]

NAME	DESCRIPTION	ANESTHETIC IMPLICATIONS
William's syndrome (elfin facies syndrome)[1]	Supravalvar aortic stenosis, hypercalcemia, mental retardation, elfin facies. Fixed cardiac output and myocardial ischemia leading to dyspnea and angina. Therapy: low-calcium diet, steroids; cardiac surgery.	Antibiotic prophylaxis preoperatively. Check history of steroids. Monitor serum Ca pre- and perioperatively. Do not use cardiac depressants.[142]
Wilson's disease (hepatolenticular degeneration)[3]	Decreased ceruloplasmin; copper deposits, especially in liver and CNS motor nuclei. Renal tubular acidosis; hepatic failure due to fibrosis.	Thiopental can be used in small doses. Muscle relaxants: succinylcholine—apnea rare, despite pseudocholinesterase reduction; d-tubocurarine—short action due to globulin binding. Care with drugs excreted by kidneys.[5,143]
Wilson–Mikity syndrome[144]	Prematurity (<1,500 g birth weight); severe chronic lung disease leading to generalized fibrosis with cystic areas, repeated chest infection, aspiration, right ventricular failure. Steroids may be given to try to prevent pulmonary fibrosis. Pathogenesis unknown; possibly a form of O_2 toxicity on lung tissue.	Check respiratory status carefully and assess cardiac function.[144,145] May have a history of steroid therapy.
Wiskott–Aldrich syndrome[2,3]	Decreased production of platelets; hypersusceptibility to severe herpes	Antibiotic prophylaxis preoperatively. Transfusions of

	simplex infections (disordered immune mechanism), eczema, asthma. May have RES malignancies. Most die before 10 yr, many from generalized herpes or opportunistic infection.	blood and platelets may be required; bone marrow transplantation has been used. All blood products must be irradiated (3,000 rads) to prevent graft-vs-host reaction. Use sterile technique (reverse isolation).[73]
Wolff–Parkinson–White (WPW) syndrome[2,146]	Anomalous conduction path between atria and ventricles. ECG: Short P-R interval; prolonged QRS with phasic variation in 40%. Prone to paroxysmal supraventricular tachycardia (SVT). May have other cardiac defects. Infants, especially preterm, with WPW are very prone to SVT.[147]	If CHD present: antibiotic prophylaxis preoperatively. Prone to arrhythmias. Paroxysmal SVT on induction of anesthesia has been reported; treat with countershock. Avoid atropine, halothane, or pancuronium. Thiopental, isoflurane, and vecuronium are suitable agents. Avoid use of neostigmine.
Wolman's disease (familial xanthomatosis)[3]	Failure to thrive due to xanthomatous visceral changes; adrenal calcification. Resembles Niemann–Pick disease, with hepatosplenomegaly, hypersplenism, and foam cell infiltration (of all tissues, including myocardium). Death usually by 6 months of age.	Treatment entirely supportive. Platelet transfusion successful only after splenectomy.[71]
Zellweger's syndrome	See Cerebrohepatorenal syndrome.	

GENERAL SOURCES OF INFORMATION

1. Gorlin RJ, JJ Pindborg, and MM Cohen Jr (eds): Syndromes of the Head and Neck, 2nd ed. New York, McGraw-Hill, 1976.
2. McKusick VA: Mendelian Inheritance in Man, 5th ed. Baltimore, Johns Hopkins University Press, 1983.
3. Stanbury JB, JB Wyngaarden, and DS Fredrickson (eds): The Metabolic Basis of Inherited Disease, 4th ed. New York, McGraw-Hill, 1978.
4. Katz J, J Bewumof, and LB Kadis (eds): Anesthesia and Uncommon Diseases, 2nd ed. Philadelphia, Saunders, 1981.
5. McKusick VA: Heritable Disorders of Connective Tissue, 8th ed. Baltimore, Johns Hopkins, 1988.
6. Warkany J: Congenital Malformations. Chicago, Year Book Medical Publishers, 1971.
7. Smith DW: Recognizable Patterns of Human Malformation, 4th ed. Philadelphia, Saunders, 1988.
8. Behrman BE, VC Vaughan, and RJ McKay (eds): Nelson's Textbook of Pediatrics, 13th ed. Philadelphia, Saunders, 1987.
9. Rudolf AM, J Hoffman, and S Axelrod (eds): Pediatrics, 18th ed. East Norwalk, CT, Appleton-Century-Crofts, 1987.

REFERENCES

10. Mayhew JF, M Miner, and ID Hall: Anaesthesia for the achrondroplastic dwarf. Can Anaesth Soc J 33:216–221, 1986.
11. Bongiovanni AM, and AW Root: The adrenogenital syndrome. N Engl J Med 268:1283, 1342, 1391, 1963.
12. Morris RC Jr: Renal tubular acidosis: mechanisms, classification and implications. N Engl J Med 281:1405, 1969.
13. Mann JB, S Alterman, and AG Hills: Albright's hereditary osteodystrophy, comprising pseudohypoparathyroidism and pseudo-pseudohypoparathyroidism: with a report of two cases representing the complete syndrome occurring in successive generations. Ann Intern Med 56:315, 1962.
14. Perkoff GT: The hereditary renal diseases. N Engl J Med 277:129, 1967.
15. Ellis FR: Neuromuscular disease and anaesthesia. Br J Anaesth 46:603, 1974.
16. Wislicki L: Anesthesia and postoperative complications in progressive muscular dystrophy: tachycardia and acute gastric dilatation. Anesthesia 17:482, 1962.
17. Editorial: Anesthetic problems in hereditary muscular abnormalities. NY State J Med 72:1051, 1972.
18. Cobham IG, and Davis HS: Anesthesia for muscle dystrophy patients. Anesth Analg 43:22, 1964.
19. Rosenbaum KJ, JL Neigh, and GE Strobel: Sensitivity to non-de-

polarizing muscle relaxants in amyotrophic lateral sclerosis: report of two cases. Anesthesiology 35:638, 1971.

20. Frank MM, JA Gelfand, and JP Atkinson (NIH conference): Hereditary angioedema: the clinical syndrome and its management. Ann Intern Med 84:580, 1976.

21. Hopkinson RB, and AJ Sutcliffe: Hereditary angioneurotic oedema: treatment of angioedema. Anesthesia 34:183, 1979; Br Med J 590, 1970.

22. Gibbs PS, AM LoSasso, SS Moorthy, and CE Hutton: The anesthetic and perioperative management of a patient with documented hereditary angioneurotic edema. Anesth Analg 56:571, 1977.

23. Gelfand JA, RJ Sherins, DW Alling, and MM Frank: Treatment of hereditary angioedema with danazol. N Engl J Med 295:1444, 1976.

24. Abada RP, and WD Owens: Hereditary angioneurotic edema, an anesthetic dilemma. Anesthesiology 46:428, 1977.

25. Hopkinson RB, and AJ Sutcliffe: Hereditary angioneurotic edema. Anesthesia 34:183, 1976.

26. Andersson H, and SP Gomes: Craniosynostosis: review of the literature and indications for surgery. Acta Paediatr Scand 57:47, 1968.

27. Davies DW, and IR Munro: The anesthetic management and intraoperative care of patients undergoing major facial osteotomies. Plast Reconstr Surg 55:50, 1975.

28. Friedlander HL, GW Westin, and WL Wood: Arthrogryposis multiplex congenita: a review of 45 cases. J Bone Joint Surg [Am] 50:89, 1968.

29. Peterson RDA, and RA Good: Ataxia-telangiectasia. Birth Defects 4:370, 1968.

30. Bauman ML, and GR Hogan: Laurence-Moon-Biedl syndrome. Am J Dis Child 126:119, 1973.

31. Gill JR Jr, JC Frölich, RE Bowden, AA Taylor, HR Keiser, HW Seyberth, JA Oates, and FC Bartter: Bartter's syndrome: a disorder characterized by high urinary prostaglandins and a dependence of hyperreninemia on prostaglandin synthesis. Am J Med 61:43, 1976.

32. Bowden RE, JR Gill Jr, N Radfer, AA Taylor, and HR Keiser: prostaglandin synthetase inhibitors in Bartter's syndrome: effect on immunoreactive prostaglandin E excretion. JAMA 239:117, 1978; and editorial, p. 137.

33. Ehrlich RM, and JM Martin: Diazoxide in the management of hypoglycemia in infancy and childhood. Am J Dis Child 117:411, 1969.

34. Filippi G, and VA McKusick: The Beckwith-Wiedemann syndrome (the exophthalmos-macroglossia-gigantism syndrome): report of two cases and review of the literature. Medicine 49:279, 1970.

35. Chamberlain MA: Behçet's syndrome in 32 patients in Yorkshire. Ann Rheum Dis 36:491, 1977.

36. Turner ME: Anaesthetic difficulties associated with Behçet's syndrome. Br J Anaesth 44:100, 1972.

37. Henderson D, and IT Jackson: Naso-maxillary hypoplasia—the Le Fort II osteotomy. Br J Oral Surg 11:77, 1973.
38. Diamond LK, DM Allen, and FB Magill: Congenital (erythroid) hypoplastic anemia: a 25-year study. Am J Dis Child 102:403, 1961.
39. Eng GD, BS Epstein, WK Engel, DW McKay, and R McKay: Malignant hyperthermia and central-core disease in a child with congenital dislocating hips. Arch Neurol 35:189, 1978.
40. Bowen P, CSN Lee, H Zellweger, and R Lindenberg: A familial syndrome of multiple congenital defects. Bull Johns Hopkins Hosp 114:402, 1964.
41. Leader RW: The Chediak-Higashi anomaly—an evolutionary concept of disease. Natl Cancer Inst Monogr 32:337, 1969.
42. Hammer JE III, and AS Ketcham: Cherubism: an analysis of treatment. Cancer 23:1133, 1969.
43. Beahrs JO, GA Lillington, RC Rosan, L Russin, JA Lindgren, and PJ Rowley: Anhidrotic ectodermal dysplasia: predisposition to bronchial disease. Ann Intern Med 74:92, 1971.
44. Johnston RB, and RL Baehner: Chronic granulomatous disease: correlation between pathogenesis and clinical findings. Pediatrics 48:730, 1971.
45. Stool SE, RD Eavey, NL Stein, and WG Sharrar: The chubby puffer syndrome: upper airway obstruction and obesity, with intermittent somnolence and cardiorespiratory embarrassment. Clin Pediatr 16:43, 1977.
46. Jenkins LC, and RW McGraw: Anaesthetic management of the patient with rheumatoid arthritis. Can Anaesth Soc J 16:407, 1969.
47. Drummond DS, RB Salter, and J Boone: Fat embolism in children: its frequency and relationships to collagen disease. Can Med Assoc J 101:200, 1969.
48. Diaz JH, and RH Friesen: Anesthetic management of complete heart block. Anesth Analg 58:334, 1979.
49. Steward DJ, and T Izukawa: Congenital complete heart block. Anesth Analg 59:81, 1980.
50. Tasker WG, AR Mastri, and AP Gold: Chondrodystrophia calcificans congenita (dysplasia epiphysalis punctate): recognition of the clinical picture. Am J Dis Child 119:122, 1970.
51. Smith DW: The compendium on shortness of stature. J Pediatr 70:463, 1967.
52. Wooley MM, S Morgan, and DM Hays: Heritable disorders of connective tissue: surgical and anesthetic problems. J Pediatr Surg 2:325, 1967.
53. DiGeorge AM: Congenital absence of the thymus and its immunologic consequences: concurrence with congenital hypopoparathyroidism. Birth Defects 4:116, 1968.
54. Flashburg MH, BS Dunbar, G August, and D Watson: Anesthesia

for surgery in an infant with DiGeorge's syndrome. Anesthesiology 58:479, 1983.

55. Benda CE: Down's Syndrome—Mongolism and its Management. New York, Grune & Stratton, 1969.

56. Whaley WJ, and WD Gray: Atlanto axial dislocation and Down's syndrome. Can Med Assoc 123:35, 1980.

57. Sethna NF, MA Rockoff, HM Worthen, and JM Rosnow: Anesthesia related complications in children with Duchenne muscular dystrophy. Anesthesiology 68:462–465, 1988.

58. Dolan P, F Sisko, and E Riley: Anesthetic considerations for Ehlers-Danlos syndrome. Anesthesiology 52:266, 1980.

59. Ellis RWB, and S van Creveld: A syndrome characterized by ectodermal dysplasia, polydactyly, chondrodysplasia and congenital morbus cordis: report of 3 cases. Arch Dis Child 15:65, 1940.

60. Reddy ARR, and DHW Wong: Epidermolysis bullosa: a review of anaesthetic problems and case reports. Can Anaesth Soc J 19:536, 1972.

61. James I, and H Wark: Airway management during anesthesia in patients with epidermolysis bullosa dystrophica. Anesthesiology 56:323–326, 1982.

62. Kaplan R, and B Strauch: Regional anesthesia in a child with epidermolysis bullosa. Anesthesiology 67:262–264, 1987.

63. Wise D, HJ Wallace, and EH Jellinek: Angiokeratoma corporis diffusum. Q J Med 31:177, 1962.

64. Melnick B, JL Chang, CE Larson, and RC Bedger: Hypokalemic familial periodic paralysis. Anesthesiology 58:263, 1983.

65. Gilbertson AA, and TB Boulton: Anaesthesia in difficult situations: influence of disease on pre-op preparation and choice of anesthetic. Anaesthesia 22:607, 1967.

66. Clarren SK, and DW Smith: The fetal alcohol syndrome. N Engl J Med 298:1063, 1978.

67. Finucaine BT: Difficult intubation associated with the fetal alcohol syndrome. Can Anaesth Soc J 27:574, 1980.

68. Ashley MJ: Symposium: alcohol and the fetus. Can Med Assoc J 125:141, 1981.

69. Laishley RS, and WL Roy: Freeman-Sheldon syndrome: report of three cases and the anaesthetic implications. Can Anaesth Soc J 33:388–393, 1986.

70. Duggar RG, PD DeMars, and VE Bolton: Whistling face syndrome: general anesthesia and early postoperative caudal analgesia. Anesthesiology 70:545–547, 1989.

71. Fredrickson DS: Disorders of lipid metabolism and xanthomatoses. *In*: Harrison's Principles of Internal Medicine, 8th ed. (GW Thorn, RD Adams, E Braunwald, KJ Isselbacher, and RG Petersdorf, eds). New York, McGraw-Hill, 1977, p. 670.

72. Watne A: Gardner's syndrome. *In*: Skin, Heredity and Malignant

Neoplasms (HT Lynch, ed). Flushing, Medical Examinations Publishing Co., 1972, p. 165.

73. Wintrobe M (ed): Clinical Hematology, 7th ed. Philadelphia, Lea & Febiger, 1974.

74. Beach TP, WA Stone, and W Hamelberg: Circulatory collapse following succinylcholine: report of a patient with diffuse lower motor neuron disease. Anesth Analg 50:431, 1971.

75. Smith RB: Hyperkalemia folllowing succinylcholine administration in neurological disorders: a review. Can Anaesth Soc J 18:199, 1971.

76. Roy RC, S McLain, A Wise, and LD Shaffner: Anesthetic management of a patient with Hallervorden-Spatz disease. Anesthesiology 58:382, 1983.

77. Lieberman PH, HWK Dargeon, and CF Begg: A reappraisal of eosinophilic granuloma of bone, Hand-Schüller-Christian syndrome and Letterer-Siwe syndrome. Medicine 48:375, 1969.

78. Lewis KB, RA Bruce, D Baum, and AG Motulsky: The upper limb-cardiovascular syndrome: an autosomal dominant genetic effect on embryogenesis. JAMA 193:1080, 1965.

79. Crooke JW, JF Towers, and WH Taylor: Management of patients with homocystinuria requiring surgery under general anesthesia. Br J Anaesth 43:96, 1971.

80. Jervell A, and F Lange-Nielsen: Congenital deaf-mutism, functional heart disease with prolongation of the Q-T interval and sudden death. Am Heart J 54:59, 1957.

81. Yanagida H, C Kemi, and K Suwa: The effects of stellate ganglion block on the idiopathic prolongation of the Q-T interval with cardiac arrhythmia (the Romano-Ward syndrome). Anesth Analg 55:782, 1976.

82. Zelt BA, and AM LoSasso: Prolonged nasotracheal intubation and mechanical ventilation in the management of asphyxiating thoracic dystrophy: a case report. Anesth Analg 51:342, 1972.

83. Miller RD, and MB Divertie: Kartagener's syndrome. Chest 62:130, 1972.

84. Kasabach HH, and KK Merritt: Capillary hemangioma with extensive purpura; report of a case. Am J Dis Child 59:1063, 1940.

85. Propp RP, and WB Scharfman: Hemangioma-thrombocytopenia syndrome associated with microangiopathic hemolytic anemia. Blood 28:623, 1966.

86. Quick AJ: Hemorrhagic Diseases and Thrombosis, 2nd ed. Phildelphia, Lea & Febiger, 1966.

87. Melish ME: Kawasaki syndrome (the mucocutaneous lymph node syndrome). Annu Rev Med 33:569, 1982.

88. McNiece WL, and G Krishna: Kawasaki disease—a disease with anesthetic implications. Anesthesiology 58:269, 1983.

89. Bauman ML, and GR Hogan: Laurence-Moon-Biedl syndrome. Am J Dis Child 126:119, 1973.

90. Hommes FA, HA Polman, and JD Reerink: Leigh's encephalomye-lopathy: an inborn error of gluconeogenesis. Arch Dis Child 43:423, 1968.
91. Kallo A, I Lakatos, and L Szijarto: Leprechaunism (Donohue's syn-drome). J Pediatr 66:372, 1965.
92. Larson LO, and RG Wilkins: Anesthesia and Lesch-Nyhan syn-drome. Anesthesiology 63:197–199, 1985.
93. Richards W, GN Donnell, WA Wilson, D Stowens, and T Perry: The oculocerebro-renal syndrome of Lowe. Am J Dis Child 109:185, 1965.
94. Desnick RJ, HL Sharp, GA Grabowski, RD Brunning, PG Quie, JH Sung, RJ Gorlin, and JU Ikonne: Mannosidosis: clinical, morpho-logic, immunologic, and biochemical studies. Pediatr Res 10:985, 1976.
95. Delaney A, and TJ Gal: Hazards of anesthesia and operation in maple syrup urine disease. Anesthesiology 44:83, 1976.
96. Coleman MA, RR Liberthson, RK Crone, and FH Levine: General anesthesia in a child with urticaria pigmentosa. Anesth Analg 59:704, 1980.
97. Cox JM; Anesthesia and glycogen-storage disease. Anesthesiology 29:1221, 1968.
98. Birkinshaw KJ: Anesthesia in a patient with a unstable neck: Mor-quio's syndrome. Anaesthesia 30:46, 1975.
99. Bingham RM, and DJ Wilkinson: Anesthetic management in moya moya disease. Anaesthesia 40:1198–1202, 1985.
100. Brown SC, and AM Lam: Moya moya disease—a review of clinical experience and anaesthetic management. Can J Anaesth 34:71–75, 1987.
101. Karhunen U: Serum creatine kinase levels after succinylcholine in children with "muscle, eye and brain disease." Can J Anaesth 35:90–92, 1988.
102. Davies DW, and DJ Steward: Myasthenia gravis in children and an-aesthetic management for thymectomy. Can Anaesth Soc J 20:253, 1973.
103. Dalal FY, EJ Bennett, and WS Gregg: Congenital myasthenia gravis and minor surgical procedures. Anaesthesia 27:61, 1972.
104. Crawford J: A review of 41 cases of myasthenia gravis subjected to thymectomy. Anaesthesia 26:513, 1971.
105. Ravin M, Z Newark, and G Saviello: Myotonia dystrophica—an an-esthetic hazard: two case reports. Anesth Analg 54:216, 1975.
106. Bolsin SN, and C Gillbe: Opitz-Frias syndrome; a case with poten-tially hazardous anesthetic implications. Anaesthesia 40:1189–1193, 1985.
107. King JD, and W Bobechko: osteogenesis imperfecta. J Bone Joint Surg [Br] 53:72, 1971.

108. Fraser GR, ME Morgans, and WR Trotter: The syndrome of sporadic goitre and congenital deafness. Q J Med 29:279, 1960.

109. Freeman MK, and JM Manners: Cor pulmonale and the Pierre-Robin's anomaly. Anesthesia 35:282, 1980.

110. Epstein FH: Cystic diseases of the kidneys. *In*: Harrison's Principles of Internal Medicine, 8th ed. (GW Thorn, ed). New York, McGraw-Hill, 1977, p. 1470.

111. Dunn HG: The Prader-Labhart-Willi syndrome: review of the literature and report of nine cases. Acta Paediatr Scand [Suppl] 186:3, 1968.

112. Palmer SK, and JL Atlee: Anesthetic management of the Prader-Willi syndrome. Anesthesiology 44:161, 1976.

113. Chapin JW, and J Kahre: Progeria and anesthesia. Anesth Analg 58:424, 1979.

114. Hannington-Kiff JG: Prune-belly syndrome and general anesthesia: case report. Br J Anaesth 42:649, 1970.

115. Haller JS: The enigmatic encephalopathy of Reye's syndrome. Hosp Pract 10:91, 1975.

116. Inkster JS: Anaesthesia for a patient suffering from familial dysautonomia (Riley-Day syndrome). Br J Anaesth 43:509, 1971.

117. Meridy HW, and RE Creighton: General anaesthesia in eight patients with familial dysautonomia. Can Anaesth Soc J 18:563, 1971.

118. Axelrod FB, RF Donenfeld, F Danziger, and H Turndorf: Anesthesia in familial dysautonomia. Anesthesiology 68:631–635, 1988.

119. Perks WH, RA Cooper, S Bradbury, P Horrocks, N Baldock, A Allen, W Van't Hoff, G Weidman, and K Prowse: Sleep apnea in Scheie's syndrome. Thorax 35:85, 1980.

120. Birkhan J, M Heifetz, and S Haim: Diffuse cutaneous scleroderma: an anaesthetic problem. Anaesthesia 27:89, 1972.

121. Cohen CA: Anesthetic management of a patient with the Shy-Drager syndrome. Anesthesiology 35:95, 1971.

122. Malan MD, and R Crago: Anesthetic implications in idiopathic orthostatic hypotension and the Shy-Drager syndrome. Can Anaesth Soc J 26:322, 1979.

123. Steiner AL, AD Goodman, and SR Powers: Study of a kindred with pheochromocytoma, medullary thyroid carcinoma, hyperparathyroidism and Cushing's disease: multiple endocrine neoplasia type 2. Medicine 47:371, 1968.

124. Chung F, and RR Crago: Sleep apnea syndrome and anesthesia. Can Anaesth Soc J 29:439, 1982.

125. Phillipson EA: Control of breathing during sleep. Am Rev Resp Dis 118:909, 1978.

126. Cucchiara RE, and B Dawson: Anesthesia in Stevens-Johnson syndrome: report of a case. Anesthesiology 35:537, 1971.

127. Lingham S, J Wilson, and EW Hart: Hereditary stiff baby syndrome. Am J Dis Child 135:909–911, 1981.

128. Cook WP, and RF Kaplan: Neuromuscular blockade in a patient with stiff baby syndrome. Anesthesiology 65:525–528, 1986.
129. Alexander GL, and RM Norman: The Sturge-Weber Syndrome. Bristol, Wright, 1960.
130. Hall JG, J Levin, JP Kuhn, EJ Ottenheimer, KAP van Berkum, and VA McKusick: Thrombocytopenia with absent radius. Medicine 48:411, 1969.
131. Vaghadia H, and D Blackstock: Anesthetic implications of the trismus pseudocamptodactyly (Dutch-Kentucky or Hecht Beals) syndrome. Can J Anaesth 35:80–85, 1988.
132. Lagos JC, and MR Gomez: Tuberous sclerosis: reappraisal of a clinical entity. Mayo Clin Proc 42:26, 1967.
133. Strader WJ III, HL Wachtel, and GD Landberg Jr: Hypertension and aortic rupture in gonadal dysgenesis. J Pediatr 79:473, 1971.
134. Quan L, and DW Smith: The vater association, vertebral defects, anal atresia, tracheoesophageal fistula with esophageal atresia, radial dysplasia. Birth Defects 8:75, 1972.
135. Shprintzen RJ, RB Goldberg, ML Lewin, EJ Sidoti, MD Berkman, RV Argamaso, and D Young: A new syndrome involving cleft palate, cardiac anomalies, typical facies and learning disabilities: velo-cardio-facial syndrome. Cleft Palate J 15:56, 1978.
136. Kravath RE, CP Pollak, B Borowieki, and ED Weitzman: Obstructive sleep apnea and death associated with surgical correction of velopharyngeal incompetence. J Pediatr 96:645, 1980.
137. Yamashita M, A Matsuki, and T Oyama: Anaesthetic considerations on von Recklinghausen's disease (multiple neurofibromatosis): abnormal response to muscle relaxants. Anaesthetic (Ber) 26:317, 1977.
138. Brasfield RD, and TK Das Gupta: von Recklinghausen's disease: a clinicopathological study. Ann Surg 175:86, 1972.
139. Gibbs NM, M Taylor, and A Young: von Recklinghausen's disease in the larynx and trachea of an infant. J Laryngol Otol 71:626, 1957.
140. Spivak JL, S Lindo, and M Coleman: Weber-Christian disease complicated by consumption coagulopathy and microangiopathic hemolytic anemia. Johns Hopkins Med J 126:344, 1970.
141. Wermer P: Endocrine adenomatosis and peptide ulcer in a large kindred: inherited multiple tumours and mosaic pleiotropism in man. Am J Med 35:205, 1963.
142. Fay JE, RB Lynn, and MW Partington: Supravalvular aortic stenosis, mental retardation and a characteristic facies. Can Med Assoc J 94:295, 1966.
143. Trachtenberg HA: Anesthesia for patient with hepatic disease. Int Anesthesiol Clin 8:437, 1970.
144. Wilson MG, and VG Mikity: A new form of respiratory disease in premature infants. Am J Dis Child 99:489, 1960.
145. Northway WH Jr, RC Rosan, and DY Porter: Pulmonary disease

following respirator therapy of hyaline-membrane disease: broncho-pulmonary dysplasia. N Engl J Med 276:357, 1967.

146. Hannington-Kiff JG: The Wolff-Parkinson-White syndrome and general anesthesia. Br J Anaesth 40:791, 1968.

147. Richmond MN, and PT Conroy: Anesthetic management of a neonate born prematurely with Wolff Parkinson White syndrome. Anesth Analg 67:477–478, 1988.

Suggested Drug Dosages for Pediatric Patients

PREOPERATIVE PERIOD

PERIOPERATIVE PERIOD
Induction
Maintenance
Neuromuscular blocking agents
Reversal of nondepolarizing neuromuscular blocking agents

POSTOPERATIVE PERIOD
Analgesics

ANCILLARY DRUGS
Antibiotics
Adrenocorticosteroids
Drugs acting on the cardiovascular system
Diuretics
Anticonvulsants
Bronchodilators
Local anesthetics

PREOPERATIVE PERIOD

Note: Avoid giving drugs intramuscularly (IM) if possible—IM injections are painful and children do not like them. If IM drugs are necessary and more than one has to be given, combine them in the same syringe whenever possible.

Drugs for Premedication

Atropine. 0.02 mg/kg intravenously (IV) at induction or IM 30–60 minutes preoperatively; maximum 0.6 mg. For infants less than 5 kg the minimum dose is 0.1 mg.
Chloral hydrate. 25–75 mg/kg orally (PO) or rectally (PR).
Diazepam. 0.2–0.5 mg/kg PO 1–2 hours preoperatively; maximum 15 mg.

Midazolam. 0.25 mg/kg PO, 0.3 mg/kg PR, or 0.08 mg/kg IM.
Morphine. 0.1–0.2 mg/kg IM 45–60 minutes preoperatively. (If atropine
  is to be given it can be mixed with morphine.)
Pentobarbital. 2–4 mg/kg PO, PR, or IM 2 hours preoperatively.

Antacids, H_2 Histamine Blocking Agents

Cimetidine. 10 mg/kg PO, or 30 mg/kg PR.
Ranitidine. 2.0 mg/kg PO.
Sodium citrate. 0.4 ml/kg PO.

To Speed Gastric Emptying

Metoclopramide. 0.15 mg/kg IV.
(**N.B.** Atropine blocks the effect of metoclopramide and should be withheld until induction of anesthesia.)

PERIOPERATIVE PERIOD

INDUCTION

Thiopental sodium (Pentothal). Up to 5 mg/kg IV in healthy children (if
  no contraindications). Infants from 6 months to 2 years of age may
  require higher doses up to 7 mg/kg.
Methohexital. Up to 2 mg/kg IV (if no contraindictions) or 15 mg/kg PR
  (1% solution).
Diprivan (Propofol). 2.5–3.5 mg/kg.
Ketamine. 2 mg/kg IV or 4–8 mg/kg IM.

For Intubation

Succinylcholine. Infants 2 mg/kg IV. Older children 1 mg/kg IV or 2 mg/
  kg IM.
Vecuronium. 0.1 mg/kg IV.
(**N.B.** Do not inject immediately after thiopental; the resulting precipitate
  may block the needle.)
Pancuronium. 0.1 mg/kg.
Topical Lidocaine for laryngeal spray. Total dose, up to 4 mg/kg.

MAINTENANCE

Fentanyl. 1–2 μg/kg IV to supplement analgesia or as an IV infusion for major surgery: loading dose, 5 μg/kg, and infusion at 2–4 μg/kg/hr.

Meperidine (Pethidine, Demerol). 0.2–0.4 mg/kg IV or 1.5 mg/kg IM.

Morphine. 0.01–0.03 mg/kg IV or IV infusion (for children over 5 years of age): loading dose, 100 μg/kg over 5 minutes, and infusion of 50–60 μg/kg/hr.

Droperidol. 0.1 mg/kg IV (do not repeat). To prevent vomiting following strabismus repair; 75 μg/kg IV (given *before* manipulation of the eye muscles).

NEUROMUSCULAR BLOCKING DRUGS

1. Give these drugs IV.
2. Give initial and repeat doses preferably as indicated by nerve stimulator, especially for infants (whose response to these drugs is extremely variable).
3. Remember that potent volatile agents (especially isoflurane) reduce the dose of nondepolarising drugs required.

d-Tubocurarine. Initial dose, 0.3–0.5 mg/kg; repeat doses should not exceed one-half the initial dose.

Pancuronium. Initial dose, 0.06–0.1 mg/kg; repeat doses should not exceed one-sixth the initial dose.

Metocurine. 0.2–0.3 mg/kg.

Atracurium. Initial dose, 0.3–0.5 mg/kg; repeat dose, 0.125 mg/kg.

Or by infusion:

During halothane or isoflurane anesthesia: loading dose, 0.3 mg/kg, and infusion of 5–6 μg/kg/min.

During balanced anesthesia with fentanyl: loading dose, 0.4 mg/kg, and infusion of 9–10 μg/kg/min.

Vecuronium. Initial dose for intubation, 0.1 mg/kg; incrimental doses, 0.02 mg/kg.

REVERSAL OF NONDEPOLARIZING NEUROMUSCULAR BLOCKING AGENTS

Atropine. 0.02 mg/kg or *glycopyrrolate*, 0.01 mg/kg mixed with *neostigmine*, 0.05 mg/kg. Administer slowly; use a nerve stimulator to monitor effect.

OR

Atropine. 0.02 mg/kg, followed by *edrophonium*, 1 mg/kg.

POSTOPERATIVE PERIOD
ANALGESICS

Acetaminophen (Tylenol). 10 mg/kg PO or PR.
Codeine (useful for minor surgery). 1–1.5 mg/kg IM.
(**N.B.** Codeine must not be given IV.)
Meperidine (Demerol, Pethidine). 1–1.5 mg/kg IM or 0.2–0.5 mg/kg IV.
Morphine. 0.05–0.2 mg/kg IM or 0.02 mg/kg IV.
Morphine infusion. 10–30 μg/kg/hr.
Preparation of solution: Mix

$$\frac{\text{Patients weight in kg}}{2} \times \text{mg morphine in 50 ml.}$$

Solution then contains 10 μg/kg/ml. Infuse at 1–3 ml/hr (equivalent to 10–30 μg/kg/hr).

Narcotic Antagonist

Naloxone (Narcan). 0.01–0.1 mg/kg IV.
Note: This drug should be titrated slowly until undesired narcotic effects are reversed. Rapid administration of an excessive dose will result in loss of analgesia, pain, and extreme restlessness.

Treatment of Nausea and Vomiting

Dimenhydrinate (Gravol, Dramamine). 1 mg/kg IV or 2 mg/kg PR.
Prochlorperazine (Stemetil). 0.05–0.1 mg/kg IV. (Do not give to infants <2 years.)

ANCILLARY DRUGS
ANTIBIOTICS

The dose given is for a single intraoperative IV administration; the lower dose should be given to neonates under 1 week (limited neonatal liver and renal function). The usual maximum daily dose for children is given in parentheses. Antibiotics should be infused over a period of minutes rather than by "push" to minimize the possibility of adverse reactions. Regimens for antibiotic prophylaxis against subacute bacterial endocarditis are listed on page 129.

*Ampicillin.** 50–100 mg/kg (300 mg/kg).
Cefazolin. 20–40 mg/kg (100 mg/kg).
Cefoxitin. 20–40 mg/kg (160 mg/kg).
Cefuroxime. 20–50 mg/kg (240 mg/kg).
Clindamycin. 5–10 mg/kg (30 mg/kg).
Cloxacillin. 12–25 mg/kg (100 mg/kg).
Erythromycin. 2.5–5 mg/kg (20 mg/kg).
Gentamycin. 2.0 mg/kg (7.5 mg/kg).
*Benzyl penicillin.** 30,000–50,000 iu/kg (250,000 iu/kg).
*Vancomycin.** 10 mg/kg (60 mg/kg).

ADRENOCORTICOSTEROIDS

Dexamethasone (Decadron). 0.2 mg/kg IV (maximum 10 mg).
Methylprednisolone (Solu-medrol). 5–15 mg/kg IV slowly over 10 minutes.
Hydrocortisone sodium succinate (Solu-cortef). 4–8 mg/kg IV over 8–10 minutes.

DRUGS ACTING ON THE CARDIOVASCULAR SYSTEM

Calcium chloride. 5 mg/kg.
Calcium gluconate. 10 mg/kg.
Dopamine. 5–15 μg/kg/min.
Dobutamine. 2–20 μg/kg/min.
Epinephrine. 0.1–1 μg/kg/min.
Hydralazine. 0.1–0.2 mg/kg IM. (Do not give IV as severe hypotension may occur.)
Isoproterenol (Isuprel). 0.025–0.1 μg/kg/min.
Lidocaine. 1 mg/kg.
Nitroglycerine. 1–10 μg/kg/min.
Phenoxybenzamine. Loading dose, 0.25 mg/kg × 4 over 2–4 hours; maintenance 0.25 mg/kg q6h.

---

* Caution in patients with renal failure.

Phentolamine. 0.2 mg/kg.
Procainamide. 3–6 mg/kg IV.
Propranolol. 0.05–0.1 mg/kg IV.
Prostaglandin-E^1. 0.05–01 μg/kg/min.
Sodium nitroprusside. 0.5–4 μg/kg/min.
Verapamil. 0.1–0.3 mg/kg IV.

DIURETICS

Furosemide (Lasix). 1 mg/kg.
Mannitol. 0.5–20 g/kg.

ANTICONVULSANTS

Diphenylhydantoin (Dilantin). Loading dose 10 mg/kg IV; maintenance
2.5–5 mg/kg bid IV or PO.
Phenobarbital. Loading dose, 10 mg/kg IV; maintenance, 1.5–2.5 mg/kg
bid IV.

BRONCHODILATORS

Salbutamol (Ventolin). Loading dose, 5–6 μg/kg IV; infusion, 0.1–1.0 μg/
kg/min; inhaled aerosol, 100 μg dose q6h.
Aminophylline. Loading dose, 5 mg/kg; infusion, 1 mg/kg/hr.
(Monitor blood levels—therapeutic range equals 10–12 μg/ml.)

LOCAL ANESTHETICS
Recommended Safe Maximum Doses

Lidocaine plain. 5 mg/kg.
Lidocaine with epinephrine. 8 mg/kg.
N.B. Maximum recommended dose of epinephrine to be infiltrated during
halothane anesthesia is 10 μg/kg.
Bupivacaine. 2 mg/kg.
Tetracaine. 0.2 mg/kg.

Appendix III

Cardiopulmonary Resuscitation

Cardiopulmonary resuscitation (CPR) is concerned with restoration of pulmonary, cardiovascular, and neurologic function. Initially it consists of artificial ventilation and artificial circulation by whatever means is immediately available. This is termed *basic life support*. Its object is to prevent clinical death from progressing to biological death before remedial measures (advanced life support) can be instituted to restore and maintain cardiopulmonary function.

As in adults, heroic resuscitative efforts may not be indicated in children with lethal terminal disease. This is a decision which should be made in advance by the parents in consultation with the medical team and clearly noted in the patient's file.

411

The success rate for pediatric CPR is possibly worse than for adults, especially if success is defined as long-term survival without neurologic deficit. A possible reason for this is that many cases of cardiac arrest in pediatric patients are a result of hypoxemia. In such patients it must be assumed that by the time the heart has suffered hypoxia enough to stop it, the brain has also suffered hypoxia enough to severely damage it. This being so every effort must be directed at detecting and treating respiratory arrest before it leads to serious hypoxemia.

PREVENTION OF CARDIAC ARREST

Awareness of precipitating factors may be valuable in preventing cardiac arrest in children, in whom the primary cause is usually extracardiac.
Common causes include

1. Asphyxia:
    (a) From primary respiratory disorders.
    (b) From regurgitation and vomiting.
    (c) From neurologic and neuromuscular disorders.
2. Hypovolemia.
3. Primary cardiac disorders. (These account for only a small percent of arrests on the general wards of a pediatric hospital.)
4. Toxicity (drugs, poisons, toxins).

Prevention requires

1. Awareness of possible causes, which are often multiple.
2. Constant surveillance.
3. Early recognition of respiratory failure.

HAZARDS OF SPECIAL PEDIATRIC SIGNIFICANCE

Anesthesiologists should constantly be aware of factors that may be insignificant in the adult but may be life-threatening in small patients.
At any time, the upper airway may become obstructed by

1. Small amounts of mucous.
2. Hypertrophied adenoidal tissue.
3. The relatively large tongue, associated with
    (a) Flaccidity in the anesthetized patient.

(b) Inadvertent displacement of submental soft tissue and tongue by the anesthesiologist's fingers.
(c) Inadequate head extension.
(d) Inadequate elevation of jaw.
(e) Premature removal of artificial airway.
4. Regurgitation is a common occurrence because of the frequency of feedings.
5. The infant stomach is readily inflated by
   (a) Too-high inflation pressure.
   (b) Partial obstruction of airway.

If decompression is needed use a no. 12 or 14 catheter or stomach tube— after protecting the airway with an endotracheal tube to reduce the possibility of aspiration.

Remember: infants are primarily nose-breathers. If the nasal airway is inadequate, an oral airway should be inserted.

PRECAUTIONS

Preoperative
1. Give atropine to all patients unless specifically contraindicated (very rare).
2. Endotracheal tube: select size carefully and check position. (These are critical in children.)
3. Give 100% O_2 before intubating the child. (Cyanosis develops more rapidly in children, particularly infants, than in adults.)
4. Intubate as quickly and smoothly as possible.

Perioperative
1. Maintain a patent airway and adequate ventilation.
2. Monitor constantly:
   (a) Heart and lung function by stethoscope, pulse oximeter.
   (b) Body temperatures.
   (c) Fluid and blood volumes.
3. Measure carefully all gases, vapors, and drugs.
4. Measure fluid losses accurately and replace as quickly as possible. (Even a small loss is significant in a small child.)
5. Avoid unintentional pressure on the chest and abdominal wall by dressings, hands, assistants' leaning on drapes, etc.
6. If problems arise, advise other members of the team (especially the surgeon) immediately.

Postoperative

1. All infants and all seriously ill patients; do not extubate until the patient is reacting vigorously.
2. If possible, all children should be taken to the postanesthesia room (PAR) in the lateral position, with the upper leg flexed at the hip and knee and the head moderately extended.
3. In the PAR:
   (a) Do not leave until you have handed over care of your patient to a nurse (*see* p. 98).
   (b) The patient's position is maintained.
       (i) Give 40% humidified O_2 by mask until the child is responding well.
       (ii) Ensure that vital signs are recorded.
   (c) Some neonates and infants need to be disturbed frequently to stimulate respiration.
   (d) Before assigning the child back to his ward, ensure that the danger of drug-induced respiratory depression is past and that he is fully conscious.
   (e) All preterm infants of less than 45 weeks conceptual age should be monitored on an apnea alarm for at least 24 hours.

RESUSCITATION

BASIC LIFE SUPPORT

Note: For basic life support in hospitals recommendations to use mouth-to-mouth ventilation in initial resuscitation are being replaced by advice to use an interposed plastic airway (e.g. the Brook airway) to avoid the risk of infection to hospital personnel. Make sure that such equipment is provided to all patient-care areas.

DO NOT LEAVE THE PATIENT. CALL FOR HELP!
Begin with the ABCs:

A—airway: check.
B—breathing (four ventilations).
C—cardiac activity: check.

When called to resuscitate a child, assess the situation immediately according to the following priorities:

A. Check ventilation.

1. *If there are respiratory movements:*
   (a) Position the patient to provide a clear airway.
   (b) Give O_2 by mask as soon as it becomes available.
2. *If there are respiratory movements but evidence of airway obstruction* (breath sounds absent, intercostal retraction, flaring of lateral chest margins, cyanosis):
   (a) Pull the tongue or lower jaw forward and remove any foreign matter from the pharynx, keeping the mouth slightly open.
   (b) Give O_2 by mask, 10 L/min.
   (c) Check for improved air exchange.
B. *If there is no respiratory movement or ventilation seems inadequate:*
   1. Begin positive-pressure ventilation at once.
   2. Ventilate directly, mouth-to-mouth, until resuscitation equipment is placed in your hand. (The small infant face necessitates application of your mouth to his mouth and nose. Also, an infant's tidal volumes are small [8–10 ml/kg]; therefore only puffs are necessary.)
C. *If the pulse is undetectable by femoral or carotid palpation:*
   1. Start external cardiac compression at once:
      (a) Site of compression: in an infant one finger breadth below the inter-mammary line; in a child one finger breadth above the xphisternum.
      (b) Depth of compression: one-fourth to one-third of the antero-posterior (AP) diameter of the chest.
      (c) Rate of compression:
      Infants: 100–120/min—depth 1.5–2.5 cm.
      Children: 80–100/min—depth 2.5–4.0 cm.
      Adolescents: 80/min.
      (d) Rate of ventilation: Having selected the appropriate rate for cardiac compression (see above), maintain the same ratio of ventilation to cardiac compressions regardless of age or size.
         (i) Two-person technique: 1 ventilation to 5 compressions.
         (ii) Single-person technique: 2 ventilations to 15 compressions.
         (iii) In small infants one person may be able to maintain a 1:5 ratio, because it is not necessary to move from mouth to chest.
         (iv) For anesthetized patients who are already intubated, a ratio of 1 cardiac compression to 2 ventilations with 100% O_2 should be initiated immediately.
      (e) If possible, and especially if the patient is on a soft bed, apply cardiac compressions to infants by encircling the chest with your hands (Fig. AIII-1). This method results in a larger cardiac output than anterior sternal compression.

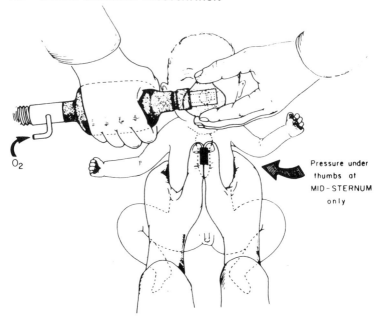

O₂

Pressure under thumbs at MID-STERNUM only

FIG. III-1. Two-handed method of external cardiac compression. Note how both hands encircle the chest and how both thumbs are used for cardiac compression. (Reproduced with permission from Todres D, and MC Rogers: Methods of external cardiac massage in the newborn infant. J Pediatr 86:781, 1975.)

    (f) Cardiac compression should occupy 50% of the cycle.
2. After the initial minute and subsequent 5-minute intervals:
    (a) Check for pulse.
    (b) Note pupil size.
    (c) Resume resuscitation within 10 seconds.

Note: All anesthesiologists should have perfected this skill to the International Heart Association Standards by practice with expert coaching on a manikin.

ADVANCED LIFE SUPPORT

    The foregoing provides only basic interim resuscitation. Most children require, in addition:

1. Ventilation with O₂ as soon as it is available. Ventilation and oxygen-

ation are the first line of therapy for the acidosis that accompanies cardiac arrest.

2. Protection of the airway by insertion of an endotracheal tube.
3. Definitive electrocardiographic (ECG) diagnosis of cardiac activity and defibrillation if indicated (rare).
4. Supportive drugs, beginning with epinephrine (see below).
5. Further pharmacologic and medical treatment, including fluid replacement, as indicated.
6. Consideration of the possibility of lung injury by aspirated acidic stomach contents.
7. Early assessment of neurologic function—plan early and continuing treatment to minimize hypoxia-induced brain damage.

Defibrillation

Ventricular fibrillation is not common in infants and children: asystole is usual. If ventricular fibrillation is present, proceed with defibrillation as soon as equipment is available.

1. For infants and children under 20 kg, use pediatric defibrillator plates (diameter of 4.5 cm for infants and 8 cm for children).
2. Set the machine to deliver shocks appropriate to the patient's size (to maximize the chance of success and minimize the danger of electrically induced myocardial damage); 2 watt-sec/kg should be the initial setting. If this is unsuccessful the dose should be doubled.
3. Patients who are digitalized should be treated with the lowest power settings initially, and the power setting gradually increased. Normal doses of countershock may cause irreversible cardiac arrest in the presence of bound digitalis in the heart muscle.

Initial Drug Therapy
Route of Administration

In the absence of normal circulation, inject epinephrine into a central line if available. Otherwise, epinephrine may be administered into the trachea via the endotracheal tube. (Intracardiac injections should not be made except as a last resort.)

Choice and Dose of Initial Drug

Although subsequent drug therapy is necessarily individualized, a standard initial protocol is advantageous.

1. *Epinephrine.* To be effective this must be given centrally (into a central vein or the trachea), and acidosis should have been at least partially corrected (as above).
   (a) Dose: 10 μg/kg (0.1 ml/kg of a 1:10,000 solution). This may be repeated every five minutes, if necessary.
2. *Dopamine infusion.* This may be required for continued hypotension and poor tissue perfusion: 5–20 μg/kg/min may be required.
3. *Sodium bicarbonate.* Administration of sodium bicarbonate should be considered for documented continuing metabolic acidosis despite adequate ventilation and oxygenation.
Note: Administration of excessive doses of $NaHCO_3$ produces hyperosmolarity and severe alkalosis after recovery.
   (a) Titration of bicarbonate dosage with serial blood gas analysis is ideal. Failing this:
   (b) If initial response to resuscitation is lacking, despite adequate ventilation and oxygenation 1 mEq/kg of sodium bicarbonate may be given, and may be repeated every 10 minutes during prolonged cardiac arrest.
4. *Calcium.* The use of calcium during resuscitation is being questioned, as intracellular calcium accumulation is known to accompany cell death. However, the use of calcium has appeared to have had a good effect in some pediatric patients. It should be given to patients suspected of having low ionized calcium levels which are contributing to continued poor cardiac action. It may also have a place as a drug of last resort in asystole.
   (a) Indication: poor cardiac action.
   (b) Dose: 20 mg/kg—may help to restore cardiac tone.

Fluid Replacement

1. Insert a large-bore IV cannula as soon as possible:
   (a) To provide a route for drug therapy.
   (b) For rapid replacement of fluid. (In cardiac arrest, hypoxic capillaries leak rapidly, diminishing the circulatory blood volume.)
2. Replace losses initially with clear fluid and later with colloid (plasma or blood) if indicated.
   Note:
   (a) Even a child previously in congestive heart failure needs infusions totalling at least 10% of the expected blood volume (EBV: approximately 1% of body weight).
   (b) With recovery, the extravasated fluid returns slowly to the vascular compartment, giving time for assessment of fluid volume and a decision whether diuretic therapy is necessary.

3. Avoid the use of dextrose containing solutions. These may cause hyperglycemia and this may compromise cerebral survival. If hypoglycemia is suspected it should be confirmed by blood glucose determination and treated accordingly.

Continuing Care

After successful cardiac resuscitation, attention must be directed to the need for further care, especially that needed to ensure maximal cerebral recovery.

1. Transfer the patient to the intensive care unit (ICU).
2. Continue artificial ventilation until the patient is fully conscious and capable of normal spontaneous ventilation.
3. Monitor cardiac status closely and arrange for therapy as indicated (e.g., inotropic drugs, antiarrythmic agents).
4. If cerebral status is in doubt nurse the patient in a 30° head up position, and
   (a) Continue with controlled ventilation to produce a $PaCO_2$ of 30–35 mmHg.
   (b) Continue to ventilate with 100% oxygen to ensure the best possible cerebral oxygenation.
   (c) Maintain blood pressure at normal or slightly elevated levels to ensure optimal cerebral perfusion—treat hypotension.
   (d) Maintain normothermia—prevent the hyperthermia which usually follows a cerebral insult.
   (e) Restrict fluid replacement: avoid large infusions of crystalloid solutions once cardiovascular stability is ensured.
   (f) Treat seizure activity with phenobarbital and/or phenytoin (dilantin).
   (g) Obtain an early full neurologic consultation.
   (h) If necessary arrange to transfer the patient to an ICU with experience in treating pediatric patients.

Suggested Additional Reading

Chameides L, GE Brown, JR Raye, D Todres, and PH Viles: Guidelines for defibrillation of infants and children. Circulation 56:(Suppl)502A–503A, 1977.

Feinberg WM, and PC Ferry: A fate worse than death. Am J Dis Child 138:128–130, 1984.

Holbrook PR, J Mickell, MM Pollack, and AI Fields: Cardiovascular resuscitation drugs for children. Crit Care Med 8:588–589, 1980.

Orlowski JP: The effectiveness of pediatric cardiopulmonary resuscitation. Am J Dis Child 138:1097–1098, 1984.

Orlowski JP: Cardiopulmonary resuscitation in children. Ped Clin North Am 27:495–512, 1980.

Redmond AD: Postresuscitation care. Br Med J 292:1444–1446, 1986.

Safar P: Resuscitation from clinical death: pathophysiological limits and therapeutic potentials. Crit Care Med 16:923–941, 1988.

Standards and guidelines for cardiopulmonary resuscitation and emergency cardiac care. JAMA 255:2954–2969, 1986.

Torphy DE, MG Minter, and BM Thompson: Cardiorespiratory arrest and resuscitation of children. Am J Dis Child 138:1099–1102, 1984.

Zideman DA: Resuscitation of infants and children. Br Med J 292: 1584–1588, 1986.

NEONATAL RESUSCITATION

The anesthesiologist is frequently called upon to assist at or manage the care of the newborn immediately after birth.

Neonatal resuscitation must be based on a detailed knowledge of the normal physiologic changes which occur during transition to extrauterine life (*see* Ch. 2), and a recognition of the pathologic processes in the mother or the fetus which may influence the infant at this time.

Many infants require little help, some however will require rapid intervention if serious sequelae are to be avoided. Preexisting maternal or fetal disease and events during labor may affect the newborn infant after delivery. Frequently infants that are at risk may be recognized before birth and preparations can be made for their immediate resuscitation upon delivery.

IMMEDIATE ASSESSMENT OF THE NEWBORN

A rapid assessment must be made to determine the extent of intervention required. The heart rate and the Apgar score are the most useful guides; a heart rate under 100 or a low 1-minute Apgar score dictate the need for immediate intervention. Low 5-minute (or later) Apgar scores may indicate poor prognosis for long-term neurologic outcome.

PROCEDURES FOR NEONATAL RESUSCITATION
ROUTINE MEASURES FOR ALL INFANTS

The mouth and pharynx and nares should be suctioned as the head presents before delivery of the chest and the initiation of the first breath. After delivery the infant should be held at the level of the uterus until the cord stops pulsating and is clamped. Elevation of the infant above or below this level may result in hypo- or hypervolemia respectively.

The infant should be dried, moved to a warm environment, and carefully examined to confirm the immediate status and to detect any anomaly.

Artificial Ventilation
Infants Who Do Not Breathe Immediately (within 60 secs) or who have bradycardia:

The cord should be clamped immediately, and the infant moved to a warm environment and assessed.

Apgar scores ≥ 5: O_2 by mask plus stimulation will frequently result in initiation of spontaneous ventilation. Cord blood should be taken for pH and PCO_2 if there is any delay. All infants should be carefully observed for several hours.

Apgar score <5: If no immediate response to O_2 by bag and mask, proceed instantly to intubation and ventilation with O_2.

Apgar score <2: Perform immediate endotracheal intubation and ventilate with oxygen.

Infants With Thick Meconium in the Amniotic Fluid
Meconium aspiration is a leading cause of morbidity and mortality but is generally preventable. If thick meconium is present this should be suctioned from the pharynx, hypopharynx, and trachea before the onset of breathing.

Once the head is delivered, suction the pharynx. As soon as the baby is delivered, laryngoscopy should be performed. The trachea should be intubated, and controlled suction applied to the endotracheal tube as it is withdrawn. This should be repeated if necessary.

The Preterm Infant
Some special considerations are necessary for the very small infant.

1. Special care must be taken to prevent heat losses—immediately dry the infant and place on a warm mattress under a heating lamp; use humidified oxygen.
2. Infants over 1000 g should be given O_2, suctioned, and stimulated.
3. Infants under 1000 g are very likely to require early intubation and ventilation. Be prepared to intervene rapidly unless they are obviously satisfactory.
4. Any preterm infant displaying respiratory difficulty should be intubated, and provided with optimal ventilation and oxygenation.

CONTINUED RESUSCITATION

Patients who need continued ventilation should have the airway pressure monitored to prevent pressures over 25 cm H_2O. In addition they should have the following:

Blood gas sample from umbilical artery for analysis.
Radial artery sample if no rapid response to therapy.
Correction of respiratory acidosis by ventilation.
Correction of documented metabolic acidosis once respiratory acidosis has been corrected.
Blood pressure monitoring and correction of hypovolemia.
Blood glucose determination and therapy for levels ≤40 mg/dl.

External Cardiac Compression

Patients with a low heart rate (≤100 beats/min) despite ventilation with 100% oxygen should have in addition:

External cardiac compression—by the chest encircling method.
Compression rates: 120/min (? faster in smaller infants).

Correction of hypovolemia:
10 ml/kg of blood, albumin, or lactated Ringer solution should be given to treat persistent hypotension.

Drug Therapy

Oxygen: 100% should be given to any infant requiring intensive resuscitation until his condition is stable and a suitable inspired concentration to produce safe arterial oxygenation can be established.

Epinephrine: 10–30 μg/kg for asystole or slow heart rates despite all other efforts. Give IV or via endotracheal tube.

Naloxone: 0.02 mg/kg to treat recognized narcotic depression.

Calcium Gluconate: 10–20 ml/kg to correct hypotension which persists despite volume replacement and correction of acidosis.

Glucose: 4 ml/kg/hr of 10% solution—preferably based on repeated blood glucose measurements to avoid hyperglycemia, which may compromise cerebral resuscitation.

Sodium Bicarbonate: to correct metabolic acidosis which persists despite correction of respiratory acidosis—preferably in a dose based on blood sample. Give in dilute solution (0.5 mEq/ml) slowly to prevent the danger of hyperosmolar solution causing intracerebral bleed. Remember that sodium bicarbonate may cause hypotension—this is due to vasodilation and reduction in ionized Ca^{2+}.

POSTRESUSCITATION CARE

Following successful neonatal resuscitation the infant must be cared for in an intensive care area. Close nursing observation should be maintained and appropriate medical therapy continued to treat persisting derangements. Careful notes should be made to document the infant's condition and the therapeutic procedures undertaken.

Suggested Additional Reading

Dawes GS: Fetal and Neonatal Physiology. Chicago, Year Book Medical Publishers, 1968.

Finberg L: The relationship of intravenous infusions and intracranial hemorrhage in newborns: a commentary. J Pediatr 91:777–778, 1977.

Milner AD: Resuscitation at birth. Br Med J 292:1657–1659, 1986.

Myers RE: Four patterns of perinatal brain damage and their conditions of occurrence in primates. Adv Neurol 10:233, 1975.

Standards and guidelines for cardiopulmonary resuscitation (CPR) and emergency care (ECC). JAMA 255:2969–2973, 1986.

Ting P, JP Brady: Tracheal suction in meconium aspiration. Am J Obstet Gynecol 122:767, 1975.

Todres ID, and MC Rogers: Methods of external cardiac massage in the newborn infant. J Pediatr 86:781–782, 1975.

Tsang RC, EF Donovan, and JJ Striechen: Calcium pathology and physiology in the neonate. Pediatr Clin North Am 23:611, 1976.

Index

Page numbers followed by an f indicate figures; those with a t indicate tables.

Abdominal injuries, 330–331
  blood replacement in, 324t
Abdominal surgery. *See* General and
    thoracoabdominal surgery
Abscess, peritonsillar, 178–181
Acetaminophen, dosage of
  for analgesia, 100
  postoperative, 408
Acetate in electrolyte solutions, 90t
Achondroplasia, 340
Acid-base balance in renal function
    disorders, 300, 303
Acidity of gastric contents, reduction
    of, 219
  and dosage of antacids, 406
Acidosis
  from massive transfusions, 326
  preoperative, fluid replacement in,
    87–88
  in renal function disorders, 300
  renal tubular, with anemia, 355
Acrocephalopolysyndactyly, 347
Acrocephalosyndactyly, 344
Acute abdomen, 248–249
Adenoidectomy, 178–181
Adenomatosis, multiple endocrine
  type I, 393
  type II, 385
Adrenal glands, pheochromocytoma
    of, 244–247
Adrenogenital syndrome, 340
Adriamycin, toxic effects of, 127
Afterload reduction, postoperative, in
    cardiac surgery, 269
Airway management
  in Down syndrome, 131
  endotracheal intubation in, 67–70
  in neonates, 95
Airway obstruction
  adenoidal tissue in, 178–179
  in burns, 212, 332

cardiopulmonary resuscitation in,
    415
  in choanal atresia, 182–184
  in craniofacial defects, 214
  in croup, 194–199
  in cystic hygroma, 207–208
  in head and facial injuries, 323
  in mediastinal tumors, 241
  in pharyngoplasty, 206
  from retraction of lungs, 220
  in subglottic stenosis, 199–200
  from vascular rings, 277–279
Albers-Schönberg disease, 340
Albright-Butler syndrome, 340
Albright hereditary osteodystrophy,
    341
Albumin levels in analbuminemia, 342
Alcohol intake, and fetal alcohol
    syndrome, 356
Alfentanil, 50
Alport syndrome, 341
Alström syndrome, 341
Aminophylline, dosage of, 410
Ampicillin, dosage of, 409
Amyotonia congenita, 341
Amyotrophic lateral sclerosis, 342
Analbuminemia, 342
Analgesia
  postoperative, 99–102
    continuous epidural, 101–102
    continuous narcotic infusions in,
      101
    dosages in, 408
    epidural narcotics in, 101
    local or regional techniques in,
      99–100
    patient-controlled, 101
    systemic drugs in, 100–101
  regional
    dosage of agents in, 410
    for postoperative pain, 99–100
    for surgical procedures, 103–105

425